Organ Donation After Circulatory Death

Sanjay P. Kolte • Amol Rameshrao Bhawane
Anil Kumar • Ashish Sharma
Vivek Balkrishna Kute
Manish Ramesh Balwani
Editors

Organ Donation After Circulatory Death

Strategies for Growth in Emerging Health Systems

Springer

Editors
Sanjay P. Kolte
Department of Urology and Kidney Transplant
Max SS Hospital Nagpur
Nagpur, Maharashtra, India

Anil Kumar
National Organ and Tissue Transplant Organization (NOTTO), Directorate General of Health Services
Ministry of Health & Family Welfare, Government of India
New Delhi, Delhi, India

Vivek Balkrishna Kute
Department of Nephrology and Transplantation
IKDRC-ITS
Ahmedabad, Gujarat, India

Amol Rameshrao Bhawane
Department of Nephrology
AIIMS Nagpur
Nagpur, Maharashtra, India

Ashish Sharma
Department of Renal Transplant Surgery
PGIMER
Chandigarh, India

Manish Ramesh Balwani
Department of Nephrology
Saraswati Kidney Care Center
Nagpur, Maharashtra, India

ISBN 978-981-92-6376-9 ISBN 978-981-92-6377-6 (eBook)
https://doi.org/10.1007/978-981-92-6377-6

This Springer imprint is published by the registered company Springer Nature Singapore Pte Ltd.
The registered company address is: 152 Beach Road, #21-01/04 Gateway East, Singapore 189721, Singapore

Preface

This book is dedicated to the numerous patients with organ failure who silently perish, unknowingly mocking our conscience as we remain mute spectators to their gradual descent into the abyss. Even as the world accelerates its pursuit of organs through xenotransplantation, we have desisted from assertively stepping forward to utilise the abundantly available resource around us—the "organs of circulatory-death donors." We owe our ailing patients a sincere apology and immediate redressal.

This book is a small effort in that direction. The privilege of compiling and editing it has made me reflect on the vast body of expertise available in our country, and I am certain that the astute channelling of this knowledge through this book will stimulate productive activity across emerging healthcare systems throughout the world.

I have no words to adequately thank the authors of all the chapters in this book. Without their contributions and dedication over the past year, this book would have remained a mere vision. The chapters have been ingeniously written and thoughtfully organised in the simplest possible language, so as to enable easy understanding, extrapolation, and application of the procedures and processes necessary for the accomplishment of DCD transplantation.

I am grateful to all my fellow editors—Drs Amol Rameshrao Bhawane, Anil Kumar, Ashish Sharma, Vivek Balkrishna Kute, and Manish Ramesh Balwani, for working ardently. Despite constraints of time, demanding work schedules, and the unmapped terrains, they were required to traverse in compiling this book. I must tip my hat to them for the excellent work they have produced.

The evolution of the field of organ transplantation has progressed at a remarkable pace over the seven to eight decades of its existence. However, the transmission of this progress across continents has been painfully tardy. While the West is increasingly using DCD organs for transplantation, the Asian subcontinent is still in its fledgling stages. India, with its 1.4 billion people—17.6% of the world's population—can become a rich source of organs, even after comfortably meeting its own requirements, if DCD organs are utilised expeditiously for transplantation.

I hope this book proves to be a useful guide to everyone who is pursuing DCD transplantation in earnest.

Nagpur, Maharashtra, India

Sanjay P. Kolte

Contents

Part I

Foundational Frameworks for Donation After Circulatory Death (DCD)

1 Historical Evolution and Classification of Donation After Circulatory Death

Pranjal Kashiv, Amol Rameshrao Bhawane, and Manish Ramesh Balwani

Introduction

Clinical organ transplantation began as donation after circulatory death (DCD). Before brain death was formally defined in 1968, every deceased-donor organ recovered for transplantation came from a donor whose heart had stopped beating [1, 2]. The first successful kidney transplantation in 1954 used a living identical-twin donor [3], but the first few sustained programmes of deceased-donor kidney transplantation in the early 1960s, and the early liver and heart transplants of the late 1960s, were performed using organs retrieved after circulatory arrest [1, 2, 4]. With the publication of the Harvard Ad Hoc Committee report on the definition of irreversible coma in 1968, donation after brain death (DBD) became the dominant pathway, and what was then called non-heart-beating donation (NHBD) was largely abandoned for nearly two decades [1, 5].

The persistent gap between organ demand and supply prompted a deliberate revival of NHBD in the early 1990s. The University of Pittsburgh Medical Centre (UPMC) policy of 1992 codified, for the first time in the United States, an institutional protocol for organ donation following circulatory determination of death after planned withdrawal of life-sustaining treatment (WLST) [6, 7]. Three years later, the First International Workshop on Non-Heart-Beating Donation, held in Maastricht in 1995, produced the original four-category Kootstra classification [8]. The terminology evolved from "non-heart-beating donation" to "donation after cardiac death" and finally to "donation after circulatory death" (DCD), or more precisely "donation after circulatory determination of death" (DCDD), to

P. Kashiv (✉) · A. R. Bhawane
Department of Nephrology, AIIMS Nagpur, Nagpur, Maharashtra, India

M. R. Balwani
Department of Nephrology, Saraswati Kidney Care Center, Nagpur, Maharashtra, India

S. P. Kolte et al. (eds.), *Organ Donation After Circulatory Death*,
https://doi.org/10.1007/978-981-92-6377-6_1

convey that death was determined, not merely presumed, by circulatory criteria before organ retrieval began [9, 10].

For the Indian transplant community, an understanding of this trajectory is more than mere academics. India's deceased-donation rate remains below one per million population, standing at 0.81 per million population in 2024 and the legal, ethical, and operational frameworks that enabled DCD to flourish in Spain, the United Kingdom, the United States, the Netherlands and elsewhere have only recently begun to crystallise within the Indian context [11, 12]. The 2022 Indian consensus guidance on DCDD published by Indian transplant and critical care experts [11] has translated international best practices into a coherent operational framework for India and proposed a locally adapted classification that includes a distinct Indian Category V for unexpected cardiac arrest in the ICU. This chapter sets out the historical evolution and the present classification of DCD, defines the standardised time-interval framework, and provides the foundation on which Indian centres can build structured programmes (Fig. 1.1).

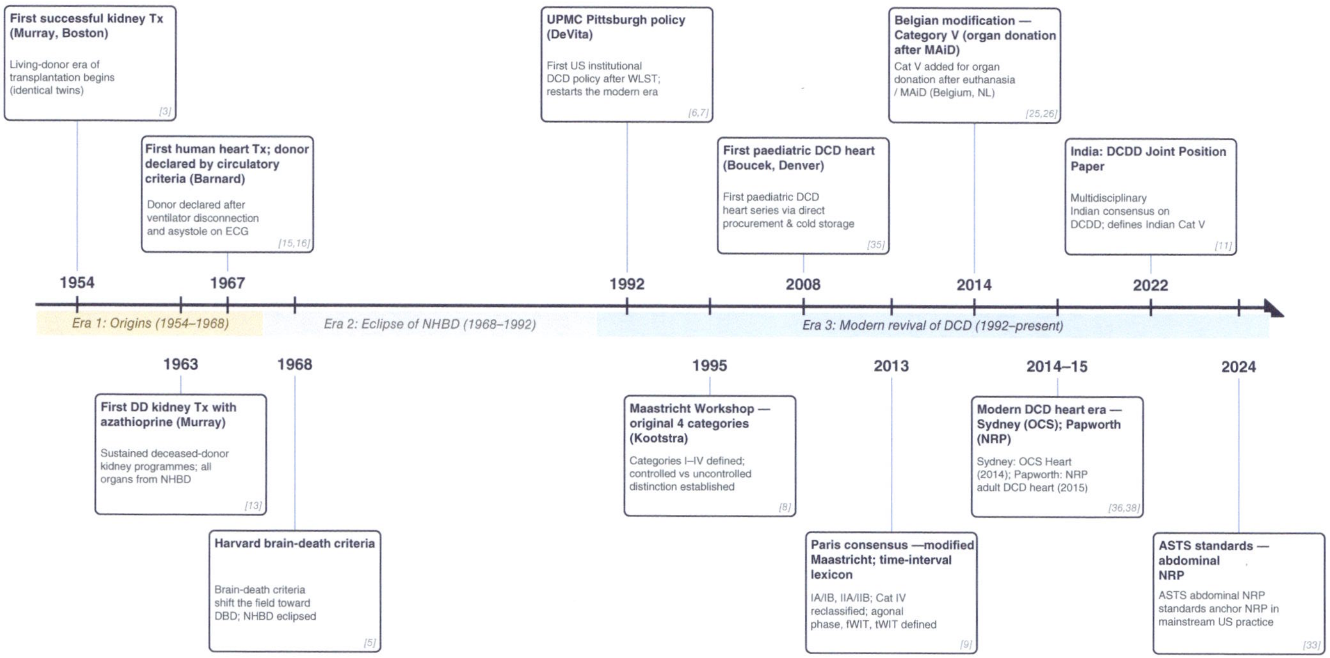

Fig. 1.1 Historical evolution of donation after circulatory death (DCD): key milestones, 1954–2024. *Reference numbers correspond to the chapter reference list.* DBD donation after brain death, DD deceased-donor, DCD donation after circulatory death, DCDD donation after circulatory determination of death, fWIT functional warm ischaemia time, MAiD medical assistance in dying, NHBD non-heart-beating donation, NRP normothermic regional perfusion, OCS Organ Care System, tWIT total warm ischaemia time, Tx transplantation, UPMC University of Pittsburgh Medical Center, WLST withdrawal of life-sustaining treatment

The Origins of Deceased-Donor Transplantation: The Era of Circulatory Death (1954–1968)

Early Kidney Transplantation

The modern history of clinical transplantation is conventionally dated to 23 December 1954, when Joseph Murray and John Merrill at the Peter Bent Brigham Hospital in Boston performed the first successful kidney transplant between the identical Herrick twins [3, 13]. Although a living donor was used in this landmark case, deceased-donor kidney transplantation followed shortly thereafter. In the early 1960s, deceased-donor kidney transplantation between genetically unrelated individuals was established at Brigham, when azathioprine was introduced as immunosuppressant [4, 13, 14]. Every deceased-donor kidney recovered during this period was procured after the cessation of circulation; the concept of donation from a heart-beating donor with neurological criteria for death had not yet entered clinical practice.

Early Heart and Liver Transplantation

The first human heart transplantation, performed by Christiaan Barnard in Cape Town on 3 December 1967, used a donor whose heart had been allowed to stop before retrieval [15, 16]. The donor, Denise Darvall, had sustained a fatal traumatic brain injury and had been certified brain dead by the neurosurgeons of Groote Schuur Hospital; nevertheless, Barnard, anticipating possible medico-legal challenge to until then unrecognised neurological criterion of death, chose to also satisfy a circulatory death criterion. He therefore disconnected the ventilator and waited until the electrocardiogram demonstrated no cardiac output, an interval of approximately six minutes, before initiating retrieval [16]. The chest was then opened, and cold oxygenated blood was perfused through the heart using cardiopulmonary bypass to protect the organ during transplantation [16]. The Barnard procedure thus represents not only the first human heart transplant but also one of the first widely publicised retrievals after circulatory determination of death. Similarly, Thomas Starzl's earliest liver transplants in 1963 and James Hardy's first lung transplant the same year all used non-heart-beating donors [1, 17].

The Eclipse of NHBD After 1968

The publication, in 1968, of the report of the Ad Hoc Committee of the Harvard Medical School to Examine the Definition of Brain Death transformed deceased donation [5]. Once neurological criteria for death were articulated and progressively codified into legislations in many jurisdictions, organs could be recovered from heart-beating donors whose circulation, oxygenation and physiological stability could be maintained until the moment of cross-clamp. Outcomes from DBD donors were superior to those from NHBDs in early series because warm ischaemia was minimised, and DBD rapidly became the dominant pathway [1, 18]. By the late 1970s, NHBD had largely vanished from the transplant landscape outside Japan, where cultural and legal factors limited the recognition of brain death and obliged centres to continue retrieving organs after circulatory arrest [1, 18].

The Revival of DCD: The Pittsburgh Protocol and the Maastricht Workshop (1992–1995)

The Pittsburgh Policy of 1992

The deliberate, institutionally sanctioned revival of NHBD in the modern era is conventionally traced to the University of Pittsburgh Medical Centre, where, under the leadership of the intensivist Michael DeVita, the institutional Ethics Committee approved in 1992 the "Policy and Procedure Manual: Management of Terminally Ill Patients Who May Become Organ Donors After Death" [6, 7, 19]. The Pittsburgh policy was the first formal institutional document in the United States to articulate a structured pathway for organ donation following planned withdrawal of life-sustaining treatment, with death declared on circulatory–respiratory criteria after a defined two-minute interval of asystole [6, 19]. Publication of this policy in 1993 generated immediate and enduring controversy, including the well-known critique by Renée Fox describing the practice as "an ignoble form of cannibalism" [20]. Despite this debate, the Pittsburgh policy crystallised the ethical and procedural template upon which subsequent international frameworks would be built [7, 19].

From NHBD to DCD to DCDD: The Evolution of Nomenclature

Over the two decades that followed the Pittsburgh policy, the terminology of the field evolved in parallel with its conceptual maturation. The term "non-heart-beating donation" was progressively replaced by "donation after cardiac death," and subsequently by "donation after circulatory death" (DCD), as it was recognised that the relevant physiological criterion is the irreversible cessation of circulation rather than mechanical cardiac standstill alone [9, 10]. More recently, the precise term "donation after circulatory determination of death" (DCDD) has gained traction in international guidelines, including the 2022 Indian consensus guidance [11], because it explicitly conveys that death has been determined—and not merely presumed—by circulatory criteria before organ retrieval begins [11, 21].

The Maastricht Classification: Original Framework, Modifications, and Time-Interval Definitions

The Original Maastricht Classification (Kootstra, 1995)

The decisive step towards an internationally accepted classification of DCD came in 1995 at the First International Workshop on Non-Heart-Beating Donation, held in Maastricht, the Netherlands, under the leadership of Gauke Kootstra and colleagues [8]. The workshop generated a four-category classification that introduced, for the first time, the central conceptual distinction between uncontrolled donation—where circulatory arrest was sudden and unexpected—and controlled donation, where it followed a planned withdrawal of life support [8, 22]. Category I ("dead on arrival") referred to donors brought to hospital after an unwitnessed cardiac arrest in whom resuscitation had not been attempted, and was uncontrolled. Category II ("unsuccessful resuscitation") referred to donors who suffered a witnessed cardiac arrest with cardiopulmonary resuscitation attempted but unsuccessful, and was likewise uncontrolled. Category III ("awaiting cardiac arrest") referred to patients in whom cardiac arrest was anticipated to follow planned withdrawal of life-sustaining treatment, and was the only controlled pathway in the original schema. Category IV ("cardiac arrest while brain dead") referred to donors who had already been declared brain dead and in whom unexpected circulatory arrest occurred before planned organ retrieval; in the original 1995 framework this was classified as uncontrolled [8, 22]. The principal contribution of the 1995 framework was conceptual: by distinguishing controlled from uncontrolled donation it allowed the transplant community to discuss, audit, and regulate the two pathways separately, recognising that they raised distinct ethical, logistical, and ischaemic concerns [8, 9, 22].

Limitations of the Original Framework and the Rationale for Revision

By the late 2000s, expanding clinical experience exposed three substantive limitations of the original four-category system [9, 23]. First, Categories I and II were defined without reference to the location of arrest, even though the operational and ischaemic profiles of out-of-hospital and in-hospital arrests differ profoundly. Second, Category IV had been classified as uncontrolled, but in clinical practice it included two distinct scenarios: a sudden, unexpected arrest in a brain-dead donor (genuinely uncontrolled), and a planned, peri-procurement arrest after brain death had already been declared and retrieval logistics arranged (functionally controlled) [9]. Third, the 1995 framework lacked a standardised lexicon for the time intervals critical to DCD practice, terms that had become essential to international audit but were used inconsistently across centres [9, 21].

The Paris Consensus: Categorical Modifications to the Maastricht Framework (2013)

Recognising these tensions, the European Working Group reconvened at the 6th International Conference in Organ Donation in Paris in 2013, and published its consensus in Transplant International in 2016 (Thuong et al.) [9]. The Paris consensus introduced four substantive categorical modifications to the original framework. First, Category I was subdivided into IA (out-of-hospital arrest, no resuscitation attempted) and IB (in-hospital arrest, no resuscitation attempted), both uncontrolled. Second, Category II was similarly subdivided into IIA (out-of-hospital arrest with unsuccessful resuscitation) and IIB (in-hospital arrest with unsuccessful resuscitation), both uncontrolled. Third, Category III was retained as a controlled pathway but reworded with greater precision as "planned circulatory arrest following withdrawal of life-sustaining treatment," replacing the original phrase "awaiting cardiac arrest." Fourth, and conceptually most important, Category IV was reclassified as either controlled or uncontrolled, depending on whether the arrest in a brain-dead donor occurred in a planned peri-procurement setting (controlled) or as a sudden, unexpected event before retrieval (uncontrolled) [9]. The full modified classification is summarised in Table 1.1.

Table 1.1 Modified Maastricht classification of donation after circulatory death [8, 9]

Category	Sub-category	Description	Pathway
I	IA	Out-of-hospital arrest, no resuscitation attempted	Uncontrolled
	IB	In-hospital arrest, no resuscitation attempted	Uncontrolled
II	IIA	Out-of-hospital arrest with unsuccessful resuscitation	Uncontrolled
	IIB	In-hospital arrest with unsuccessful resuscitation	Uncontrolled
III	–	Planned circulatory arrest following withdrawal of life-sustaining treatment	Controlled
IV	–	Cardiac arrest in a brain-dead donor before planned organ retrieval	Controlled or uncontrolled

The Standardised Time-Interval Framework Introduced by the Paris Consensus

In addition to the categorical refinements, the Paris consensus established a standardised lexicon of time intervals that is now embedded in international DCD protocols, outcome reporting, and the 2022 Indian consensus guidance [4, 9, 21]. Precise, time-stamped documentation of these intervals is the foundation of safe DCD practice; their definitions are summarised in Table 1.2 and supplemented by the broader set of commonly used DCD terms in Table 1.3.

The agonal phase is defined as the interval between WLST and circulatory arrest [9]. The duration of this phase varies widely between donors and is influenced by

Table 1.2 Standardised time intervals in donation after circulatory death: operational parameters [4, 9, 11, 21]

Interval	Start trigger	End trigger	Threshold/duration	Relevance
Agonal phase	Withdrawal of life-sustaining treatment (WLST)	Circulatory arrest	No fixed limit; duration donor-dependent. Centre-specific windows (commonly 1–3 h) define the period within which arrest must occur for organs to remain viable; failure to arrest triggers stand-down [9]	Marks onset of functional warm ischaemia; principal source of inter-donor variability
No-touch period	Circulatory arrest	Formal declaration of death	2–5 min internationally; 5 min in most contemporary protocols and in India, to exclude auto-resuscitation [4, 9, 11]	Mandatory observation confirming irreversibility before any intervention
Functional warm ischaemia time (fWIT)	Donor SBP < ~50–60 mmHg or SpO_2 < ~70%	Initiation of cold (in-situ) perfusion	Threshold values vary by guideline (some use MAP 50 mmHg or SpO_2 80%); centre cut-offs typically 30–60 min [9]	Period of true hypoperfusion injury; basis for organ acceptance decisions
Total warm ischaemia time (tWIT)	Circulatory arrest	Initiation of cold (in-situ) perfusion	Encompasses the no-touch period and any subsequent delay to perfusion; minimised by super-rapid retrieval or NRP [9, 21]	Principal determinant of graft outcome; the interval against which retrieval cut-offs are calibrated

Table 1.3 Commonly used terminology in donation after circulatory death

Term	Definition
End-of-life care (EOL)	Care provided to patients in the final stage of an irreversible illness, focused on dignity, comfort and family support; the umbrella within which WLST decisions are made
Withdrawal of life-sustaining treatment (WLST)	Planned discontinuation of mechanical ventilation, vasopressors, and other organ-supportive therapies when continued treatment is judged non-beneficial; the precondition for controlled (Category III) DCD
Agonal phase	The interval between WLST and circulatory arrest, characterised by progressive haemodynamic and respiratory deterioration. Used to define the onset of functional warm ischaemia [9]
Functional warm ischaemia time (fWIT)	Interval beginning when the donor systolic blood pressure falls below 50–60 mmHg or arterial oxygen saturation falls below 70%, and ending with the initiation of cold (in-situ) perfusion [9]. Threshold values vary across guidelines
Asystolic period	Interval from circulatory arrest to initiation of cold perfusion, encompassing the no-touch period and any subsequent delay before perfusion
No-touch period	Mandatory observation period after circulatory arrest, during which no intervention is permitted, to confirm irreversibility of cessation and exclude auto-resuscitation. Typically, 2–5 min internationally; 5 min in most contemporary protocols and in India [4, 9]
Total warm ischaemia time (tWIT)	Total interval from circulatory arrest to initiation of cold perfusion; the principal determinant of graft outcome [9]
Cold ischaemia time (CIT)	Interval from initiation of cold perfusion in the donor to organ reperfusion in the recipient
Super-rapid retrieval	Surgical technique characterised by immediate aortic cannulation and rapid cold perfusion of abdominal organs following death declaration; the foundational operational approach in DCD without normothermic regional perfusion
Normothermic regional perfusion (NRP)	Restoration of oxygenated, normothermic, in-situ perfusion to the abdominal (A-NRP) or thoraco-abdominal (TA-NRP) compartments after death declaration, using an extracorporeal circuit. Mitigates warm ischaemic injury and permits functional assessment of organs
Premortem heparinisation	Administration of intravenous heparin (typically 25,000–30,000 IU) before WLST in controlled DCD pathways, to reduce microvascular thrombosis after circulatory arrest. Requires explicit family consent
Stand-down	Return of the donor to the ICU when circulatory arrest does not occur within the time window compatible with viable organ retrieval; donation is abandoned and end-of-life care continues without donation [4]

the underlying pathology and the degree of organ-supportive therapy at the time of WLST. The no-touch period is the mandatory observation period after circulatory arrest during which no intervention occurs and which must elapse before death can be formally declared. International protocols specify durations of two to five minutes; most contemporary protocols—including those endorsed by the 2022 Indian consensus guidance [11]—adopt five minutes, on the basis that this duration reliably excludes the possibility of auto-resuscitation [4, 9, 11]. The functional warm ischaemia time (fWIT) begins when the donor systolic blood pressure falls below approximately 50–60 mmHg or arterial oxygen saturation falls below approximately 70%, and ends with the initiation of cold (in-situ) perfusion [9]. The exact thresholds vary by guideline; some centres use mean arterial pressure of 50 mmHg, others use SpO_2 thresholds of 80%. The total warm ischaemia time (tWIT) is measured from circulatory arrest to the initiation of cold perfusion and is the principal determinant of graft outcome [9, 21]. The conceptual sequence of events for controlled DCD (Category III) is: WLST → agonal phase → circulatory arrest → no-touch period → death declaration → cold perfusion (Fig. 1.2a). For uncontrolled DCD (Categories I, II), the corresponding sequence is: cardiac arrest (witnessed or unwitnessed) → cardiopulmonary resuscitation (attempted or not) → termination of resuscitation → death declaration → in-situ preservation (Fig. 1.2b) [9, 11].

The Belgian Modification and the Introduction of Category V (2012/2014)

A subsequent modification of the Maastricht classification was proposed by the Belgian DCD Working Group, led by Detry and colleagues, to accommodate organ donation following medically assisted circulatory death in jurisdictions where the practice is legal [24]. The Belgian modification added a fifth category, Category V, defined as "medically assisted cardio-circulatory death," which applies to patients who, having met the legal criteria for euthanasia or medical assistance in dying (MAiD), consent to organ donation after the resulting circulatory arrest [24, 25]. Category V is conceptually a controlled pathway, since the timing of arrest is planned, but it is ethically and procedurally distinct from Category III because the proximate cause of death is the administration of a lethal substance rather than the withdrawal of life-sustaining treatment in a patient with terminal illness [24–26]. Category V donors have been recognised in Belgium, the Netherlands, Canada and Spain; according to the international scoping review by Mulder et al. (2022), organ donation after euthanasia (ODE) had been performed 286 times across these four jurisdictions by 2021, with approximately 837 recipients having received organs from ODE donors and the practice contributing up to 14% of DCDD donors in some series [26].

The Indian Consensus Guidance and Indian Category V (2022)

The 2022 Indian consensus guidance on DCDD (Seth et al.) [11] adopts the four-category modified Maastricht/Paris framework and additionally proposes a locally defined Category V, distinct from the Belgian Category V, to address a scenario considered operationally important in Indian transplant centres. The Indian Category V is defined as organ donation following unsuccessful cardiopulmonary resuscitation of cardiac arrest occurring in the intensive care unit (an uncontrolled pathway)

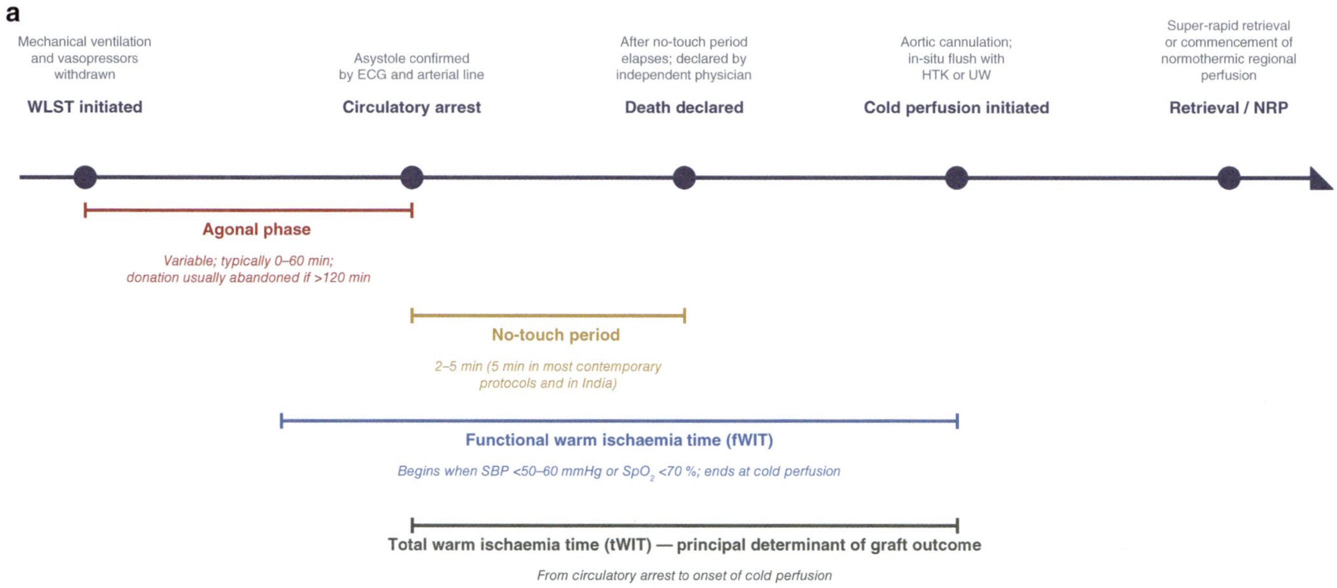

Fig. 1.2 (**a**) Time-interval framework for controlled DCD. (**b**) Time-interval framework for uncontrolled DCD. *Note: Functional warm ischaemia time (fWIT), as defined in controlled DCD, is not applicable to uncontrolled DCD because there is no agonal phase preceded by WLST. In uncontrolled DCD, total warm ischaemia time (tWIT)—from cardiac arrest to* in-situ *preservation—is the principal determinant of organ viability*

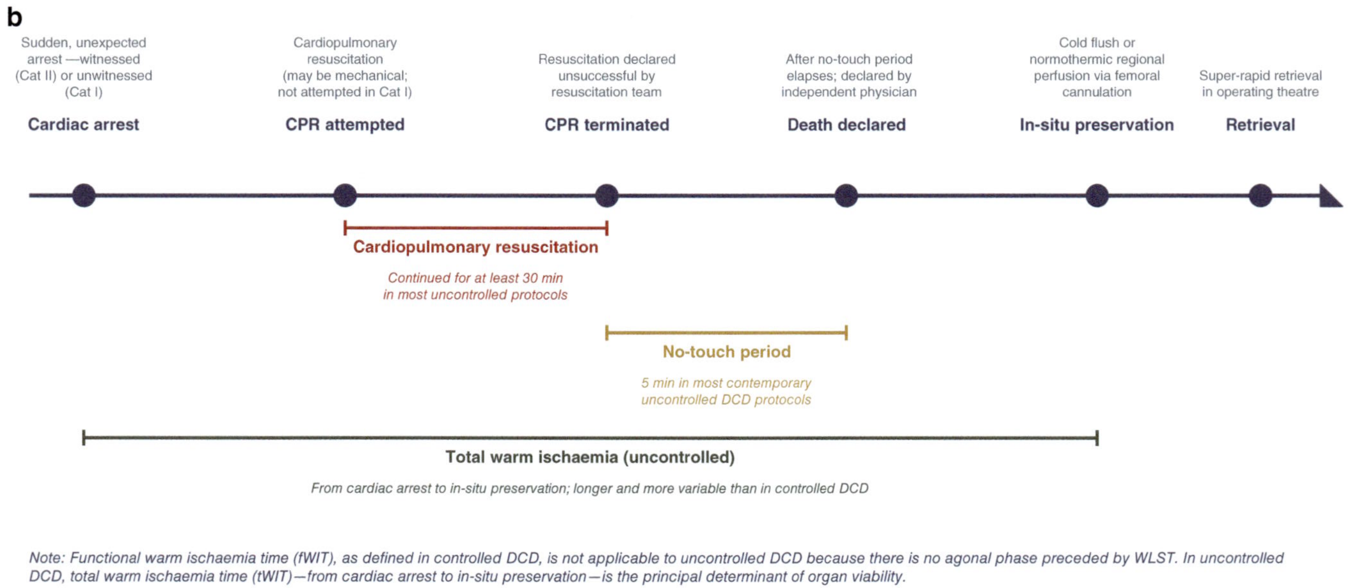

Fig. 1.2 (continued)

[11]. This terminology is therefore contrarian to the Belgian usage, in which Category V denotes medically assisted death and is a controlled pathway. The two are conceptually and ethically very different, and care is required when discussing Category V across jurisdictions. For the purposes of this volume, the modified Maastricht framework of Paris 2013 (Categories I–IV) is treated as the primary classification, while the Belgian Category V (organ donation after euthanasia) and the Indian Category V (in-ICU unsuccessful resuscitation) are described as regional adaptations applicable only within their respective jurisdictions. Active euthanasia is not legal in India under the current Bharatiya Nyaya Sanhita 2023, and the Belgian Category V is therefore not applicable to Indian practice [11, 27].

Comparative Summary of the Classifications

The stepwise evolution of the Maastricht classification, from the original 1995 Kootstra framework through the 2013 Paris modification, the 2014 Belgian addition, and the 2022 Indian adaptation, is summarised comparatively in Table 1.4. For routine international practice, the Paris 2013 modification remains the contemporary standard.

Table 1.4 Stepwise evolution of the Maastricht classification: 1995, 2013, 2014 and the 2022 Indian adaptation [8, 9, 11, 24]

Cat.	Original Maastricht (Kootstra, 1995)	Modified Maastricht (Paris/Thuong, 2013)	Belgian Modification (Detry, 2012/2014)	Indian Consensus (Seth, 2022)
I	Dead on arrival (uncontrolled)	Subdivided: IA (out-of-hospital), IB (in-hospital); no resuscitation attempted	Retained	Retained
II	Unsuccessful resuscitation (uncontrolled)	Subdivided: IIA (out-of-hospital), IIB (in-hospital); unsuccessful resuscitation	Retained	Retained
III	Awaiting cardiac arrest (controlled)	Reworded: planned arrest after WLST (controlled)	Retained	Retained
IV	Cardiac arrest while brain dead (uncontrolled only)	Cardiac arrest in a brain-dead donor— now either controlled or uncontrolled	Retained	Retained

(continued)

Table 1.4 (continued)

Cat.	Original Maastricht (Kootstra, 1995)	Modified Maastricht (Paris/Thuong, 2013)	Belgian Modification (Detry, 2012/2014)	Indian Consensus (Seth, 2022)
V	*Not present*	*Not present*	Medically assisted cardio-circulatory death (organ donation after euthanasia/ MAiD; controlled). Used in Belgium, the Netherlands, Canada and Spain	Defined locally as organ donation following unsuccessful CPR for cardiac arrest in the ICU (uncontrolled). Distinct from Belgian Category V

Global Expansion of DCD and the Maturation of Perfusion Technology

National Experience: Heterogeneous Adoption

Following the Maastricht Workshop and the Pittsburgh policy, DCD programmes expanded heterogeneously. Spain emerged as the global leader in uncontrolled DCD (Category II), supported by integrated emergency medical and procurement infrastructure that enabled rapid in-situ preservation and, increasingly, normothermic regional perfusion [23, 28]. The United Kingdom built its DCD programme largely around controlled (Category III) donation integrated within intensive-care end-of-life pathways; controlled DCD now accounts for approximately 40% of UK deceased-donor activity [29]. The United States expanded controlled DCD steadily from fewer than 200 transplants in 2001 to more than 2200 by 2015, and DCD now accounts for roughly 30% of deceased-donor organs in the United States [30, 31].

Normothermic Regional Perfusion: A Brief Introduction

Normothermic regional perfusion (NRP) is the single most influential technical advance of the past decade in DCD. In brief, after death has been declared and the no-touch period has elapsed, an extracorporeal circuit restores oxygenated, normothermic perfusion to the abdominal compartment (A-NRP), or to both the abdominal and thoracic compartments (TA-NRP), with effective vascular isolation above the diaphragm to prevent cerebral reperfusion [32, 33]. NRP mitigates warm ischaemic injury, permits in-situ functional assessment of organs, and substantially expands the spectrum of organs that can be utilised from DCD donors [32, 33]. The American Society of Transplant Surgeons issued formal standards for abdominal NRP in 2024 [33], and NRP has been associated with improved liver utilisation and outcomes [34]. A detailed account of NRP technique, vascular access, and clinical outcomes is beyond the scope of this historical and classification chapter, and is provided in a dedicated chapter of this volume.

The Reintroduction of DCD Heart Transplantation

The first human heart transplant, by Barnard in 1967, was technically a DCD heart transplant [15, 16]. Cardiac DCD then disappeared from clinical practice for nearly half a century, returning only after major advances in ex-situ machine perfusion. The first paediatric series of DCD heart transplants using direct procurement and cold storage was reported by Boucek and colleagues in 2008 [35]. The modern adult era of DCD heart transplantation was inaugurated in July 2014 by the team led by Kumud Dhital at St Vincent's Hospital, Sydney, who introduced the use of the TransMedics Organ Care System for ex-vivo normothermic preservation following direct procurement [36, 37]. Royal Papworth Hospital, Cambridge, performed the first European adult DCD heart transplant in February 2015, integrating NRP into its protocol [38]. DCD heart transplantation has since been adopted in centres across the United Kingdom, the United States and Belgium, with outcomes broadly comparable to DBD heart transplantation [36, 38, 39].

DCD Beyond Kidney Transplantation: Liver, Lung and Pancreas

Although kidney transplantation has historically been the dominant application of DCD organs, the contemporary scope of DCD extends across multiple solid organs. The 2022 Indian consensus guidance provides organ-specific recommendations for kidney, liver, heart and lung transplantation following DCDD [11]. DCD liver transplantation is now well established, with outcomes approaching those of DBD liver transplantation when warm ischaemia is minimised and NRP is employed to mitigate biliary injury [11, 34]. DCD lung transplantation, originally pioneered by Steen and colleagues using ex-vivo lung perfusion, has demonstrated outcomes comparable to DBD lung transplantation in large series, and is now performed routinely in mature programmes including those in Australia, the United Kingdom and Spain [11, 28]. DCD pancreas transplantation is technically feasible and is reported in selected centres, although the absolute numbers remain small [11]. For Indian centres beginning DCD activity, kidney-only programmes provide the lowest-threshold entry point, with liver and thoracic organ retrieval introduced progressively as institutional capability and NRP infrastructure mature [11].

The Indian Trajectory: From Constraint to Feasibility

The Legal and Infrastructural Backdrop

India enacted the Transplantation of Human Organs Act (THOA) in 1994, recognising both brain death and circulatory death as valid bases for deceased donation [11, 40]. THOA has therefore never prohibited DCD; the practical barrier was the absence of a legally and ethically secure framework for the withdrawal of life-sustaining treatment, without which controlled (Category III) DCD could not safely proceed [11]. The Bharatiya Nyaya Sanhita 2023 retains the prohibition on active euthanasia (Sections 100 and 101); withdrawal of life-sustaining treatment in patients with futile prognosis is, however, recognised as ethically and legally permissible under defined procedural safeguards [11, 27].

Early Indian DCD Experience

Despite these constraints, two Indian centres pioneered cautious DCD activity. The Institute of Kidney Diseases and Research Centre (IKDRC), Ahmedabad, performed a substantial series of controlled DCD kidney transplants from the late 1990s through the early 2010s, accounting for a notable proportion of its deceased-donor activity, with withdrawal of life support in the operating theatre, a defined no-touch period, premortem heparinisation, femoral cannulation and rapid retrieval, and reported acceptable medium-term patient and graft survival [41]. The Postgraduate Institute of Medical Education and Research (PGIMER), Chandigarh, subsequently reported a small series of predominantly Maastricht category IV donors, with a single category V donor, demonstrating that uncontrolled donation could be feasible in a tertiary public-sector setting when coupled with continued chest compressions after death declaration and rapid in-situ perfusion [42]. These early reports established proof-of-concept for both controlled and uncontrolled DCD in India.

The 2022 Indian Consensus Guidance and the Contemporary Landscape

In 2022, a multidisciplinary group of Indian experts published consensus guidance on DCDD under the auspices of the Indian Society of Critical Care Medicine, the Liver Transplant Society of India and other professional bodies [11]. This guidance translated international best practice into operational clinical recommendations, defined the categories of DCDD applicable in India (including the locally adapted Category V), and outlined the institutional, ethical and procedural prerequisites for safe implementation [11]. AIIMS Nagpur reported uncontrolled Category IV DCD kidney transplants from December 2023 onwards. In November 2025, a centre in Delhi performed the first reported use of post-mortem NRP in Asia, retrieving a liver and two kidneys from a controlled DCD donor. In 2024, the Armed Forces

Medical Services performed their first DCD organ retrieval at Command Hospital, Chandimandir [12]. Although the absolute numbers remain small, these milestones together signal the emergence of DCD as a viable second pillar of deceased donation in India.

Classification in Indian Practice: Practical Implications

Category III: The Structured Controlled Pathway

For Indian centres with the requisite ICU governance, end-of-life care infrastructure and operating-theatre coordination, controlled (Category III) DCD provides a legally defensible, ethically structured pathway for programme expansion [11]. It is the dominant pathway internationally and offers the most predictable warm ischaemic profile, the most robust audit trail, and the clearest separation between end-of-life decisions and donation decisions [9, 29].

Category IV: The Most Immediately Deployable Pathway in India

Category IV—cardiac arrest in a donor in whom brain death has already been declared—occupies a distinctive position in the Indian context. Because consent for donation has typically already been obtained, donor evaluation is complete, and ICU and theatre teams are already mobilised, an unexpected arrest in such a donor can be converted into a successful retrieval without invoking the WLST framework [11, 12]. Category IV uncontrolled DCD therefore represents the most immediately deployable pathway for Indian programmes that wish to commence DCD activity while controlled-DCD governance structures mature, and is the pathway through which several recent Indian centres have entered the DCD field [11, 12].

Categories I, II and V: Limited or Context-Specific Applicability

Categories I and II (uncontrolled out-of-hospital and in-hospital arrests) require prehospital and emergency-department infrastructure that exists at scale only in a small number of mature programmes worldwide, most notably in Spain and France [23, 28]. These categories are, at present, of limited applicability in routine Indian practice, although they may become relevant in selected metropolitan centres as emergency medical services and NRP capability mature. The Belgian Category V (organ donation after euthanasia) is not applicable in India, where active euthanasia remains a criminal offence [11, 27]. The Indian Category V (unsuccessful resuscitation of cardiac arrest in the ICU), as defined in the 2022 Indian consensus guidance [11], is potentially applicable in Indian transplant-centre ICUs but requires the same operational discipline as Categories I and II, including rapid in-situ preservation and pre-arrest recipient mobilisation.

Conclusion

The history of DCD is, in important respects, the history of clinical organ transplantation itself. From its origins in the 1950s and the 1960s, through its eclipse after the formal recognition of brain death in 1968, its deliberate revival at Pittsburgh in 1992 and Maastricht in 1995, and its contemporary expansion driven by NRP and ex-situ machine perfusion, DCD has progressed from a contested practice to an integral component of mature deceased-donation systems. The Maastricht classification has evolved across four distinct stages: the original Kootstra framework of 1995, the modified Paris classification of 2013 (with subdivision of Categories I and II and reclassification of Category IV), the Belgian addition of Category V in 2012/2014, and the locally adapted Indian Category V proposed in the 2022 Indian consensus guidance. The standardised time-interval framework of Paris 2013—agonal phase, no-touch period, functional warm ischaemia time, and total warm ischaemia time—provides the operational vocabulary within which contemporary DCD practice is audited and refined. For India, the convergence of THOA 1994, the 2022 Indian consensus guidance, and a growing portfolio of institutional experience now permits structured engagement with both controlled and uncontrolled DCD pathways. An understanding of the historical evolution and the current classification is therefore not a peripheral concern but the foundation on which Indian programmes—legally defensible, ethically transparent, and operationally rigorous—can be built.

Conflict of Interest The author(s) declare no conflict of interest.

Ethical Declaration This chapter is a narrative review of previously published literature and publicly available policy documents; no original human or animal research was undertaken, and ethical committee approval was therefore not required.

Competing Interests The author(s) has no competing interests to declare that are relevant to the content of this manuscript.

Ethics Approval The author(s) declares that this manuscript does not include primary research with human participants.

The author(s) declares that this manuscript does not include primary studies involving animals.

References

1. Manara A, Procaccio F, Domínguez-Gil B. Expanding the pool of deceased organ donors: the ICU and beyond. Intensive Care Med. 2019;45(3):357–60. https://doi.org/10.1007/s00134-019-05546-9.
2. Wijdicks EFM. The history of donation after circulatory death (DCD): backlash and boomerang. Neurocrit Care. 2024;40(2):425–35. https://doi.org/10.1007/s12028-023-01919-7.
3. Murray JE, Merrill JP, Harrison JH. Renal homotransplantation in identical twins. Surg Forum. 1955;6:432–6.
4. Abdi R. John Putnam Merrill: the unsung hero behind the first successful renal transplantation. Front Transplant. 2025;4:1620534. https://doi.org/10.3389/frtra.2025.1620534.

5. Ad Hoc Committee of the Harvard Medical School to Examine the Definition of Brain Death. A definition of irreversible coma. JAMA. 1968;205(6):337–40. https://doi.org/10.1001/jama.1968.03140320031009.
6. DeVita MA, Snyder JV. Development of the University of Pittsburgh Medical Center policy for the care of terminally ill patients who may become organ donors after death following the removal of life support. Kennedy Inst Ethics J. 1993;3(2):131–43. https://doi.org/10.1353/ken.0.0175.
7. University of Pittsburgh Medical Center. Policy and procedure manual: management of terminally ill patients who may become organ donors after death (May 1992). Kennedy Inst Ethics J. 1993;3(2):A1–15.
8. Kootstra G, Daemen JH, Oomen AP. Categories of non-heart-beating donors. Transplant Proc. 1995;27(5):2893–4.
9. Thuong M, Ruiz A, Evrard P, et al. New classification of donation after circulatory death donors: definitions and terminology. Transpl Int. 2016;29(7):749–59. https://doi.org/10.1111/tri.12776.
10. Bernat JL. The whole-brain concept of death remains optimum public policy. J Law Med Ethics. 2006;34(1):35–43. https://doi.org/10.1111/j.1748-720X.2006.00006.x.
11. Seth AK, Mohanka R, Navin S, et al. Organ donation after circulatory determination of death in India: a joint position paper. Indian J Crit Care Med. 2022;26(4):421–38. https://doi.org/10.5005/jp-journals-10071-24198.
12. Indian Society of Organ Transplantation. National updates on deceased donation activity in India: NOTTO/ROTTO/SOTTO data. New Delhi: National Organ and Tissue Transplant Organisation; 2024. Available from: https://www.notto.gov.in.
13. Murray JE, Merrill JP, Harrison JH, et al. Prolonged survival of human-kidney homografts by immunosuppressive drug therapy. N Engl J Med. 1963;268:1315–23. https://doi.org/10.1056/NEJM196306132682401.
14. Sayegh MH, Carpenter CB. Transplantation 50 years later: progress, challenges, and promises. N Engl J Med. 2004;351(26):2761–6. https://doi.org/10.1056/NEJMon043418.
15. Barnard CN. The operation. A human cardiac transplant: an interim report of a successful operation performed at Groote Schuur Hospital, Cape Town. S Afr Med J. 1967;41(48):1271–4.
16. Cooper DKC. Christiaan Barnard — the surgeon who dared: the story of the first human-to-human heart transplant. Glob Cardiol Sci Pract. 2018;2018(2):11. https://doi.org/10.21542/gcsp.2018.11.
17. Starzl TE, Marchioro TL, Vonkaulla KN, et al. Homotransplantation of the liver in humans. Surg Gynecol Obstet. 1963;117:659–76.
18. Daemen JWHC, de Wit RJ, Bronkhorst MWGA, et al. Non-heart-beating donor program contributes 40% of kidneys for transplantation. Transplant Proc. 1996;28(1):105–6.
19. DeVita MA, Snyder JV, Grenvik A. History of organ donation by patients with cardiac death. Kennedy Inst Ethics J. 1993;3(2):113–29. https://doi.org/10.1353/ken.0.0147.
20. Fox RC. "An ignoble form of cannibalism": reflections on the Pittsburgh protocol for procuring organs from non-heart-beating cadavers. Kennedy Inst Ethics J. 1993;3(2):231–9. https://doi.org/10.1353/ken.0.0070.
21. Manara AR, Murphy PG, O'Callaghan G. Donation after circulatory death. Br J Anaesth. 2012;108(Suppl 1):i108–21. https://doi.org/10.1093/bja/aer357.
22. Kootstra G, van Heurn E. Non-heartbeating donation of kidneys for transplantation. Nat Clin Pract Nephrol. 2007;3(3):154–63. https://doi.org/10.1038/ncpneph0426.
23. Domínguez-Gil B, Haase-Kromwijk B, Van Leiden H, et al. Current situation of donation after circulatory death in European countries. Transpl Int. 2011;24(7):676–86. https://doi.org/10.1111/j.1432-2277.2011.01257.x.
24. Detry O, Le Dinh H, Noterdaeme T, et al. Categories of donation after cardiocirculatory death. Transplant Proc. 2012;44(5):1189–95. https://doi.org/10.1016/j.transproceed.2012.05.001.
25. Bollen J, Ten Hoopen R, Ysebaert D, et al. Legal and ethical aspects of organ donation after euthanasia in Belgium and The Netherlands. J Med Ethics. 2016;42(8):486–9. https://doi.org/10.1136/medethics-2015-102898.

26. Mulder J, Sonneveld H, Van Raemdonck D, et al. Practice and challenges for organ donation after medical assistance in dying: a scoping review including the results of the first international roundtable in 2021. Am J Transplant. 2022;22(12):2759–80. https://doi.org/10.1111/ajt.17198.
27. Government of India. The Bharatiya Nyaya Sanhita, 2023 (Act No. 45 of 2023). Sections 100 and 101. New Delhi: Ministry of Law and Justice; 2023.
28. Domínguez-Gil B, Duranteau J, Mateos A, et al. Uncontrolled donation after circulatory death: European practices and recommendations for the development and optimization of an effective programme. Transpl Int. 2016;29(8):842–59. https://doi.org/10.1111/tri.12734.
29. NHS Blood and Transplant. Organ donation and transplantation: activity report 2023/24. Bristol: NHS Blood and Transplant; 2024. Available from: https://www.odt.nhs.uk
30. Israni AK, Zaun DA, Gauntt K, et al. OPTN/SRTR 2022 annual data report: deceased organ donation. Am J Transplant. 2024;24(2 Suppl 1):S457–88. https://doi.org/10.1016/j.ajt.2024.01.018. https://www.odt.nhs.uk.
31. O'Rourke J, Crowe G, Turner R, et al. Donation after circulatory death: a narrative review of current controversies, attitudes, and the evolving role of regional perfusion technology. AME Med J. 2024;9:9. https://doi.org/10.21037/amj-23-65.
32. Croome KP, Barbas AS, Whitson B, et al. American Society of Transplant Surgeons Scientific Studies Committee. American Society of Transplant Surgeons recommendations on best practices in donation after circulatory death organ procurement. Am J Transplant. 2023;23(2):171–9. https://doi.org/10.1016/j.ajt.2022.10.009.
33. Croome K, Bababekov Y, Brubaker A, et al. American Society of Transplant Surgeons normothermic regional perfusion standards: abdominal. Transplantation. 2024;108(8):1660–8. https://doi.org/10.1097/TP.0000000000005114.
34. Sellers MT, Nassar A, Alebrahim M, et al. Early United States experience with liver donation after circulatory determination of death using thoraco-abdominal normothermic regional perfusion: a multi-institutional observational study. Clin Transpl. 2022;36(6):e14659. https://doi.org/10.1111/ctr.14659.
35. Boucek MM, Mashburn C, Dunn SM, et al. Pediatric heart transplantation after declaration of cardiocirculatory death. N Engl J Med. 2008;359(7):709–14. https://doi.org/10.1056/NEJMoa0800660.
36. Dhital KK, Iyer A, Connellan M, et al. Adult heart transplantation with distant procurement and ex-vivo preservation of donor hearts after circulatory death: a case series. Lancet. 2015;385(9987):2585–91. https://doi.org/10.1016/S0140-6736(15)60038-1.
37. Dhital K, Ludhani P, Scheuer S, et al. DCD donations and outcomes of heart transplantation: the Australian experience. Indian J Thorac Cardiovasc Surg. 2020;36(Suppl 2):224–32. https://doi.org/10.1007/s12055-020-00998-x.
38. Messer S, Page A, Axell R, et al. Outcome after heart transplantation from donation after circulatory-determined death donors. J Heart Lung Transplant. 2017;36(12):1311–8. https://doi.org/10.1016/j.healun.2017.10.021.
39. Schroder JN, Patel CB, DeVore AD, et al. Transplantation outcomes with donor hearts after circulatory death. N Engl J Med. 2023;388(23):2121–31. https://doi.org/10.1056/NEJMoa2212438.
40. Government of India. Transplantation of Human Organs Act, 1994 (Act No. 42 of 1994), as amended by the Transplantation of Human Organs and Tissues (Amendment) Act, 2011. New Delhi: Ministry of Health and Family Welfare; 2011.
41. Kute VB, Vanikar AV, Shah PR, et al. Outcome of renal transplantation from deceased donors after cardiac death: a single-center experience from a developing country. Transplant Proc. 2013;45(6):2147–51. https://doi.org/10.1016/j.transproceed.2013.02.128.
42. Singh S, Kumar S, Dasgupta S, et al. A single-center experience of kidney transplantation from donation after circulatory death: challenges and scope in India. Indian J Nephrol. 2017;27(3):205–9. https://doi.org/10.4103/0971-4065.202843.

Establishing a DCD Programme: Infrastructure, Feasibility and Institutional Preparedness

2

Pranjal Kashiv, Ashish Saharia, and Sanjay Kolte

Introduction

At mature transplant systems DCD is a routine rather than exceptional practice. Controlled DCD now contributes approximately 40% of deceased-donor activity in the United Kingdom [1], while DCD accounts for approximately 30% of deceased-donor organs in the USA [2], and Spain has built a high-volume uncontrolled DCD programme on the foundation of an integrated pre-hospital and procurement network. India, by contrast, has a deceased-donation rate that remains below one per million population, and DCD has historically contributed only a small fraction of that activity. The principal constraint has rarely been the law since the Transplantation of Human Organs Act, 1994, has always permitted retrieval after circulatory determination of death; the binding constraint has been the absence of the institutional infrastructure required to translate legal permission into safe and reproducible clinical practice [3].

The legal foundation for withdrawal of life-sustaining treatment (WLST) in India is the judgement of the Supreme Court in Common Cause v. Union of India, delivered on 9 March, 2018, which recognised advance medical directives and the right of patients to refuse life-sustaining treatment [4]. The procedure laid down in that judgement proved unworkable in practice, and on 24 January,

P. Kashiv (✉)
AIIMS Nagpur, Nagpur, Maharashtra, India

A. Saharia
Liver Transplantation at Houston Methodist J.C. Walter Jr. Transplant Center and Surgical Director of Liver Transplantation in the Department of Surgery, Houston, TX, USA
e-mail: asaharia@houstonmethodist.org

S. Kolte
Department of Urology and Kidney Transplant, Max SS Hospital Nagpur, Nagpur, Maharashtra, India

S. P. Kolte et al. (eds.), *Organ Donation After Circulatory Death*,
https://doi.org/10.1007/978-981-92-6377-6_2

2023, the Supreme Court issued a clarificatory order in Miscellaneous Application No. 1699 of 2019 that substantially simplified the dual-medical-board pathway and removed the requirement of prior judicial approval [5]. The 2020 ICMR Consensus Guidelines on Do Not Attempt Resuscitation [6] and the AIIMS New Delhi institutional end-of-life care policy of 2022 [7] together provided the earliest Indian operational templates for the bedside translation of these rights, and the AIIMS document remains a practical reference that other centres can adapt to local practice. The 2022 Joint Position Paper of Indian transplant and critical-care societies subsequently adapted international DCD best practice to Indian medico-legal realities and introduced category-specific operational checklists for controlled and uncontrolled pathways [3], and the 2024 expert consensus of the Indian Society of Critical Care Medicine and the Indian Association of Palliative Care set out the contemporary bedside framework for end-of-life care in the intensive care unit consistent with the 2023 order [8]. The 2024 multi-society DCD consensus statement published in the Indian Journal of Transplantation, endorsed by the Indian Society of Organ Transplantation along with multiple other Indian scientific societies, collated these strands into a single procedural reference for the Category III pathway [9]. The primary legal source remains the 2018 judgement as simplified by the 2023 order; the position papers cited in this chapter are consequential documents that translate that source into bedside operational form.

The historical evolution and classification of DCD are addressed in Chap. 1, and the present chapter takes that material as its starting point. The focus here is on operational implementation, including the architecture of the intensive care unit and operating theatre, the coordination and consent pathways, the documentation and audit systems and the workforce competencies that determine whether a centre can move from policy to first case and from first case to a sustainable programme. The pathway-specific operational sequences for controlled and uncontrolled DCD are summarised in Figs. 2.1 and 2.2a, b, and category-specific readiness checklists are presented in Table 2.1.

Throughout the chapter, the modified Maastricht classification (Paris 2013) is used uniformly, namely IA, IB, IIA, IIB, III and IV, in order to maintain alignment with Chap. 1 and to enable direct cross-reference between the two chapters [10]. Where the Indian context introduces a locally specific consideration, for example, the operational status of a donor in whom brain-stem-death testing has not been formally completed, that consideration is annotated explicitly rather than absorbed into a new category.

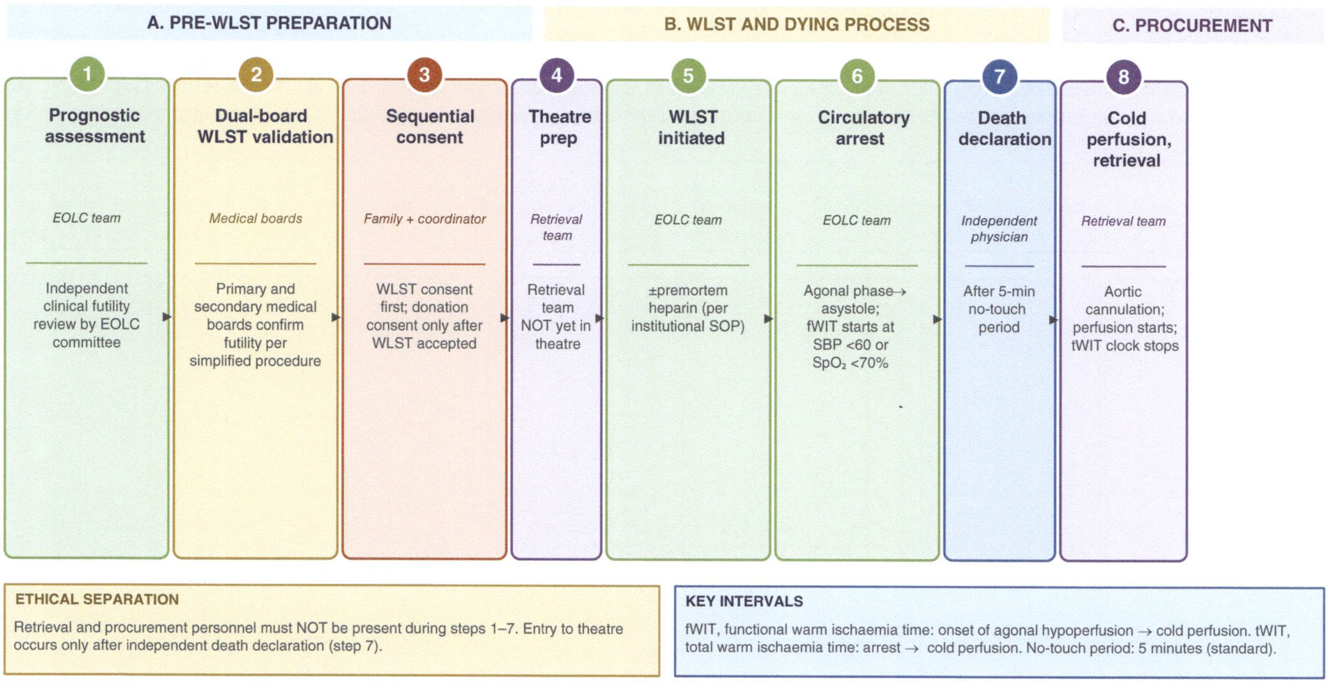

Fig. 2.1 Operational pathway for controlled (Category III) donation after circulatory death, from the end-of-life decision through to retrieval. The pathway is depicted as a swimlane diagram with five parallel actor roles: the EOLC team (intensivist, palliative care); the institutional medical boards; the family and consent process; the transplant coordinator and the retrieval and recipient teams. The key time-stamped events are indicated along the central time axis, namely the WLST decision, sequential consent, transfer to the operating theatre, initiation of WLST, the agonal phase, circulatory arrest, the no-touch period, declaration of death and initiation of cold perfusion

a

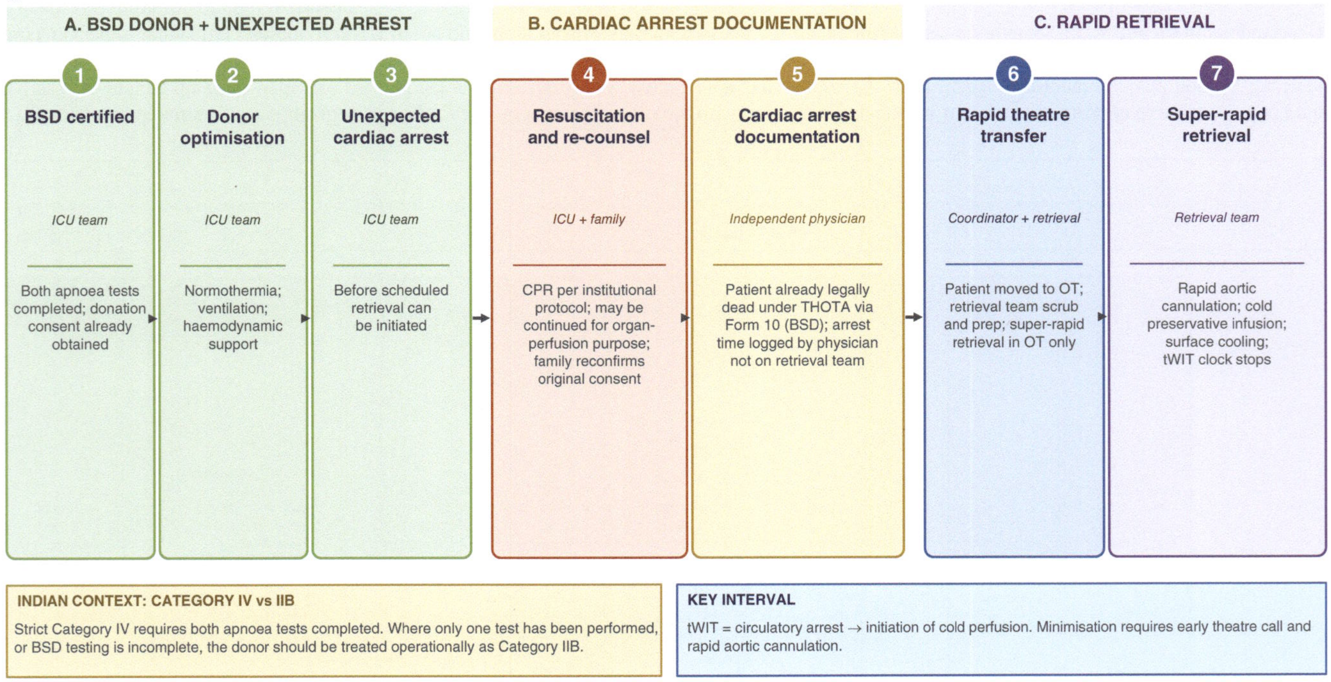

Fig. 2.2 (**a**) Operational pathway for uncontrolled DCD, Category IV (donor-salvage following completed brain-stem-death declaration). The pathway is depicted as a swimlane diagram, beginning at the moment of unexpected cardiac arrest in a fully certified BSD donor and proceeding through resuscitation (continued, in selected cases, for organ-preservation purposes), documentation of circulatory arrest in the already-declared brain-dead donor (no additional no-touch period required), rapid transfer to the operating theatre, super-rapid retrieval and initiation of cold perfusion. Where brain-stem-death certification is incomplete (for example, only one apnoea test performed), the donor is operationally re-classified as Category IIB, and the standard 5-min no-touch period applies before retrieval is initiated. (**b**) Operational pathway for uncontrolled DCD, Categories I and II (cardiac arrest without preceding brain-stem-death declaration). The pathway is depicted as a swimlane diagram, beginning at the moment of cardiac arrest (out-of-hospital for IA and IIA, in-hospital for IB and IIB) and proceeding through unsuccessful resuscitation, the no-touch period, declaration of death, the acute family-consent conversation, in situ preservation (with or without NRP) and surgical retrieval

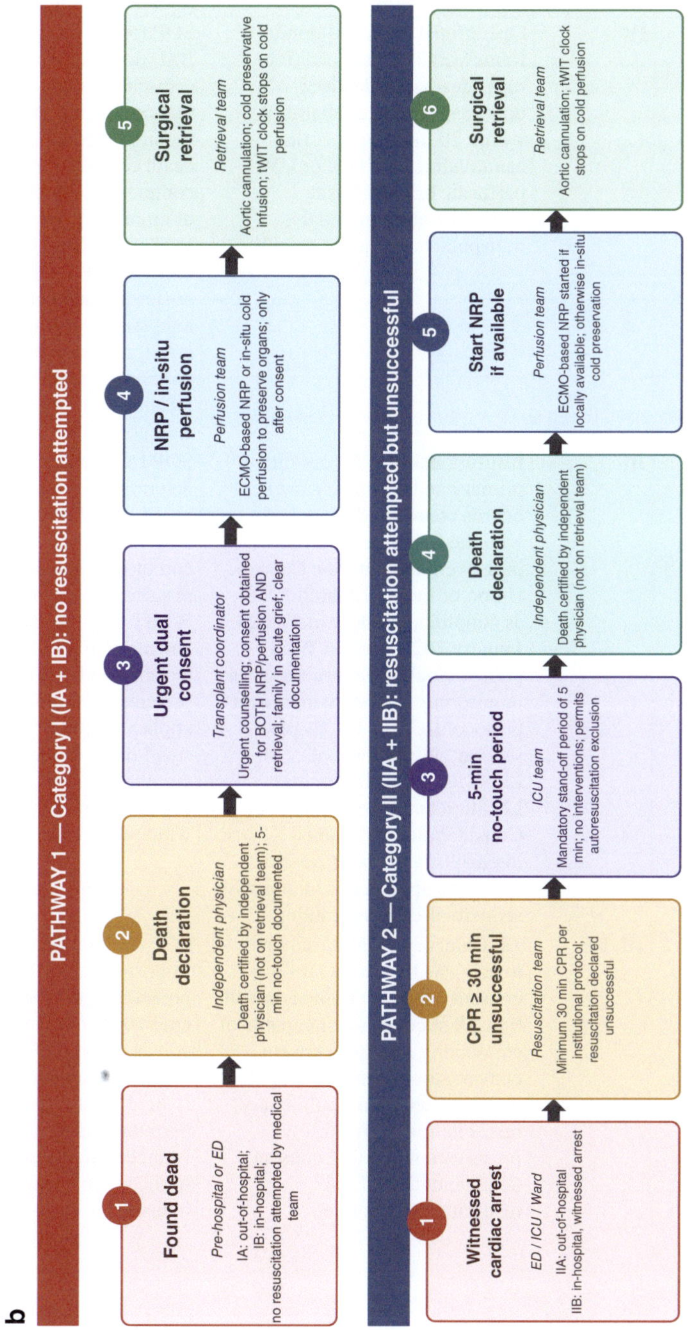

Fig. 2.2 (continued)

Table 2.1 Category-specific operational readiness for DCD pathways

Pathway	Categories	Minimum readiness	Mandatory SOPs
Uncontrolled, post-BSD	IV	Operational deceased-donor framework; trained team for rapid death certification; operating theatre availability within 30 min; rapid aortic-cannulation set; HTK or UW perfusate primed; basic surface-cooling materials; transplant coordinator on call	SOP for cardiac arrest in a BSD donor (covering resuscitation, recognition that no-touch period is not required where brain-stem-death certification is complete and documentation of circulatory arrest in the already-declared brain-dead donor); SOP for super-rapid retrieval; documentation template recording time of arrest, no-touch period (where applicable), surgical incision and initiation of cold perfusion
Controlled, WLST-based	III	Institutional EOLC committee; primary and secondary medical boards constituted in accordance with the Supreme Court's judgement in Common Cause v. Union of India (9 March 2018) as simplified by the order of 24 January 2023; written WLST policy; clock-synchronised event monitoring; defined withdrawal protocol (ICU or OT, as per section "Withdrawal of Life-Sustaining Treatment: Location and Operational Considerations"); trained intensivist and palliative-care team; transplant coordinator with sequential-consent training	SOP for futility determination and dual-board WLST validation; SOP for family communication and sequential consent; SOP for WLST procedure and antemortem interventions (specifying heparin dose and pre-emptive cannulation if applicable); SOP for stand-down in the event that circulatory arrest does not occur within the viability window
Uncontrolled, in-hospital, no BSD	IB, IIB	All Category IV requirements together with a rapid family-consent pathway; trained on-call transplant coordinator capable of conducting an acute consent conversation; institutional policy on continued cardiopulmonary resuscitation or in situ preservation pending consent; documentation of the resuscitation timeline	SOP for unexpected in-hospital arrest in a potential donor; SOP for the emergency consent conversation; SOP for continued resuscitation (where institutionally permitted) until consent and cannulation; documentation of the warm ischaemia interval

(continued)

Table 2.1 (continued)

Pathway	Categories	Minimum readiness	Mandatory SOPs
Uncontrolled, out-of-hospital	IA, IIA	All of the above together with an integrated pre-hospital emergency-medical-services link; double-balloon catheter or in situ NRP capability; ECMO or extracorporeal circuit; trained perfusionist; established referral pathway from the receiving emergency department.	SOP for pre-hospital identification and transport; SOP for in situ preservation pending consent; SOP for handover between the emergency department and the operating theatre; SOP for NRP initiation and decanting; family-communication SOP adapted to acute bereavement.

Intensive Care Unit Readiness

End-of-Life Care Governance and the WLST Framework

Controlled donation after circulatory death originates in the intensive care unit, and the strength of institutional end-of-life care (EOLC) governance therefore determines whether a Category III programme is operationally feasible. Each centre should constitute a standing EOLC committee with representation from critical care, neurology or neurosurgery, palliative medicine and an ethics or hospital-administration nominee. The committee's role is threefold: prognostic confirmation, determination of futility and oversight of decisions on withdrawal of life-sustaining treatment (WLST). The dual primary and secondary medical board structure that operationalises these functions in Indian practice derives directly from the Supreme Court's judgement in Common Cause v. Union of India (9 March, 2018), as simplified by the clarificatory order of 24 January, 2023, which removed the requirement of prior approval from a Judicial Magistrate of the First Class and reduced the procedure to intimation alone [4, 5]. The AIIMS New Delhi institutional EOLC policy of 2022 [7], the 2024 ISCCM and IAPC expert consensus [8] and the 2024 multi-society DCD consensus statement (IJT 2024) endorsed by ISOT and multiple Indian scientific societies [9] each provide bedside templates for family communication, sequential consent and dual-board validation that translate the simplified procedure into clinical workflow.

Three principles govern the EOLC pathway and must be observed without exception. First, the decision to withdraw or withhold treatment must rest exclusively on clinical futility and the patient's best interests, and the prospect of organ donation must not influence that determination at any stage. Second, the conversation regarding WLST and the conversation regarding organ donation must remain separated in both time and personnel, such that the treating intensivist typically conducts the former and a transplant coordinator the latter and only after the family has accepted the WLST plan [3, 8]. Third, the do-not-attempt-resuscitation (DNAR) order, structured along the lines of the 2020 Indian Council of Medical Research consensus, must be coherent with the WLST plan to avoid contradictory orders within the same admission [6]. Adherence to these three principles secures both the ethical defensibility of the pathway and the medico-legal protection of the institution.

Clinical Monitoring and Event Documentation

The DCD pathway is, more than anything else, a documented sequence of time-stamped events. The minimum clinical-monitoring infrastructure therefore comprises continuous arterial blood-pressure monitoring (or, where invasive access is impractical, non-invasive blood pressure measured at intervals of no longer than 1 min), continuous electrocardiography, pulse oximetry and a clock-synchronised event logger that records the agonal phase, the no-touch period, the moment of death declaration and the time of cold-perfusion initiation to the minute [3, 10]. Functional warm ischaemia time (fWIT) is defined as the interval beginning when the systolic blood pressure falls below 50 to 60 mmHg or arterial oxygen saturation falls below 70%, and total warm ischaemia time (tWIT) is measured from circulatory arrest to the initiation of cold perfusion [3, 10]. These two intervals are the principal determinants of graft outcome, and accurate time-stamping is therefore a substantive clinical requirement rather than an administrative formality. The full conceptual sequence for controlled DCD is shown in Fig. 2.1, and the corresponding sequences for the two principal uncontrolled scenarios, namely Category IV (donor-salvage following completed brain-stem-death declaration) and Categories I and II (cardiac arrest without preceding brain-stem-death declaration), are shown in Fig. 2.2a and b, respectively.

Antemortem Interventions in Controlled DCD

Several pre-withdrawal interventions in controlled DCD improve graft viability without compromising the ethical separation between EOLC and donation, provided that each is performed under explicit family consent. Premortem heparinisation is the most consistently practised intervention. Indian centres have generally used a fixed dose of 10,000 units at the time of WLST, in keeping with the protocol of the Institute of Kidney Diseases and Research Centre at Ahmedabad [11]. International guidance favours a higher dose, with the British Transplantation Society recommending approximately 25,000 IU based on a weight-adjusted dose of 300 IU per kilogramme administered in the preservation solution [12], and the American Society of Transplant Surgeons recommending either a fixed dose of 30,000 units or a weight-based dose of 100 to 300 units per kilogramme administered 3 to 5 min before WLST in order to permit adequate circulation [13]. A multicentre observational study has shown no significant association between heparin dose and renal graft outcomes [14], although higher doses may be more clearly relevant when liver or thoracic organs are retrieved. The dose used at a given centre should therefore be specified in institutional policy, supported by an appropriate reference and disclosed transparently to the family, rather than presented as a universal recommendation.

Maintenance of physiological stability until the point of WLST, including normothermia, adequate ventilation and haemodynamic support, preserves organ quality and shortens the post-withdrawal agonal phase. Pre-emptive femoral arterial and venous cannulation, where used, requires comprehensive family counselling, documented informed consent and a clearly defined procedural rationale (typically the planned use of in situ normothermic regional perfusion). It is not a routine practice and should not be presented to families as such [3, 13].

Operating Theatre Infrastructure

Sterile Readiness and Team Positioning

The operating theatre must be fully prepared before WLST, with clear physical and procedural boundaries separating the end-of-life care team from the procurement team [3, 13]. The retrieval team must not be present in the theatre during WLST, the no-touch period or death declaration and must enter the theatre only after death has been formally certified by an independent physician. This separation is non-negotiable and protects both the patient's family and the procurement team from any perception, however unfounded, of a conflict of interest. Where liver retrieval is planned, the donor may be transferred to the theatre, positioned and draped before WLST, provided that all procurement personnel leave the theatre before withdrawal commences; this approach permits immediate surgical access on death declaration and is critical for limiting hepatic warm ischaemia. In kidney-only programmes, draping may follow death declaration, although prepositioning is encouraged wherever logistics permit, in order to shorten the interval to aortic cannulation [3, 13, 15].

Equipment and Perfusion Readiness

A DCD-capable theatre requires an unobstructed transfer pathway from the intensive care unit, pre-primed cold preservation solution (histidine-tryptophan-ketoglutarate or University of Wisconsin solution), ice slush and surface-cooling materials, a rapid aortic-cannulation set and femoral-access capability for centres planning normothermic regional perfusion (NRP) [3, 13, 15]. Where NRP is to be employed, additional infrastructure is required, including an extracorporeal circuit with oxygenator and heat exchanger, an occlusive thoracic-aortic balloon for abdominal NRP and a trained perfusionist on standby. NRP is increasingly regarded as a recommended adjunct in mature DCD programmes; the British Transplantation

Society guideline recommends abdominal NRP in all DCD retrievals where a competent team is available [12] and the 2024 American Society of Transplant Surgeons standards for abdominal NRP provide the procedural framework for current United States practice [15]. NRP is not, however, a prerequisite for programme initiation, and most Indian centres beginning DCD activity will operate without it, relying instead on super-rapid retrieval with rapid cold perfusion.

The Retrieval Team

The minimum retrieval team comprises a retrieval surgeon proficient in super-rapid retrieval and rapid aortic cannulation; an assistant surgeon for kidney mobilisation and back-table preparation; an anaesthetist for comfort-focused care during WLST, who is explicitly excluded from death determination and from any role in retrieval; a perfusionist where NRP is planned; one or two scrub nurses and a transplant coordinator who oversees documentation and inter-team coordination. Theatre staff must be familiar with the time pressures that are peculiar to DCD since the interval from death declaration to cold perfusion is the principal determinant of graft outcome, and a rehearsed sequence between teams is operationally more important than the addition of further personnel.

Withdrawal of Life-Sustaining Treatment: Location and Operational Considerations

The optimal location for WLST in controlled DCD is one of the most consequential operational decisions a programme will make, and there is no single answer that is correct in all circumstances. The choice between the intensive care unit and the operating theatre depends on four interacting factors, namely family preference, the planned use and modality of NRP, the organs intended for retrieval and local logistical feasibility. Each is addressed below.

Family Preference and Presence During Withdrawal

Many families wish to be present at the moment of death and to remain with the donor until shortly before retrieval. This is more naturally accommodated in the intensive care unit, where the environment is familiar to the family and where palliative-care staff are typically available. Counselling regarding the location of withdrawal and the option of family presence should therefore precede the operational decision rather than follow it. Where a family expresses a strong preference for ICU-based withdrawal, that preference should be respected wherever it is logistically compatible with the planned retrieval, and the implications of each option for the timing of subsequent steps should be explained in clear terms.

Normothermic Regional Perfusion Planning

Where NRP is not planned, theatre-based WLST is generally preferable because it minimises the interval between circulatory arrest and the initiation of cold perfusion, and it is therefore associated with shorter functional and total warm ischaemia times. Where ECMO-based in situ NRP is planned, WLST may feasibly occur in either the intensive care unit or the operating theatre because perfusion is restored rapidly after death declaration, and the additional minutes of cold-perfusion delay are of reduced consequence for graft outcome. Where cardiopulmonary-bypass-based NRP is planned, the operating theatre is generally more suitable for practical reasons related to circuit setup and cannulation. Some centres employ super-rapid retrieval followed by ex situ normothermic machine perfusion, for example, using the Organ Care System or comparable platforms; in such centres, the trade-off between ICU comfort and theatre proximity is altered, and the optimal withdrawal location may differ from the default.

Organ-Specific Considerations

Heart and lung retrieval is, in almost all current protocols, performed in the operating theatre, with WLST conducted there in order to minimise warm ischaemia. Liver retrieval without NRP similarly favours theatre-based WLST. Kidney-only retrieval is more flexible: where transfer from the intensive care unit to the operating theatre can be accomplished rapidly and reliably, ICU-based WLST is acceptable and may, at some institutions, be preferable for reasons related to family experience.

Logistical Feasibility

Theatre-based WLST, although ideal from the perspective of ischaemia time, is not feasible at all centres at all times. Some institutions cannot reliably ring-fence an operating theatre for a procedure of indeterminate duration, and some lack the transport infrastructure required to move a ventilated patient with grieving family from the intensive care unit to the operating theatre. Each institution should therefore formalise its preferred WLST location for each organ-specific pathway in a written protocol, with an explicit fallback in the event that the preferred option is unavailable. Dignity, privacy and the family's right to be with the donor must be preserved irrespective of the location chosen.

Transplant Coordination and Consent

Notification and Allocation

The framework of the National, Regional and State Organ and Tissue Transplant Organisations (NOTTO, ROTTO, SOTTO) requires early notification of potential DCD donors, ideally at the point of WLST decision in controlled pathways or immediately after death declaration in uncontrolled Category IV pathways [3]. Early notification permits cross-verification of the registry, recipient identification, initiation of crossmatch testing and logistical preparation in advance of retrieval. Recipient mobilisation in advance of retrieval has been emphasised in controlled DCD practice, including the IKDRC controlled DCD programme, where the timing of WLST is itself controlled, and recipient teams can therefore be assembled in parallel [11]. In uncontrolled pathways, by contrast, the timing of arrest is by definition unanticipated, and death determination must remain procedurally and ethically distinct from any preparatory step directed at donation; in such settings, recipient mobilisation can be initiated only after death has been declared, and cold ischaemia is minimised through pre-existing on-call infrastructure rather than through pre-arrest preparation [3].

Sequential Consent Pathway

Consent for WLST and consent for organ donation must be sequential, transparent and independently documented, and donation must be discussed only after WLST has been finalised and accepted by the family [3, 8]. A defined hierarchy of family decision-makers reduces conflict, and explicit confirmation of the absence of any financial exchange, recorded within the donation consent form, protects the credibility of the programme. Family counselling should make clear that WLST is a decision to avoid non-beneficial treatment rather than a step towards donation. The 2024 ISCCM and IAPC consensus and the 2024 multi-society DCD consensus statement (IJT 2024, endorsed by ISOT and multiple Indian scientific societies) together provide culturally appropriate templates for the consent conversation in Indian practice [8, 9].

Recipient-Side Preparation

The recipient side of the pathway requires the same operational discipline as the donor side. Indian DCD kidney series has reported delayed graft function (DGF) rates of 31% to 80%, with the precise rate depending on the pathway used and on whether perfusion technology was employed [11, 16]. Recipients should be selected with this consideration in mind, counselled explicitly regarding DGF and the possibility of prolonged early dialysis and given the opportunity to decline a DCD allograft in favour of remaining on the standard deceased-donor list. Crossmatch laboratories should be on standby from the time of donor notification, surgical teams should be pre-mobilised and the operating theatre for the recipient transplant should be booked in advance, with the explicit recognition that the actual time of incision is contingent on the donor pathway proceeding to cold perfusion.

Operational Pathways for Uncontrolled DCD

Most of the international literature, and most of the discussion in the preceding sections, concerns controlled (Category III) DCD. For Indian centres beginning DCD activity, however, the uncontrolled pathways are operationally important, and in several centres, they are the dominant pathway. The reason is practical: a controlled programme requires a fully operational WLST framework, whereas Category IV donor-salvage in a donor in whom brain-stem death has already been declared can be initiated within existing deceased-donation infrastructure, without the additional WLST machinery. AIIMS Nagpur entered the DCD field by precisely this route in late 2023, and the early institutional experience illustrates the practical importance of the Category IIB pathway. Between December 2023 and 2025, the centre managed four potential brain-stem-dead donors in whom haemodynamic instability and cardiac arrest supervened while brain-stem-death certification was being attempted: in one donor, only the first apnoea test had been performed before arrest, and in the remaining three donors, not even the first apnoea test could be completed. Brain-stem-death certification was therefore incomplete in all four cases, and the centre operationally classified each donor as Category IIB and proceeded along the uncontrolled DCD pathway, with the standard 5-min no-touch period observed before retrieval. This pragmatic use of the Category IIB window converted what would otherwise have been four lost potential donors into four DCD donations, yielding eight DCD kidney transplants—every retrieved kidney utilised in-house and together accounting for a substantial proportion of the institution's deceased-donor kidney activity during that period [3, 17].

The operational requirements differ substantially between two broad uncontrolled scenarios, and they are therefore best treated separately. The first scenario, addressed in section "Category IV: Cardiac Arrest in a Donor with Completed Brain-Stem-Death Declaration", concerns the donor in whom brain-stem death has been declared, and in whom unexpected cardiac arrest then occurs before retrieval, which is the classical Category IV donor. The second scenario, addressed in section "Categories I and II: Cardiac Arrest Without Preceding Brain-Stem Death Declaration", concerns the donor in whom brain-stem death has not been declared, and in whom cardiac arrest has occurred without preceding brain-stem-death certification, corresponding to Categories I (resuscitation not attempted) and II (resuscitation attempted but unsuccessful), with subcategories A and B denoting out-of-hospital and in-hospital location, respectively. The consent pathway, documentation, legal considerations and infrastructural requirements differ between these two situations, and each is described in turn.

Category IV: Cardiac Arrest in a Donor with Completed Brain-Stem-Death Declaration

Category IV applies where brain-stem death has been formally certified, that is, where both apnoea tests have been completed, and the donor has been declared brain-dead under the Transplantation of Human Organs Act, and where cardiac arrest then occurs before retrieval can be initiated. This is the most immediately deployable DCD pathway available to Indian centres because consent for donation has typically already been obtained, donor evaluation is complete and ICU and theatre teams are already mobilised. The clinical question therefore becomes one of speed since the interval from cardiac arrest to cold perfusion must be minimised.

The pathway is summarised in Fig. 2.2. Where arrest occurs, the standard operational sequence comprises resuscitation according to institutional protocol (continued, where the family has been counselled and has consented, for the purpose of preserving organ perfusion), documentation of circulatory arrest in the already-declared brain-dead donor (no additional no-touch period required), rapid transfer to the operating theatre, super-rapid retrieval and initiation of cold perfusion. A conceptual clarification is required at this point. Under the Transplantation of Human Organs and Tissues Act (THOTA), death has already been legally certified through Form 10, once brain-stem death has been declared by two apnoea tests, and the donor is therefore already legally dead before the circulatory arrest occurs. A second determination of death after circulatory arrest is, in this setting, logically and legally redundant since a person already certified dead cannot be re-declared dead. The Indian position statement of 2022 accordingly recognises that a mandatory 5-min no-touch period is not required in this scenario, and the event at arrest is therefore most accurately described as documentation of circulatory arrest in an already-declared brain-dead donor rather than a fresh death declaration [3]. The PGIMER, Chandigarh series demonstrated an Indian uncontrolled DCD pathway in a public-sector tertiary setting between 2011 and 2015, employing rapid aortic cannulation, infusion of cold preservative solution and immediate surface cooling of the kidneys at the time of retrieval; continued cardiopulmonary resuscitation in three of five donors was associated with better early graft function in those kidneys, although the series was small [16]. Prior femoral cannulation was not used at PGIMER, and the operative technique was therefore super-rapid surgical retrieval rather than in situ NRP.

Two interrelated caveats apply to the use of the Category IV designation in the Indian context, and both have practical consequences for documentation, audit and medico-legal defensibility. The first concerns the completeness of brain-stem-death certification. Recognising that the binary Category IV/Category IIB distinction is too coarse for the heterogeneous clinical situations actually encountered in Indian intensive care units, the 2022 position statement of Indian transplant and critical-care societies introduced a scenario-based schema that more accurately describes practice [3]. In Scenarios 1 and 2 of that schema, both apnoea tests have been completed, Form 10 has been signed, brain-stem-death certification is therefore complete and consent for donation has been obtained (Form number 8); cardiac arrest occurring at this point constitutes a Category IV event, 5 min no-touch period is not required and the donor proceeds to retrieval (with or without normothermic regional perfusion). In Scenario 3, both apnoea tests have been completed, and Form 10 has been signed, so brain-stem death is established, but consent in Form 8 has not yet been obtained; the only pending step is completion of Form 8 consent, and because death has already been determined neurologically, no 5 min no-touch period is required. In Scenarios 4 and 5, by contrast, only one apnoea test has been performed (Scenario 4), or even the first apnoea test has not been completed (Scenario 5); brain-stem-death certification is therefore incomplete, the donor is operationally re-classified as Category IIB as per modified Maastricht classification (Or category 5 as per 2022 Indian position statement paper) and a 5-min no-touch period is then required because death is determined by circulatory criteria rather than neurologically. This scenario-based framework is the most accurate available descriptor of contemporary Indian DCD activity and should be adopted in institutional documentation [3]. The second caveat concerns the conceptual gap between legal death determination and operational transplant classification. Under THOTA, death may be determined either by irreversible cessation of circulatory and respiratory function or by certification of brain-stem death, but the Act does not provide detailed statutory guidance regarding circulatory determination of death or mandatory no-touch periods in donors already certified brain-dead. Consequently, in Category IV (Scenarios 1 and 2 above), a donor is legally dead under THOTA from the time of brain-stem-death certification, and the subsequent circulatory arrest does not constitute a new death event requiring repeat determination or an additional no-touch period; at the same time, the modified Maastricht–Paris classification operationally treats such donors as Category IV because circulatory arrest before retrieval has substantive implications for warm ischaemia, preservation strategy and graft outcomes. The legal determination of death and the operational transplant classification therefore address different questions and should not be conflated in case documentation. Related ethical questions, including whether cardiopulmonary resuscitation following arrest in an already brain-stem-dead donor may transiently restore some degree of cerebral perfusion despite the donor being legally dead, remain unresolved and merit institutional deliberation [3].

Categories I and II: Cardiac Arrest Without Preceding Brain-Stem Death Declaration

Categories I and II concern donors in whom brain-stem death has not been declared, and in whom death is determined by circulatory criteria alone. The primary axis that distinguishes Category I from Category II is whether resuscitation was attempted: Category I refers to donors in whom resuscitation was not attempted at all (donors brought in dead or found dead), whereas Category II refers to donors in whom resuscitation was attempted but failed. The secondary sub-axis denotes the location of cardiac arrest, with IA and IIA referring to out-of-hospital arrest and IB and IIB referring to in-hospital arrest. The operational requirements differ markedly from those of Category IV.

The first practical difficulty is consent. The donor is dead at the point of identification, and the family is typically in acute grief without prior preparation. Consent must therefore be obtained urgently, by a transplant coordinator rather than by a member of the treating team, and must be unambiguously documented before any retrieval-related intervention is undertaken. The second practical difficulty is logistical. The warm ischaemic clock is already running, and the interval between cardiac arrest and the initiation of cold perfusion is often the principal determinant of whether retrieval is feasible at all. In international practice, Categories IA and IIA and a substantial proportion of IIB activity depend on integrated pre-hospital and emergency-department infrastructure of the kind that exists at scale in Spain and France but has not yet been established in most of India [18].

The pathway is summarised in Fig. 2B. The standard operational sequence, where feasible, begins at the moment of cardiac arrest (out-of-hospital for IA and IIA, in-hospital for IB and IIB) and proceeds through unsuccessful resuscitation, the no-touch period, declaration of death, the acute family-consent conversation, in situ preservation (with or without NRP) and surgical retrieval. Some centres maintain continued chest compressions or extracorporeal cardiopulmonary resuscitation from the point of cardiac arrest until aortic cannulation in order to preserve organ perfusion; this is an ethically contested practice and is appropriate only where institutional policy and family consent have been clearly established. For Indian centres, Categories I and II activity is currently realistic only in metropolitan tertiary centres with strong emergency-medical-services links, and even there it is likely to constitute only a small fraction of overall DCD activity. The infrastructural prerequisites are summarised in Table 2.1.

Category-Specific Institutional Readiness

Institutional readiness is not uniform across DCD categories. A centre may be operationally ready for Category IV donor-salvage without being ready for Category III WLST-based retrieval, and a centre that has implemented both may not yet be ready for Category I or II uncontrolled activity. The 2022 Joint Position Paper provides category-specific checklists, and these are condensed in Table 2.1 as a practical ready-reference for centres planning or auditing their DCD activity [3]. Each centre should formalise its preferred pathway in a written standard operating procedure (SOP), with the relevant checklist appended.

Governance, Documentation and Audit

Documentation

The medico-legal defensibility of a DCD programme rests on rigorous documentation. The minimum dataset for each case comprises the following five elements: the WLST deliberation, including the basis for the futility determination and the certifications of the primary and secondary medical boards; precise time-stamps for the initiation of WLST, circulatory arrest, completion of the no-touch period, declaration of death, surgical incision and initiation of cold perfusion; the donation consent form, recording the family hierarchy that was used and the absence of any financial exchange; the DNAR order where applicable; and a post-retrieval debrief recording any deviation from protocol [3, 8, 9]. These records together constitute the regulatory audit trail and the substrate for programme improvement, and they should be stored in a structured institutional registry.

Quality Metrics and Continuous Improvement

Continuous audit is the most important single determinant of programme longevity. Recommended quality metrics include the conversion rate from potential to actual DCD donor; mean functional and total warm ischaemia times; the distribution of no-touch intervals; the proportion of controlled DCD donors progressing to retrieval within 60 to 90 min of WLST; rates of kidney delayed graft function and primary non-function and one-year and five-year graft and patient survival [1, 3, 13]. Periodic multidisciplinary case review, ideally conducted on a quarterly basis in an active programme, surfaces the process bottlenecks and inter-team communication failures that are not detectable from individual case audits alone. The IKDRC long-term outcomes, with one-year and ten-year patient survival of 87.3% and 72.8% respectively, demonstrate that an auditable Indian DCD programme can achieve outcomes consistent with international benchmarks; the published series also indicates that this level of performance is attainable with relatively modest infrastructure, provided that audit and review processes are sustained over time [11].

Workforce Competency and Training

A trained multidisciplinary team is a more reliable determinant of DCD success than advanced technology. Intensive care nurses and intensivists must be competent in WLST communication, end-of-life symptom control and the documentation of the agonal phase [3, 8]. Retrieval surgeons must be proficient in super-rapid retrieval and rapid aortic cannulation, and familiarity with femoral cannulation and NRP is required only in centres that plan to employ those techniques [12, 15]. Anaesthetists provide comfort-focused care during WLST but must remain excluded from death determination and from any role in organ recovery, which is the ethical core of the team structure. Perfusionists are essential in centres that employ NRP, and they require formal training in flow, pressure, temperature and circuit-integrity management [15]. Transplant coordinators discharge the integrative function within the team, holding together the ethical, documentary, communication and inter-team threads from notification through allocation.

Structured simulation, incorporating ICU-to-operating-theatre transfers, time-stamped event recording and post-simulation debrief, is the most effective method of building team-level competence and should precede the first DCD case at every centre. The investment is modest, and the return, in terms of protocol fluency, early identification of process bottlenecks and team confidence, is substantial.

Phased Implementation in Indian Centres

Most Indian institutions presently lack at least one of the components required for full multi-organ DCD, whether pre-emptive cannulation infrastructure, NRP capability, dedicated DCD operating theatres or fully protocolised WLST systems. A phased approach is therefore appropriate, beginning with the pathway that is immediately deployable within existing infrastructure and progressing towards more resource-intensive techniques as institutional capability matures. Table 2.2 sets out a four-phase model that the present authors regard as realistic for most Indian centres.

Table 2.2 Phased model for DCD programme implementation in Indian centres

Phase	Pathway	Prerequisites	Anticipated yield
1	Kidney-only Category IV (donor-salvage in a fully certified BSD donor with unexpected arrest before retrieval)	Existing deceased-donor framework; rapid recognition of arrest; trained rapid-cannulation surgical team; cold perfusate primed; no WLST infrastructure required	Two kidneys per donor; immediate programme initiation; lowest infrastructural threshold
2	Controlled Category III, kidney-first	Institutional WLST policy with primary and secondary medical boards; ICU and OT coordination protocol; trained transplant coordinator; SOPs for sequential consent and stand-down	Two kidneys per donor; predictable warm ischaemia times; structured audit feasible; foundation for subsequent expansion

(continued)

Table 2.2 (continued)

Phase	Pathway	Prerequisites	Anticipated yield
3	Liver-inclusive Category III DCD, with selective use of abdominal NRP	Perfusion expertise; ECMO or extracorporeal circuit; trained surgical and perfusion team; theatre-based WLST capability	Liver and two kidneys per donor; reduced biliary complications via NRP
4	Multi-organ DCD including thoracic organs (thoraco-abdominal NRP or ex situ machine perfusion)	Thoraco-abdominal NRP capability or ex situ machine perfusion infrastructure (e.g., Organ Care System); co-located cardiothoracic and abdominal retrieval teams.	Heart, lung, liver, kidneys and pancreas where applicable; organ utilisation approaching DBD benchmarks

Reported Indian Institutional Experience

Three published Indian series, together with the early reports from AIIMS Nagpur and the first post-mortem NRP procedure in Asia performed at a Delhi centre in November 2025 [19], now establish proof of concept across diverse Indian institutional settings (Table 2.3). Each is summarised briefly here because the operational details of each, and in particular, the differences in retrieval technique are instructive for centres planning to begin DCD activity.

Two operational observations emerge from this collective Indian experience. The first is that the dominant pathway in Indian practice to date has been kidney-only DCD, achieved through either super-rapid retrieval or premortem femoral cannulation, both of which can be implemented within existing institutional infrastructure. The second is that the Delhi NRP procedure, the AIIMS Nagpur activity and the AFMS retrieval together indicate that the field is now beginning to diversify across pathway types, institutional sectors and geographies. A separate Indian point of reference is the documented withdrawal-of-life-sustaining-treatment case at AIIMS New Delhi (the Harshit Rana case), which remains, to the knowledge of the present authors, the only Indian case in which formal WLST under the simplified Common Cause procedure was carried out and followed by organ or tissue donation; in that case, only corneal donation occurred, and no solid organs were retrieved. The Indian Category III solid-organ pathway therefore remains, as of writing, without a fully documented published exemplar, and the operational scaffolding outlined in sections "Intensive Care Unit Readiness" to "Phased Implementation in Indian Centres" is intended to support its diversification.

Table 2.3 Reported Indian institutional experience with donation after circulatory death

Centre	Period	Pathway	Technique and outcomes
IKDRC-ITS, Ahmedabad	1999 to 2012	Controlled (III, IV)	Thirty-three DCD kidney transplants, representing approximately 10% of deceased-donor activity over the study period; WLST conducted in the operating theatre with a 5 to 10 min no-touch period; premortem heparin 10,000 U; femoral cannulation, HTK perfusion and ice-slush surface cooling; warm ischaemia under 20 min; one-year and ten-year patient survival of 87.3% and 72.8% respectively; death-censored graft survival of 90.9% in donors younger than 70 years; DGF rates of 31 to 36% [11]
PGIMER, Chandigarh	2011 to 2015	Predominantly uncontrolled (II, IV)	Five DCD donors from which ten kidneys were retrieved and nine transplanted, one kidney being discarded after the recipient withdrew consent; cardiopulmonary resuscitation was continued in 3 of 5 donors until the time of retrieval. Operative technique consisted of super-rapid retrieval with rapid aortic cannulation, infusion of cold preservative solution and immediate surface cooling at the time of retrieval. Prior femoral cannulation was not used in any donor. Continued resuscitation was associated with better early graft function in this small series. The experience demonstrated the feasibility of uncontrolled DCD in an Indian public-sector tertiary centre [16]
AIIMS Nagpur	2023 onwards	Uncontrolled (Category IIB)	The first DCD kidney retrieval in the state of Maharashtra was performed on 3 December 2023. Between December 2023 and 2025, four DCD donations yielded eight DCD kidney transplants, with every retrieved kidney utilised in-house and together accounting for a substantial proportion of the institution's deceased-donor kidney activity during that period. All four donors were potential brain-stem-dead donors in whom cardiac arrest supervened while brain-stem-death certification was being attempted: the first apnoea test had been performed in only one donor, and in the remaining three not even the first apnoea test could be completed. Brain-stem-death certification was therefore incomplete in all four cases, and each donor was operationally classified as Category IIB and managed along the uncontrolled DCD pathway with a 5-min no-touch period applied before retrieval. This pragmatic use of the Category IIB window converted four otherwise-lost potential donations into eight functioning kidney transplants [3, 17]

(continued)

Table 2.3 (continued)

Centre	Period	Pathway	Technique and outcomes
Delhi (private-sector centre)	November 2025	Uncontrolled (Category IIB), with abdominal NRP	The first reported use of post-mortem abdominal normothermic regional perfusion via femoral cannulation in Asia, facilitating retrieval of one liver and two kidneys [19]. The publicly available account does not document a formal withdrawal-of-life-sustaining-treatment process with primary and secondary medical board certification; in the absence of documented WLST, the case cannot be classified as controlled Category III DCD, and for documentation purposes, it is most accurately characterised as an uncontrolled Category IIB retrieval with abdominal NRP—the first Asian post-mortem NRP procedure rather than a fully documented Category III controlled DCD. The case nevertheless established the technical feasibility of NRP-based abdominal multi-organ retrieval in India [3]
Command Hospital, Chandimandir	2024	Service-sector DCD	The first DCD organ retrieval performed by the Armed Forces Medical Services [20]

Cultural and Communication Considerations

Family communication is, in practice, the variable that most often determines whether a DCD pathway proceeds to retrieval. Three points warrant emphasis for Indian practice. The first is that the WLST conversation must never carry, in language or in tone, the implication that the decision is linked to organ donation. The structured separation recommended by the 2024 ISCCM and IAPC consensus, involving different personnel and a defined temporal interval between the two conversations, is a robust safeguard and should be adopted as the institutional default [8]. The second is that culturally appropriate framing of WLST varies across regions, religions and families, and transplant coordinators who are skilled in this conversation are not interchangeable with intensivists; centres should therefore invest in formal coordinator training. The third is that families require a clear understanding of the practical sequence of events, including the agonal phase, the no-touch period, the moment of death and the family's opportunity to be present and subsequently to take leave of the donor. This information should be conveyed in clear terms, in the family's preferred language and without medical jargon. In published Indian series in which this conversation has been conducted well, conversion rates have been considerably higher than the international average; where it has been conducted poorly, even fully consented cases have collapsed at the bedside.

Conclusion

The establishment of a DCD programme in India is now a matter of disciplined institutional preparation rather than of waiting for further legal or technological developments. The legal foundation is settled: the Transplantation of Human Organs and Tissues Act of 1994 has always permitted retrieval after circulatory determination of death, and the Supreme Court's judgement in the case 'Common Cause v. Union of India (9 March 2018), as simplified by the order of 24 January 2023' now provides a workable bedside procedure for withdrawal of life-sustaining treatment, while the 2020 ICMR DNAR consensus, the 2022 AIIMS New Delhi institutional EOLC policy, the 2022 Joint Position Paper of Indian transplant and critical-care societies, the 2024 ISCCM and IAPC end-of-life care consensus and the 2024 multi-society DCD consensus statement (IJT 2024, endorsed by ISOT and multiple Indian scientific societies) together translate that framework into bedside procedural detail, which the present chapter has condensed and operationalised for the centre planning a programme. The published Indian experience confirms that outcomes consistent with international benchmarks are achievable with the infrastructure that most tertiary centres already possess, and four priorities follow: institutional EOLC committees and the primary and secondary medical board structure required by the simplified WLST procedure should function as a working bedside system rather than a theoretical one; structured simulation should precede the first DCD case at every centre; prospective registries capturing warm ischaemia times, no-touch intervals, conversion rates, delayed graft function and survival should be established from the outset and shared through NOTTO and, where Category III governance is not yet in place, the Category IV donor-salvage pathway offers an immediately deployable entry point that yields two kidneys per donor and requires no new legal infrastructure. On these foundations, DCD is likely, over the next several years, to expand the deceased-donor pool meaningfully, to reduce waiting-list mortality and to align Indian practice with the established international standard.

Conflict of Interest The author(s) declare no conflict of interest.

Ethical Declaration This chapter is a narrative review of previously published literature, judicial documents and institutional reports. No original human or animal research was undertaken, and ethical committee approval was therefore not required.

Competing Interests The author(s) has no competing interests to declare that are relevant to the content of this manuscript.

Ethics Approval The author(s) declares that this manuscript does not include primary research with human participants.

The author(s) declares that this manuscript does not include primary studies involving animals.

References

1. NHS Blood and Transplant. Organ donation and transplantation activity report 2023/24. Bristol: NHS Blood and Transplant; 2024. Available from: https://www.odt.nhs.uk [accessed 2026 May 20].
2. Israni AK, Zaun DA, Gauntt K, et al. OPTN/SRTR 2022 annual data report: deceased organ donation. Am J Transplant. 2024;24(2 Suppl 1):S457–88. https://doi.org/10.1016/j.ajt.2024.01.018.
3. Seth AK, Mohanka R, Navin S, et al. Organ donation after circulatory determination of death in India: a joint position paper. Indian J Crit Care Med. 2022;26(4):421–38. https://doi.org/10.5005/jp-journals-10071-24198.
4. Common Cause (A Regd. Society) v. Union of India and Another. Writ Petition (Civil) No. 215 of 2005. Supreme Court of India, judgment dated 9 March 2018. Available from: https://main.sci.gov.in/supremecourt/2005/9123/9123_2005_Judgement_09-Mar-2018.pdf [accessed 2026 May 20].
5. Common Cause (A Regd. Society) v. Union of India. Miscellaneous Application No. 1699 of 2019 in Writ Petition (Civil) No. 215 of 2005. Supreme Court of India, order dated 24 January 2023 (simplifying the procedure for advance medical directives and withdrawal of life-sustaining treatment laid down in the 2018 judgment).
6. Mathur R. ICMR consensus guidelines on "Do Not Attempt Resuscitation". Indian J Med Res. 2020;151(4):303–10. https://doi.org/10.4103/ijmr.IJMR_395_20.
7. Bhatnagar S, Biswas S, Kumar A, et al. Institutional end-of-life care policy for inpatients at a tertiary care centre in India: a way forward to provide a system for a dignified death. Indian J Med Res. 2022;155(2):232–42. https://doi.org/10.4103/ijmr.IJMR_902_21.
8. Mani RK, Bhatnagar S, Butola S, et al. Indian Society of Critical Care Medicine and Indian Association of Palliative Care expert consensus and position statements for end-of-life and palliative care in the intensive care unit. Indian J Crit Care Med. 2024;28(3):200–50. https://doi.org/10.5005/jp-journals-10071-24661.
9. Seth AK, Mohanka R, Mani RK, et al. Organ donation after circulatory determination of death — consensus statement. Indian J Transplant. 2024;18(3):247–56. https://doi.org/10.4103/ijot.ijot_37_24.
10. Thuong M, Ruiz A, Evrard P, et al. New classification of donation after circulatory death donors: definitions and terminology. Transpl Int. 2016;29(7):749–59. https://doi.org/10.1111/tri.12776.
11. Kute VB, Vanikar AV, Shah PR, et al. Outcome of renal transplantation from deceased donors after cardiac death: a single-center experience from a developing country. Transplant Proc. 2013;45(6):2147–51. https://doi.org/10.1016/j.transproceed.2013.02.128.
12. Phillips B, Asgari E, Berry M, et al. British Transplantation Society guidelines on abdominal organ transplantation from deceased donors after circulatory death. Transplant Rev (Orlando). 2024;38(1):100801. https://doi.org/10.1016/j.trre.2023.100801.
13. Croome KP, Barbas AS, Whitson B, et al. American Society of Transplant Surgeons Scientific Studies Committee. American Society of Transplant Surgeons recommendations on best practices in donation after circulatory death organ procurement. Am J Transplant. 2023;23(2):171–9. https://doi.org/10.1016/j.ajt.2022.10.009.
14. Kramer AH, Holliday K, Keenan S, et al. Premortem anticoagulation timing and dose in donation after circulatory death: multicentre study of associations with graft function. Can J Surg. 2022;65(4):E474–84. https://doi.org/10.1503/cjs.023120.
15. Croome K, Bababekov Y, Brubaker A, et al. American Society of Transplant Surgeons normothermic regional perfusion standards: abdominal. Transplantation. 2024;108(8):1660–8. https://doi.org/10.1097/TP.0000000000005114.

16. Singh S, Kumar S, Dasgupta S, et al. A single-center experience of kidney transplantation from donation after circulatory death: challenges and scope in India. Indian J Nephrol. 2017;27(3):205–9. https://doi.org/10.4103/0971-4065.202843.
17. Deshpande C. State's 1st DCD transplant done in city. The Times of India [Internet]. 2023 Dec 4 [cited 2026 May 20]. Available from: https://timesofindia.indiatimes.com/city/nagpur/states-1st-dcd-transplant-done-in-city/articleshow/105712716.cms.
18. Domínguez-Gil B, Duranteau J, Mateos A, et al. Uncontrolled donation after circulatory death: European practices and recommendations for the development and optimization of an effective programme. Transpl Int. 2016;29(8):842–59. https://doi.org/10.1111/tri.12734.
19. Delhi doctors restart blood flow post death for organ donation, 1st in Asia. Business Standard [Internet]. 2025 Nov 8 [cited 2026 Jun 7]. Available from: https://www.business-standard.com/health/delhi-doctors-restart-blood-flow-post-death-for-organ-donation-1st-in-asia-125110801388_1.html.
20. Transplant team of Western Command successfully harvest organs post-cardiac death into needy recipients. Asian News International (ANI) [Internet]. 2024 Jul 11 [cited 2026 Jun 7]. Available from: https://aninews.in/news/national/general-news/transplant-team-of-western-command-successfully-harvest-organs-post-cardiac-death-into-needy-recipients20240711062623/.

Legal and Ethical Aspects of Organ Donation After Circulatory Death in India

3

Avnish Kumar Seth, Ravi Mohanka, and Philip G. Thomas

Introduction

Progress in medical science and technology, availability of life-sustaining therapies and organ support systems have constantly redefined conditions that were previously regarded as not treatable, reversible, or curable. It has also made the definition of death a moving goalpost.

In medieval times when our understanding about heart and circulation was limited, death was diagnosed when breathing visibly ceased in an unconscious individual. In some innovative places, at the time of burial, a bell would be placed at ground level attached to a string inside the buried coffin, so that if someone were buried alive, they could ring and be dug up! With the availability of stethoscope and ECG, absence of cardiac electrical activity was widely used to determine death.

With medical advances disease-related deaths became potentially reversible. Artificial life support systems were developed including ventilators, pacemakers, aortic counter-pulsation balloons, and dialysis. Despite apparent recovery from acute conditions, some patients developed neurological damage leading to coma, brain death or persistent vegetative state. Neurological status is now considered the most important determinant of prognosis, deciding the likelihood of a satisfactory outcome with meaningful life beyond the intensive care unit.

It has been shown that in patients who die following devastating brain injury, 30% follow the brain death pathway, while circulatory death is seen in 70% [1].

A. K. Seth (✉)
Manipal Hospitals, Manipal Organ Sharing & Transplant, Delhi, New Delhi, India

R. Mohanka
Department of Liver Transplantation and HPB Sciences,
Sir HN Reliance Foundation Hospital, Mumbai, India

P. G. Thomas
Texas Organ Sharing Alliance, San Antonio, TX, USA

S. P. Kolte et al. (eds.), *Organ Donation After Circulatory Death*,
https://doi.org/10.1007/978-981-92-6377-6_3

While donation after brain death (DBD) is well understood by transplant professionals in India, it's awareness and acceptance by the public and physicians not associated with transplant may be patchy. However, circulatory death is well understood and accepted by the population at large. There is a huge opportunity to increase organ donation by the donation after circulatory death (DCD) pathway.

Advances in medicine not only challenged how death should be defined but also reshaped our understanding of when artificial organ support systems may be futile and lead to withdrawal of life-sustaining treatment (WLST). In today's era, with the availability of advanced life sustaining measures, and invasive interventions such as extracorporeal membrane oxygenator (ECMO) and ventricular assist devices, it may be possible to support circulation and oxygenation for prolonged times. Patients on these advanced life-sustaining therapies and organ support systems may have irreversible organ damage that may be incompatible with life without them. There is no support device to reverse neurological damage. However, the decision to declare futility of treatment and discontinuing medical treatment has always been a difficult one. A focused drive to increase DCD transplants following WLST can substantially increase the inadequate deceased organ donation rates in India and address the very long waiting time and waiting list mortality. To make WLST routine practice and to enable DCD in India, we must adopt an ethical approach consistent with our laws and cultural beliefs, with buy-in of all stakeholders.

Newer Technologies Enabling DCD

Traditionally, the outcomes of DCD transplants are considered inferior to DBD. However, in the last decade, two new technologies have not only enabled better organ assessment and preservation but made the outcomes of DCD transplants equivalent to DBD.

- *Normothermic regional perfusion (NRP):* Following WLST and declaration of death by circulatory criteria, the circulation to abdominal/thoracic organs is restored in situ. It reverses ischemic damage to the organs and allows assessment of their functional status.
- Ex vivo *machine perfusion* (XVMP): Rapid explantation of organs is followed by ex vivo circulation on a perfusion machine:
  (a) Hypothermic machine perfusion (HMP): perfusion of organ preservative fluid with or without oxygen at hypothermic temperature (4–8 °C).
  (b) Normothermic machine perfusion (NMP): circulation of blood with oxygen at body temperature.

Several countries have witnessed a surge in number of DCD transplants and improved outcomes, fueled by the availability and clinical use of these technologies.

Is DCD Legal in India?

It was in 2015 that the initial steps on DCD were taken in India during a national summit at National Capital Region, Delhi. Upon scrutiny of THOA 1994, legality of DCD in India was established. The law clearly stated that for the purpose of organ donation, 'deceased person means a person in whom permanent disappearance of all evidence of life occurs, by reason of brainstem death or in a cardio-pulmonary sense, at any time after live birth has taken place' [2]. While the former referred to brainstem death, the latter part of the statement clearly referred to circulatory determination of death, thus establishing the legality of DCD in India.

It was also noted that 'Form 8,' used for consent of near relative for organ donation in brain death could also be used for DCD as it was stated that 'I have been informed that my relative has been declared brainstem dead/dead.'

While THOA detailed the legislative and administrative framework and process for brain death certification and organ donation, it does not describe the process for DCD.

History and Events Related to DCD in India

So far there have been close to 70 DCD kidney transplants in Gujarat [3], Chandigarh [4], Maharashtra and Delhi. Recently, the first successful DCD liver transplant was done in Delhi. Some events related to DCD in India along with timelines are shown in Table 3.1.

Table 3.1 Landmarks in organ transplantation, end-of-life care, palliative care, withdrawal of life-sustaining treatment and donation after circulatory determination of death in India

Year	Landmark
1994	THOA passed by Indian parliament
1995	THOA rules published
1999	First DCD kidney transplant performed at IKDRC, Ahmedabad
2011	First DCD kidney transplant performed at PGIMER, Chandigarh
2011	THOTA, amendment to THOA passed by the parliament
2011	Supreme Court Judgment on Aruna Shanbaug case: in an incompetent person, parents, spouse, other close relatives or "next friend" were allowed to withdraw nutrition, water or WLST with court's approval. Withdrawal of cardiorespiratory support in BD was also brought out
2014	THOTA amended rules published
2014	EOLC guidelines published by ISCCM and IAPC

(continued)

Table 3.1 (continued)

Year	Landmark
2015	ELICIT constituted by ISCCM, IAPC and IAN
2015	National Summits held on DCD in Fortis Hospital, Gurugram and Apollo Hospital, Delhi
2017	The supreme court ruled in Justice K S Puttaswamy (Retd.) versus Union of India case that the right to privacy included the right to refuse life-sustaining treatment
2017	EOLC guidelines published by IAP
2017	First national symposium on death and dying held in Mathura resulting in "The Mathura declaration" Medical professionals across multiple specialties and intelligentsia from Law, Bureaucracy, Sociology, Academia, Writing, Journalism, Psychology, Religion and Social work declared Universal concern for improving EOLC in India "CANDID", a citizens' advocacy platform was formed Intersection of universal definition of death, EOLC and WLST with transplantation was discussed
2018	Supreme Court Judgment in common cause Vs. The union of India case validated AMD and WLST, prescribing conditions and procedures for the same, including a safeguard and oversight mechanism
2019	FICCI and ELICIT published a guide to improve EOLC
2020	DNAR consensus guidelines published by ICMR
2020	Guidelines for EOLC published by AIIMS, New Delhi
2021	A model legal framework version 2.0 published for EOLC in India by Vidhi Centre Center for legal policy
2022	A joint position paper on organ donation after circulatory death in India was published by Indian Journal of Transplantation
2023 2023	Supreme Court Judgment Common Cause vs. The Union of India. Legal provisions for advance directives, withdrawal, and withholding decisions in terminal care. First DCD kidney transplantation performed in AIIMS Nagpur
2024	Consensus statement on organ donation after circulatory death was published by Indian Journal of Transplantation

(continued)

Table 3.1 (continued)

Year	Landmark
2025	Meeting of the National Consortium on Normothermic Regional Perfusion (NRP) for Donation after Circulatory Death (DCD)
2025	First successful NRP-DCD in India at Manipal Hospital Delhi leading to liver transplantation at ILBS, New Delhi

Categories of DCD

The legal pathway, challenges, and documentation for each category of DCD as per the modified Maastricht classification, applicable to India are discussed below.

Category I: A patient who suffers circulatory arrest in the community and is declared dead on arrival at the emergency room (ER) of a hospital may donate organs after formal declaration of death and family's consent. However, this is often not feasible because the downtime before arrival at the hospital may be unknown, precluding organ donation. Furthermore, the suddenness and unexpectedness of events generally makes it difficult for families to accept mortality, as they may not have had adequate time to go through the grieving process and are often not prepared to consider or even discuss organ donation. In countries such as Spain with pre-hospital extracorporeal-CPR (ECPR) program, very high level of awareness on organ donation, presumed consent, and availability of NRP, HMP and NMP technologies and expertise, conversion to DCD is more likely, especially if the patient is transferred to the ER of a transplant hospital.

Category II: A patient who suffers cardio-circulatory arrest either in the community or ER and could not be successfully resuscitated could be an organ donor after formal declaration of death and family's consent. Challenges with conversion to DCD are like category I, though the duration of significant hypoxic-ischemic injury may be better discerned. Even though DCD category II is unlikely in India due to opt-in policy, let us consider a failed resuscitation following cardiac arrest in an individual from a motivated family highly committed to the cause of organ donation. Even if they readily sign the consent for DCD, most hospitals may be medically incapable of retrieving organs successfully. However, given the increasing applicability of ECPR, the possibility of DCD category II in India should not be completely discounted. A determined unit that is fully prepared for this situation may be able to fulfill the wishes of the family.

Category III: Some patients sustain irreversible brain damage not amounting to brainstem death. These individuals may not be expected to survive despite continuation of life-sustaining therapies and organ support systems or lead a meaningful life without them. In such situations, WLST may allow end of life care (EOLC) and a dignified death. Determination of futility of medical care is complex, and although there are several published criteria in neurological and non-neurological conditions, most experienced intensivists have good instincts for what constitutes futile medical care.

On 24th January 2023, the honorable Supreme Court of India (SC) stated that the right to life guaranteed under Article 21 of the Constitution encompassed the right to die with dignity and clarified the validity of WLST in terminally ill patients and laid down a simplified procedure for the same. It involved constituting primary and secondary Medical Boards to determine futility of care. If futility of medical care was established, WLST could be done with the consent of the family. State Governments in Karnataka, Goa, Maharashtra, and others have issued guidelines for implementation of this judgment, that also paves the way for DCD. The judgment has provided much needed clarity on the legal framework for WLST and helped the clinicians to navigate difficult discussions around the care of dying patients [5].

In India, where the staggering cost of intensive care interventions is difficult to bear or sustain, intensivists have developed one of two common approaches:

- A passive one where nothing is changed until death occurs. In such situations currently, the terminally ill patient is often discharged or leaves against medical advice (DAMA/LAMA). The practice of DAMA/LAMA is an undignified way to diagnose and act upon futility without giving opportunity to the family for organ donation.
- A proactive one where EOLC is considered, discussed, and next-of-kin are informed and consented for 'do not attempt resuscitation' (DNAR) or WLST. Despite willingness for this approach, there is many a slip between the cup and the lip. Even when a few clinicians are inclined toward WLST, approval for Secondary Medical Board is not being given by Chief Medical Officers due to lack of awareness. The Health Secretaries of each state must be made aware of the protocol for WLST and they in turn pass suitable instructions to CMOs. Karnataka has passed an effective Govt Order where-in the members of Brain Death certification Committee are required to function as Secondary Medical Board.

WLST must become a routine part of clinical practice before DCD category III can happen in the country. It must be emphasized that no single physician should have to bear alone the crushing responsibility of life and death decisions. Prior identification of a group of peers in the hospital, palliative care specialists and ethicists, to serve as a consultative body to assist decision-making for an individual patient is perhaps the single most important measure that will make the process transparent, establish good faith, and consolidate experience going forward.

When the family of a terminally ill patient, wishing to avoid resuscitation and futile care, opts for WLST, DCD is possible when it is anticipated that the patient will progress to circulatory arrest within a short period of time (usually 2 h). This situation contributes to almost 90% of all DCD donations globally and may be a successful strategy in India [6]. There is sufficient time for documentation of all interactions between the medical teams, hospital administration and patient's family members in addition to documentation of death and consent for organ donation. Just like we speak about 'decoupling' in brain death pathway, where-in declaration of brain death and the ask for organs are never done simultaneously; in DCD pathway, the talk about organ donation should be 'delinked' from and should happen only after the family has consented to WLST.

Death is declared after permanent cessation in circulatory function, typically established by a 5 min asystole observation period. Controversy persists over which terminology is appropriate!

- "permanent" (will not resume spontaneously), or
- "irreversible" (cannot be restored by any means)

In practice, situations in which WLST is contemplated the use of "any means possible" to restore circulation after it has ceased are precluded. The diagnosis of "Permanent cessation of circulation" in DCD, requires a reliable arterial line to monitor the pulse, systolic (SBP) and diastolic blood pressure, and mean arterial pressure, after WLST has been instituted.

'Agonal phase' is diagnosed when the SBP shows a sustained drop below 70 mmHg. Cessation of circulation is diagnosed after the pulse wave forms flat lines, and heart sounds are not audible to two separate observers. The "circulatory time of death" (CTOD) is then recorded. Continuous EKG monitoring is not typically required for diagnosis of CTOD. Individual physicians or hospitals might require this and should pulseless electrical activity (PEA) be encountered, CTOD might have to be postponed till this also ceases.

The progress of the patient is meticulously documented minute to minute. It should also be explained that in 20% patients, the heart may not stop within 2 h of WLST, thus precluding DCD and warranting a return to palliative care.

Currently, WLST is rarely practiced in ICUs in India, limiting this potential pathway for DCD. However, DNAR-DCD was done recently in Delhi and is an option that may be exercised with less cumbersome documentation. The differences between WLST-DCD and DNAR-DCD are shown in Table 3.2.

A simplified checklist of documentation for DCD category III is shown in Table 3.3.

Category IV: In India, the occurrence of cardiac arrest during the process of BD declaration is not uncommon. In eligible donors, where brain death has been certified after both sets of tests, CPR and no-touch period are not required and donation can be performed as category IV. In potential donors where no formal testing or

Table 3.2 Difference between DCD following withdrawal of life sustaining treatment (WLST-DCD) and do not attempt resuscitation (DNAR-DCD)

	WLST-DCD	DNAR-DCD
Process	Active	Passive
Action	"Pulling the plug"	"Letting him/her go"
Time taken to cardiac standstill	Short	Maybe longer
Legal and ethical	Yes	Yes
Emotional difficulty for family	++	+
Willingness by critical care teams	±	+

Table 3.3 List of documents needed for DCD category III (WLST-DCD and DNAR-DCD)

	WLST-DCD	DNAR-DCD
Daily counseling forms	Yes	Yes
DNAR	Yes	Yes
Primary Medical Board	Yes	No
Secondary Medical Board	Yes	No
Consent from family	Yes	Yes
Information to JMFC	Yes	No
Consent for DCD	Yes	Yes
Death certificate (Form 4)	Yes	Yes

Table 3.4 Summary of legal processes and expected challenges for DCD donation for Maastricht categories in India

Category/type/situation	Pathway/documentation	Challenges
I / *Uncontrolled*: Circulatory arrest in the community. Dead on arrival to the emergency room	Medical Certificate of Cause of Death (Form 4, Registration of Births and Deaths Act, 1969) Consent for organ donation (in Form 8, THOA Rules)	Unknown hypoxic/ ischemic injury to organs Low likelihood of consent due to suddenness of events
II / *Uncontrolled*: Unsuccessful resuscitation	Form 4, 8	Low likelihood of consent due to suddenness of events
III / *Controlled*: Anticipated cardiac arrest (When family wishes DNAR/WLST)	Form 4, 8 Documentation of family counseling: diagnosis, daily assessments/progress notes with prognosis (life expectancy and quality of life), names of individuals present in each meeting Documentation of WLST/DNAR Consent for pre-mortem heparinization, cannulation and NRP	WLST practice in ICUs is uncommon Legal validity of DNAR should be clarified
IV / *Controlled*: Cardiac arrest in a brain-dead donor	Form 4, 8	Organ procurement may have to expedited
V / *Uncontrolled*	Form 4, 8	ICU at a transplant center

only one set of brainstem death tests have confirmed BD, CPR should be performed for 30 min. However, if DNAR has been signed, CPR is not required but 5-min no-touch period remains a mandatory requirement [7].

Category V: Patients in the ICU who unexpectedly suffer circulatory arrest could be organ donors if resuscitation is unsuccessful. This situation is similar to category I and II, but resuscitation efforts in the hospital are prompt and duration of down-time is well-known, limiting ischemic/hypoxic injury to them. If the patient is put on extracorporeal membrane oxygenator (ECMO) during resuscitation, determination of futility of care and WLST may be more nuanced.

Each category of DCD has different documentation and procedural challenges (Table 3.4).

Ethical Considerations in WLST

Ethical considerations governing WLST span the four core principles of bioethics: autonomy, beneficence, non-maleficence, and justice. Withdrawing and withholding life-sustaining therapy are generally considered equivalent when the trajectory toward death is anticipated, even though this might be a challenge to an individual physician's moral understanding, or emotional situation. When a patient's known values and preferences are unknown; when there is no legally executed 'Advanced Directive'; and when the patient lacks capacity to make his or her own decision regarding WLST, it becomes necessary to incorporate family cultural, and spiritual traditions into decisions regarding end-of-life care [8]. WLST represents a shift in goals, not abandonment of the patient. Protocolized approaches to symptom management including opioids and sedation for comfort, are recommended to ensure the patient does not experience pain or suffering [9].

Clinician moral distress is recognized worldwide as an important issue surrounding WLST. It is usually the result of conflating WLST with euthanasia or Medical Aid in Dying (MAID) which are morally repugnant to many. The involvement of Palliative Care specialists and ethics consultation can mitigate this [10]. Disagreements between families and the healthcare team are to be anticipated and planned for. Constituting in advance an institutional review process will help prevent the appearance of an ad hoc approach when such a situation is encountered in the ICU.

Ethical Considerations in Donation After Circulatory Death (DCD)

The Dead Donor Rule (DDR): The DDR mandates that organ recovery must not cause the donor's death. It is essential therefore that the decision for WLST should be made independently of, and prior to, any consideration of organ donation [8–10].

A systematic review of ICU healthcare professionals found that while support for DCD is generally positive, it remains lower than for donation after brain death (DBD). Common barriers include insufficient training, lack of standardized protocols, and ethical uncertainty surrounding death determination [11].

Ethical issues in DCD have always been spoken about and have been largely overcome in the last 30 years. In 1993, Renne Fox, a bioethicist called DCD 'An ignoble form of cannibalism. Doctors and nurses put death in an accelerated time clock and then race frantically to beat the clock' [12]. The same team of doctors who are there to save lives switch gears toward declaration of death and enable DCD. The rushed decision-making required by treating teams may lead to a prognostic fog. This conflict of interest in critical care teams comes to the fore in a situation of DCD, where one has to be careful to avoid accusation of over-reaching for organ donation and being trigger happy. In 1995, Fox and Christakis discouraged DCD by saying that 'We would like to propose that medical journals attach less value and priority to publishing articles related to non-heart beating donors' [13].

With the advent of NRP, new ethical issues emerged [14]. When we place inguinal arterial and venous lines and administer IV Heparin ante-mortem are we violating the Dead Donor Rule (DDR)? When we are re-animating the heart by machine perfusion or NRP and transplanting the same, are we not questioning the very definition of death? What if cerebral circulation is restored with NRP in a person who has been declared dead? By clamping the great vessels above the aorta are we murdering the not so dead? If they were dead in the first place, why bother to clamp the great vessels? The science of EOLC and the art of declaring futility have developed enough over the last 30 years to paint the canvas of organ transplantation where-in DCD accounts for 30% of the world's organ transplants [12]. We don't have to re-invent the wheel of DCD in India. It is already up and running like a well-oiled machine in some parts of the world. The process of DCD is not kind toward the emotions and feelings of the donor family. A hurried goodbye to a loved one in the medicalized, impersonal setting of ICU or OT lacks privacy. Their feeling of deprivation of intimacy with a loved family member is like a 'stolen death'. Our transplant coordinators have no exposure to the nuances of handling a grieving family in WLST-DCD-NRP interphase and much training will be required.

Conflict Between Advance Directive and Being an Organ Donor

An interesting conflict has emerged with more and more people signing up for advance directives. What if that individual has also signed up to be an organ donor? The latter requires one to be in the ICU on ventilatory support while the former is meant to keep one away from ICU and life support. How does one handle this dichotomy? The language in advance directives needs to be modified to mention that one has signed up to be an organ donor and that while one does not want life support for prolonging life, the use of ECMO and other procedures required for organ preservation during the process of dying and immediately after, may be carried out for the purpose of organ preservation.

Case Report of First Successful DNAR-DCD-NRP in India

In November 2025, a 55 years female, bedridden with motor neuron disease for 2 years was admitted to Manipal Hospital New Delhi, 6 h after developing labored breathing and dullness of sensorium. On admission Glasgow coma scale (GCS) was E4V1M5, respirations 30/min, pulse 115/min, BP 110/70, afebrile, and with pupils equal and reacting to light. ABG showed severe respiratory acidosis; and lactate was 0.3 mmol/L. The family wanted no invasive interventions, and signed a DNAR order, before shifting the patient to ICU on non-invasive ventilation (NIV).

Over next 24 h, the condition worsened with progressive deterioration in mental status. The family requested organ donation be considered in accordance with their knowledge of the patient's wishes. A supplementary consent form, designed by the National Consortium for Normothermic Regional Perfusion (NRP) in India, that incorporates consent for DCD, NRP, pre-mortem interventions, use of Heparin, placement of sheaths in both femoral arteries and right femoral vein and shifting to OT for organ retrieval was filled out in addition to 'Form 8' [15]. NIV was discontinued at 8.13 pm, resulting in immediate fall in BP t0 73/41 mmHg, and cardiac arrest occurred at 8.33 pm. Following observation for autoresuscitation and a 'no-touch' period of 5 min, low-cost hybrid ECMO was started via the femoral access, with an intra-aortic occlusion balloon positioned in the descending aorta. Abdominal NRP was established with a flow of 2-3 L/min. Peak lactate, of 3.6 was noted 30 mins into the NRP run which was continued for 4 h and 10 mins, at which time lactate dropped to 1.6. AST/ALT remained normal, and urine output was 50–60 ml/h. Liver and both kidneys were recovered and transplanted successfully. The total cost of consumables was only Rs 92,165/−. This patient falls in DCD category III(A) of the new classification proposed for India [16].

Conclusion

The DCD pathway has the potential to significantly increase organ donation in India and with the availability of technologies such as NRP, HMP and NMP the same can be achieved with very good outcomes. DCD following DNAR, as shown in the case described above, adds to the donor pool by including patients with Motor Neuron Disease and Interstitial Lung Disease.

Acknowledgement: Ms Sukhvinder Lal, Senior Officer, Manipal Organ Sharing & Transplant (MOST), for helping in preparing the manuscript.

Competing Interests The author(s) has no competing interests to declare that are relevant to the content of this manuscript.

Ethics Approval The author(s) declares that this manuscript does not include primary research with human participants.

The author(s) declares that this manuscript does not include primary studies involving animals.

References

1. Seth AK, Nambiar P, Joshi A, Ramprasad R, Choubey R, Puri P, et al. First prospective study on brain stem death and attitude towards organ donation in India. Liver Transpl. 2009;15:1443–7.
2. The Transplantation of Human Organs Act (THOA). 1994. Available from: https://main.mohfw.gov.in/sites/default/files/Act%201994.pdf.
3. Kute VB, Vanikar AV, Shah PR, Gumber MR, Patel HV, Modi PR, et al. Outcome of renal transplantation from deceased donors after cardiac death: a single-center experience from a developing country. Transplant Proc. 2013;45(6):2147–51. https://doi.org/10.1016/j.transproceed.2013.02.128.
4. Singh S, Kumar S, Dasgupta S, Kenwar DB, Rathi M, Sharma A, et al. A single-center experience of kidney transplantation from donation after circulatory death: challenges and scope in India. Indian J Nephrol. 2017;27(3):205–9. https://doi.org/10.4103/0971-4065.202843.

5. Mani RK. End-of-life care in India: a care paradigm whose time has come. Curr Med Res Pract. 2026;16(1):4–6. https://doi.org/10.4103/cmrp.cmrp_9_26.
6. Seth AK, Mohanka RM, Mani RK, Asthana S, Attawar S, Dhital KK. Organ donation after circulatory determination of death-consensus statement. Indian Journal of Transplantation. 2024;18:247–56.
7. Seth AK, Mohanka R, Navin S, Gokhale AG, Sharma A, Kumar A, et al. Organ donation after circulatory determination of death in India: a joint position paper. Indian J Crit Care Med. 2022;26:421–38.
8. Elmer J, Atkins DL, Daya MR, Del Rios M, Fry JT, Henderson CM, et al. American Heart Association Guidelines for Cardiopulmonary Resuscitation and Emergency Cardiovascular Care. Circulation. 2025;152(16_suppl_2):S323–52. https://doi.org/10.1161/CIR.0000000000001371. Epub 2025 Oct 22. PMID: 41122890.
9. Pope TM, Bennett J, Carson SS, Cederquist L, Cohen AB, al DeMartino ES e. Making Medical Treatment Decisions for Unrepresented Patients in the ICU. An Official American Thoracic Society/American Geriatrics Society Policy Statement. Am J Respir Crit Care Med. 2020;201(10):1182–92. https://doi.org/10.1164/rccm.202003-0512ST. PMID: 32412853; PMCID: PMC7233335.
10. Marshall MF, Davis FD, Fogelman PA, Oczkowski S, Reid JC, Arellano D, et al. Society of Critical Care Medicine clinical practice guidelines on adult end-of-life care in the ICU. Crit Care Med. 2025;53(12):e2734–46. https://doi.org/10.1097/CCM.0000000000006856. Epub 2025 Dec 2. PMID: 41342842.
11. Domínguez-Gil B, Ascher N, Capron AM, Gardiner D, Manara AR, Bernat JL, et al. Expanding controlled donation after the circulatory determination of death: statement from an international collaborative. Intensive Care Med. 2021;47(3):265–81. https://doi.org/10.1007/s00134-020-06341-7. Epub 2021 Feb 26. Erratum in: Intensive Care Med. 2021 Sep;47(9):1059–1060. https://doi.org/10.1007/s00134-021-06435-w. PMID: 33635355; PMCID: PMC7907666.
12. Fox RC. "An ignoble form of cannibalism": reflections on the Pittsburgh protocol for procuring organs from non-heart-beating cadavers. Kennedy Inst Ethics J. 1993;3(2):231–9.
13. Fox RC, Christakis NA. Perish and publish: non-heart-beating organ donation and unduly iterative ethical review. Kennedy Inst Ethics J. 1995;5(4):335–42.
14. Gries CJ, White DB, Truog RD, Dubois J, Cosio CC, Dhanani S, et al. American Thoracic Society Health Policy Committee. An official American Thoracic Society/International Society for Heart and Lung Transplantation/Society of Critical Care Medicine/Association of Organ and Procurement Organizations/United Network of Organ Sharing Statement: ethical and policy considerations in organ donation after circulatory determination of death. Am J Respir Crit Care Med. 2013;188(1):103–9. https://doi.org/10.1164/rccm.201304-0714ST. PMID: 23815722.
15. Seth AK, Mohanka R, Haji JY, Dhital K, Banker A, Sharma A, et al. Consensus statement of the national consortium on normothermic regional perfusion for organ donation after circulatory determination of death in India. Indian J Transplant. 2026;20:23–35.
16. Seth AK. 30-ABC and the first DCD-NRP in India. Indian Transplant Newsletter. 2025;24(4):4–5. https://doi.org/10.64384/ITN.2025.063.

Part II

Donor Management, Organ Retrieval and Technical Considerations in DCD

ICU Workflow in DCD: From Donor Identification to Organ Retrieval

4

Shrikanth Srinivasan and N. Dileep

Abbreviations

ABG	Arterial blood gas
ACLS	Advanced cardiac life support
ALT	Alanine aminotransferase
AST	Aspartate aminotransferase
ATP	Adenosine triphosphate
cDCD	Controlled donation after circulatory determination of death
CI	Cardiac index
CIT	Cold ischaemia time
CO	Cardiac output
CPB	Cardiopulmonary bypass
CVP	Central venous pressure
DCDD	Donation after circulatory determination of death
EBOA	Endovascular balloon occlusion of aorta
ECMO	Extracorporeal membrane oxygenation
FiO_2	Fraction of inspired oxygen
fWIT	Functional warm ischaemia time
GFR	Glomerular filtration rate
HbA1c	Glycated haemoglobin
HCT	Haematocrit
HR	Heart rate
ICU	Intensive care unit
IMV	Inferior mesenteric vein
IVC	Inferior vena cava
IVS	Interventricular septum

S. Srinivasan (✉) · N. Dileep
Manipal Institute of Critical Care Medicine, Manipal Hospitals, New Delhi, Delhi, India

S. P. Kolte et al. (eds.), *Organ Donation After Circulatory Death*,
https://doi.org/10.1007/978-981-92-6377-6_4

JMFC	Judicial Magistrate First Class
LVEF	left ventricular ejection fraction
MAP	Mean arterial pressure
MDT	Multidisciplinary team
NRP	Normothermic regional perfusion
NOTTO	National Organ and Tissue Transplant Organisation
OHCA	Out-of-hospital cardiac arrest
OPO	Organ procurement organisation
OR	Operating room
P:F ratio	PaO_2:FiO_2 ratio
PA	Pulmonary artery
PAP	Pulmonary arterial pressure
PCWP	Pulmonary capillary wedge pressure
PEEP	Positive end-expiratory pressure
PFO	Patent foramen ovale
PRBCs	Packed red blood cells
PV	Pulmonary vein
PVR	Pulmonary vascular resistance
RAP	Right atrial pressure
REBOA	Resuscitative endovascular balloon occlusion of the aorta
SBP	Systolic blood pressure
SC	Supreme Court
SpO_2	Peripheral oxygen saturation
SRR/DP	Super rapid recovery/direct procurement
SvO_2	Mixed venous oxygen saturation
TA-NRP	Thoracoabdominal normothermic regional perfusion
TEE	Transoesophageal echocardiography
THOTA	Transplantation of Human Organs and Tissues Act
TV	Tidal volume
uDCD	Uncontrolled donation after circulatory determination of death
UW DCD Score	University of Wisconsin DCD Donor Score
UW solution	University of Wisconsin preservation solution
VSD	Ventricular septal defect
WIT	Warm ischaemia time
WLST	Withdrawal of life-sustaining therapy

Pre-WLST Optimisation and Planning

Withdrawal of Life Support (WLST) may be considered for terminally ill patients whose care is deemed futile, according to the Supreme Court Judgement of 2023 [1]. The WLST decision must be reached on clinical grounds alone, without reference to organ donation. Everything that follows is ethically valid only if that prerequisite is satisfied. It is also, in practice, the condition most frequently compromised, usually not by bad intent but by timing: the organ transplant coordinator in the room too early, or the retrieval team asking questions before the family has consented to organ donation. Having a protocol built into the standard operating procedures (SOP) prevents collapsing what should be two separate distinct conversations into one and is the only reliable safeguard.

The Legal Framework for WLST Initiation

India's WLST pathway changed fundamentally in January 2023, when the Supreme Court gave effect to the Common Cause judgement in a form that removed the requirement for Judicial Magistrate (JMFC) approval before WLST could proceed [1]. For years, that requirement had made DCD programmes operationally impossible. The ruling replaced it with a dual-tier Hospital Medical Board. The Primary Board consists of the treating physician and two specialist colleagues, each with over 5 years of post-qualification experience. Their task is to certify irreversibility on clinical and investigational grounds. The Secondary Board independently validates that determination within 48 h. The family provides written consent on the statutory form, and the competent District Authority is notified, though hospitals do not await administrative clearance to proceed. Karnataka became the first state to formally integrate this into its medical governance framework in January 2025 [2]. Other states are yet to implement it fully in their programmes, which means the dual-board model is implemented in some institutions by an institutional initiative rather than state mandate.

Standardised WLST documentation templates do not yet exist nationally. Also, the competency requirements for Medical Board members are undefined in statute. There is no nationally mandated protocol for resolving family dissent after board certification of futility. Individual programmes must fill each gap themselves, and the resulting inconsistency creates medicolegal exposure without any shared standard to defend against it.

The Identification Trigger

The workflow begins with the identification of patients with irreversible catastrophic illness, who do not meet the criteria for brain death. Some of the common aetiologies/conditions where medical care might be futile are:

(a) Severe irreversible neurological injury (not meeting the stringent BSD criteria) due to brain haemorrhage, ischaemic stroke, anoxia (post-resuscitation after cardiac arrest) and other uncommon/rare conditions after a trial of salvage therapies and a reasonable period of complete intensive care.

(b) Non-neurological triggers include patients on multiorgan supports with prolonged ICU care who are unlikely to make a meaningful recovery.

In neurological determination of death, aggressive hormonal resuscitation (vasopressin, methylprednisolone, thyroxine, insulin) is directed at reversing the catecholamine storm, hypothalamic-pituitary disruption and systemic inflammatory cascade that characterise brainstem death. The controlled donation after circulatory death (cDCD) donor, by contrast, retains an intact neurohumoral regulation until the moment of WLST. Management is therefore conservative: the idea being to sustain what is already working, while adding nothing that compromises comfort. Vasopressors are continued at existing doses. Fluid resuscitation follows haemodynamic indices, with deliberate avoidance of hypervolaemia.

At this stage, absolute contraindications to organ donation must be formally excluded (active malignancy, uncontrolled sepsis, cause of death being unknown, etc).

Decoupling WLST from Donation

The sequence is non-negotiable, with the treating intensivist conducting the futility assessment, following which the family reaches a decision on WLST. Multiple evaluations, multidisciplinary discussions and treatment response evaluations may be needed before a consensus can be reached. Once medical futility is established and WLST consents are documented, the intensive care team notifies the hospital transplant coordinator. It is only after that decision is documented does the transplant coordinator approaches the family regarding donation.

Conflating the two discussions even by implication, by introducing the coordinator prematurely, exposes the consent framework to legal challenge. In practice, time pressure from the organ retrieval team is the most common factor by which this sequencing collapses.

Programmes should build this into their SOPs, with separate personnel for each conversation, proper documentation of timestamps, and a defined minimum interval between the two discussions.

Preparation of the Teams

There should also be a clear SOP in place delineating the individual members of the WLST team and the organ procurement team, and their roles and responsibilities.

The WLST Team (treating intensivist/primary) has the sole authority over WLST, palliative care, and the Declaration of Death. The caveat is that they should not be involved in the transplant surgery or the process of organ allocation.

The organ procurement team (transplant coordinator, retrieval surgeons and staff) must not enter the room, touch the patient or influence management in any way until after death is declared and the 5-min stand-off is complete.

Ante-mortem Cannulation

Invasive arterial blood pressure monitoring is essential for accurate assessment of functional warm ischaemia time. Under local anaesthesia and with specific additional surrogate consents, an upper limb arterial line is cannulated for the purpose of confirmation of aortic occlusion. Also, femoral arterial and venous cannulas are placed for perfusion, and the contralateral femoral artery is cannulated for the placement of aortic occlusion balloon placement, before death is declared. This exploits the window of intact cardiac output to accomplish vascular access under controlled haemodynamic conditions, reducing the interval between the end of the no-touch period and normothermic regional perfusion (NRP) initiation; this reduces the gap after no-touch period to re-establishing circulation to under 2 min. Alternatively, in view of ethical considerations and not causing any pain to donor, smaller vascular access lines may be placed before death and exchanged over a guidewire for larger NRP cannulas immediately afterwards.

Where neither option has been consented or is feasible, a post-mortem rapid surgical cut-down at the femoral vessels is performed immediately following the 5-min no-touch period [4].

Systemic Heparinisation

Heparin at 300 to 500 IU/kg administered intravenously just prior to WLST, or at the onset of the agonal haemodynamic threshold (usually a systolic blood pressure of <80 mmHg), this interrupts the activation of the coagulation cascade and prevents microvascular thrombosis via antithrombin III activation. Without heparinisation, incidence of primary non-function of the liver and delayed graft function of the kidneys increases substantially, though the magnitude of this effect in the era of NRP has not been precisely quantified [3].

Heparin provides no therapeutic benefit to the dying donor and carries a risk of haemorrhage, particularly in patients with intracranial pathology where blood–brain barrier disruption makes even modest anticoagulation clinically significant, and hence, it requires a separate, specific surrogate consent. That consent must be explicitly distinguished in the medical record from general WLST consent. In practice, this means a second consent form, obtained in the same conversation window, which most families find confusing and which programmes have no standardised template for. In patients with active uncontrolled haemorrhage, heparin is withheld.

Whether heparin's net benefit outweighs its haemorrhagic risk in donors with intracranial pathology is yet to be researched in any powered prospective trial. Programmes make this call on institutional inference.

NRP Circuit Preparation

The circuit, whether a cardiopulmonary bypass (CPB) system with integrated heater-cooler or a modified ECMO configuration, must be fully assembled, primed, and functionally tested before WLST begins [4]. The prime is Plasmalyte at one litre, an isotonic pH-buffered base that avoids the hyperchloraemic acidosis generated by normal saline. Heparin at 50,000 IU is incorporated to prevent thrombosis at oxygenator membrane and heat-exchanger surfaces. Sodium bicarbonate at 50–100 mEq buffers the predictable reperfusion acidosis as ischaemic organ beds discharge their accumulated lactate load into the circuit. A broad-spectrum antibiotic is incorporated to reduce the risk of circuit contamination from enteric organism translocation across the ischaemia-compromised intestinal mucosal barrier. Packed red cells are added to achieve a reservoir haematocrit above 20%, below which oxygen-carrying capacity is insufficient at the moment of reperfusion when injured mitochondria are most dependent on substrate delivery for aerobic ATP resynthesis.

The heater-cooler is pre-set to 37 °C to preserve enzyme kinetics in the reperfused parenchyma. Oxygen is routed through a Sechrist blender to deliver FiO2 of 0.21 at 2 L/min. Hyperoxic perfusate at this stage generates reactive oxygen species that exacerbate reperfusion injury and is avoided. A portable battery-powered ECMO is deployed when NRP must be initiated in the ICU and the donor transferred to the OR on circuit. Transfer time is a live warm ischaemia exposure with every unnecessary corridor minute having profound influence on organ acceptance decisions.

Withdrawal of Life-Sustaining Treatment (WLST)

WLST Process

WLST is ideally performed in the operating room or an adjacent recovery area. Each additional metre of hospital corridor between asystole and the surgical team accrues warm ischaemia time that can be detrimental. However, this scenario is not always feasible for a critically ill patient on multi-organ supports in the ICU.

Withdrawal involves the sequential cessation of mechanical ventilation, vasopressors, inotropes, renal replacement therapy and cardiac pacemakers. Palliative analgesia is titrated by the WLST intensive care team for dyspnoea and air hunger, and anxiolysis is added for distress and agitation. The Doctrine of Double Effect provides the ethical and legal protection when opioid doses required for adequate symptom control may incidentally accelerate the agonal phase, provided the intent is symptom-directed and dosing is proportionate to a quantifiable symptom state.

There are a few caveats to be kept in mind at this stage. No pharmacological agent whose primary mechanism precipitates asystole is permissible (potassium chloride, neuromuscular blocking agents without concurrent deep sedation). Also, no withdrawn intervention may be reinstated for operational convenience, regardless of retrieval team scheduling pressure. The Dead Donor Rule has to be mandatorily upheld at all times [3].

The Agonal Phase

This phase begins when WLST is withdrawn. However, organs are not considered 'ischaemic' right from the point of WLST, as organ damage occurs only when the perfusion pressure and oxygenation fall below a certain threshold (SBP < 50 mmHg, or SpO2 < 70%).

Approximately 20% of referred cDCD donors fail to progress to cardiac arrest within the permissible window (90 to 120 min), in the case of which the cDCD programme is aborted.

The University of Wisconsin (UW) DCD Donor Score was developed specifically to stratify stand-down risk before team commitment is made [5]. The key predictors of early asystole are a spontaneous respiratory rate below 12 breaths per minute, reflecting profound impairment of central respiratory pattern generation; vasopressor dependency at norepinephrine doses above 0.5 mcg/kg/min, indicating exhaustion of endogenous sympathetic vasomotor reserve; and a PaO_2:FiO_2 ratio below 150 mmHg, signifying ventilation-perfusion mismatch that cannot be corrected by residual respiratory effort after extubation. The inverse profile—the slow-die phenotype—is characterised by brisk spontaneous respiratory drive (>20/min), no vasopressor requirement and preserved gas exchange, with stand-down rates approaching 40% to 50% in some series, which is worth stating explicitly to families before any commitment is made. The family, which has said their goodbyes in the context of organ donation, find themselves back at the bedside. The mental toll of this situation is not to be understated, and most teams experience their first stand-down unprepared.

Documentation of the minute-by-minute vitals during the agonal phase is the primary data on which organ acceptance decisions are made.

The Five-Minute No-Touch Period and Death Certification

Following asystole, confirmed by a flat arterial waveform on the invasive monitor and electrical silence on the ECG, a mandatory 5-min no-touch period is advocated. No contact, cannulation or preparatory manoeuvre by any member of either team is permissible during this time interval, the main concern being auto-resuscitation, i.e. the Lazarus phenomenon. It is rare but documented: spontaneous return of cardiac electrical automaticity after global ischaemia has been reported, and it would invalidate death certification if it occurred undetected.

It is also to be noted that no prospective human study has established 5 min as the biological threshold beyond which auto-resuscitation cannot occur. The figure comes from expert consensus and sparse case reports. Teams should keep in mind that this is the regulatory minimum for legal protection, and not a calibrated physiological safety margin.

Death is certified by the WLST intensivist and never by a member of the retrieval team. Under THOTA and its amendments, this is a statutory requirement and not an institutional preference.

Retrieval Pathways and Optimal Donor Management

After WLST consent is documented, the ICU team is managing two processes simultaneously, the end-of-life care, and an organ procurement. The common failure is institutional where teams treat them as if they conflict, leading to either inadequate circuit preparation or undocumented ante-mortem interventions, either of which can abort or legally compromise the entire programme.

The Modified Maastricht Classification

DCDD is broadly divided into controlled DCD (cDCD) and uncontrolled DCD (uDCD) and is further sub-classified into different categories [4] (Table 4.1):

Pathways of Organ Retrieval

Donor retrieval is done by one of the following techniques:

(a) *Super Rapid Recovery (SRR)/ Direct Procurement (DP):* After certification of death and the no-touch period, organs are perfused using an ice-cold preservative solution via ante-mortem percutaneous femoral cannulas or via aortic cannulas placed intraoperatively. A rapid thoracoabdominal laparotomy is done and surface cooling with ice is initiated. Surgical dissection and organ retrieval are carried out in this cold phase [3]. The logistics for SRR/DP are tricky and need pinpoint coordination between the surgical and anaesthesia teams, which is difficult to consistently achieve.

(b) *Normothermic Regional Perfusion (NRP)*: This is the new standard where, after certification of death and the no-touch period, the donor's abdominal (or thoracoabdominal) circulation is re-established using a cardiopulmonary bypass (CPB) or a modified extracorporeal membrane oxygenator (ECMO) in a circuit that excludes cerebral circulation. Abdominal NRP may be started in the ICU once hospital SOPs for ante-mortem cannulation and systemic heparinisation are in place. Thoracoabdominal NRP is required if DCD heart retrieval is planned. If lung retrieval is planned, re-intubation and reinitiation of mechanical ventilation,

Table 4.1 Maastricht categories of donors

Type	Organs that can be donated	Location
I Dead on arrival *(uncontrolled)*	Tissues (cornea, heart valves)	Out of hospital
II Unsuccessful resuscitation (*uncontrolled*)	Lungs Liver Kidney Pancreas	Emergency room
III Anticipated cardiac arrest (withdrawal of life sustaining treatment) *(controlled)*	Heart Lungs Liver Kidney Pancreas	Scenario 1: Operation theatre (thoracoabdominal NRP)
		Scenario 2: Operation theatre (peripheral/abdominal ± cold perfusion for lungs)
		Scenario 3: Intensive care unit (peripheral/abdominal ± cold perfusion for lungs)
IV Cardiac arrest in a brain-dead donor *(controlled)*	All organs	Intensive care unit
V Unexpected In-hospital witnessed cardiac arrest *(uncontrolled)*	Lungs Liver Kidney Pancreas	Intensive care unit

along with bilateral pleural cold perfusion, is started. To maintain normothermia, warming blankets with heat exchanger blankets may be needed [4].

NRP Circuit Dynamics: The Reperfusion Surge

The first 15 to 20 min of NRP are characteristically destabilising. As ischaemically vasodilated splanchnic and hepatic capillary beds reconnect to the circuit and discharge an accumulated metabolic debt, both lactates and CO2 rise sharply. Teams encountering this for the first time may misread it as circuit failure or donor unsuitability. Sweep gas is increased to augment CO_2 clearance across the oxygenator membrane. Sodium bicarbonate corrects pH below 7.2, preventing acidosis-driven inhibition of citric acid cycle enzymes. Volume replacement (blood or albumin 5% or 20%) addresses reperfusion vasoplegia, which is mediated by nitric oxide and prostacyclin released from the ischaemically primed splanchnic endothelium upon restoration of shear stress.

Stabilising blood flows in the NRP circuit may take up to 90–120 min. NRP is typically run for 30 min to 2 h (sometimes up to 4 h by unanimous MDT). Target NRP parameters are a pump flow 2.0 to 2.5 L/min (approximately 2.4 L/min/m^2); FiO_2 0.21 at 2 L/min sweep gas; SvO_2 60 to 80%; arterial pCO_2 35 to 45 mmHg; temperature 37 °C; haematocrit above 20%. Arterial blood gas, lactate, AST and ALT are measured every 15 min [3].

Warm Ischaemia Timelines

At least three distinct intervals govern organ viability in cDCD and treating them as the same generates systematic errors in organ acceptance decisions.

Total WIT versus fWIT: Why the Distinction Is Not Pedantic

Total warm ischaemia time runs from the cessation of effective circulation to the initiation of organ preservation. It is the metric most cited in early DCD literature and the most misleading in cDCD, because it includes the early agonal phase during which a diminished but non-zero cardiac output sustains partial end-organ perfusion above the threshold of irreversible mitochondrial injury. Counting this sub-critical period as frank ischaemia overstates the true ischaemic burden and drives unnecessary organ decline decisions.

Functional warm ischaemia time (fWIT) corrects for this assumption. The clock is triggered when systolic blood pressure falls to or below 50 mmHg, at which point autoregulatory reserve in the hepatic and renal circulations is exhausted and perfusion pressure falls below the critical closing pressure of the microvasculature, or when peripheral oxygen saturation falls to or below 70%. Some programmes use MAP below 60 mmHg as the SBP surrogate, which better captures the true driving pressure across the systemic vasculature. The clock stops at the initiation of organ preservation. The invasive arterial line is the only permissible instrument for recording the haemodynamic trigger and oscillometric readings are inadmissible for this determination (Table 4.2).

Table 4.2 Organ-specific warm ischaemia thresholds, cold ischaemia tolerances and NRP viability assessment criteria

Organ	Max fWIT (cDCD)	Max CIT	fWIT trigger	NRP assessment period	Key viability parameters on NRP	Critical note
Heart	<30 min	4–6 h	SBP ≤ 50 mmHg or SpO_2 < 70%	30–45 min wean test on TA-NRP	MAP > 60 mmHg; CI > 2.5 L/min/m^2; LVEF > 50% on TEE; HR < 120 bpm; CVP 4–6 mmHg; PCWP <12 mmHg	TEE mandatory. DC cardioversion permissible. Most ischaemia-sensitive organ—creatine phosphate reserves last seconds
Lungs	<60–90 min	6–8 h	Asystole (not haemodynamic threshold)	P:F ratio assessed post re-ventilation	P:F ratio > 3 (300 mmHg); individual pulmonary venous blood gas on FiO_2 1.0 + PEEP 8 after 5 min; bilateral bronchoscopy clear	Re-intubation mandatory with TA-NRP. Bilateral intercostal drains + cold saline if fWIT >60 min with peripheral NRP
Liver	<30 min	<12 h	SBP ≤ 50 mmHg or SpO_2 < 70%	Up to 2 h (max 4 h by unanimous MDT)	Lactate stable or falling; AST < 500 U/L; ALT <1000 U/L; bile production and biliary pH; gross appearance at laparotomy	Biliary epithelium is the rate-limiting structure. Sub-ischaemic hypotension before fWIT trigger can cause occult cholangiocyte injury not captured by fWIT alone
Kidneys	<120 min	24–36 h	SBP ≤ 50 mmHg or SpO_2 < 70%	Continuous throughout NRP	Gross perfusion and cortical appearance; biopsy if age > 60 or pre-existing renal disease; urine output supportive but not a stand-alone criterion	Most resilient organ. Tubular epithelium regenerates—primary non-function from WIT alone is uncommon in donors <65 y with intact baseline renal function
Pancreas	<30 min	10–12 h	SBP ≤ 50 mmHg or SpO_2 < 70%	Gross assessment at laparotomy	Amylase, lipase, HbA1c pre-operatively; gross appearance at laparotomy for oedema, haemorrhagic change, or necrosis	Any haemorrhagic or necrotic change at laparotomy terminates procurement regardless of pre-operative biochemistry

[a] *For lungs, the fWIT clock starts at asystole rather than at the haemodynamic threshold (SBP ≤ 50 mmHg / SpO_2 ≤ 70%). Residual alveolar oxygen sustains aerobic pulmonary parenchymal metabolism for several minutes after circulatory arrest, making the conventional haemodynamic trigger inapplicable to this organ*

[b] *The 30-min hepatic fWIT threshold is a statistical risk inflection point, not a biological boundary. Biliary injury may occur below this threshold in donors with steatosis, advanced age, or prolonged sub-ischaemic agonal phases. NRP-based multiparametric metabolic assessment—lactate trajectory, biliary pH, bile production, transaminase trend—is the definitive viability determination and not fWIT alone*

cDCD Versus uDCD Pathways

Definitions

A controlled DCD is donation that occurs when death is anticipated and follows the planned Withdrawal of Life-Sustaining Treatment (WLST), whereas uncontrolled DCD is the donation that occurs after an unexpected cardiac arrest where resuscitation has been attempted but was unsuccessful and the organ preservation must often begin while mechanical CPR is ongoing or immediately after death is declared, often before full family consent is finalised.

In controlled DCD, the clinical team retains temporal control over the dying process. WLST is planned, the retrieval team is pre-positioned, and the circuit is primed. Uncontrolled DCD operates under fundamentally different constraints because the ischaemic exposure cannot be modulated prospectively.

Both controlled and uncontrolled DCD share the Dead Donor Rule, the 5-min no-touch period, mandatory cerebral exclusion during NRP and the priority of ethical consent. Beyond those foundations, the two pathways diverge substantially in operational architecture, ischaemic burden, recoverable organ complement and consent framework (See Table 4.3.).

The uDCD Pathway

The trigger is a refractory cardiac arrest—out-of-hospital in Maastricht Category II or witnessed in-hospital in Category V. In case of unexpected cardiac arrest, if the family is strongly inclined towards organ donation or if the patient had expressed his wishes for organ donation via an advanced medical directive or a donor card, etc. counselling may be initiated even during the process of cardiopulmonary resuscitation [6].

The operative metric shifts from fWIT to total WIT, beginning at the moment of collapse, because the entire interval from arrest to preservation represents a period of accumulating ATP deficit in organ parenchyma, with no sub-threshold haemodynamic period to exclude.

Total WIT beyond 45 to 60 min precludes liver retrieval in most programmes. Kidneys remain viable up to 90 to 120 min if CPR was effective; proximal tubular regeneration partially mitigates the consequences of ischaemia-reperfusion injury over the post-transplant recovery period. Lungs can be assessed on NRP if total WIT is under 90 min and TA-NRP is feasible.

The Consent Problem in uDCD

This model operates in a legislative gap in India. THOTA and the 2023 Supreme Court guidance contain no provision that explicitly authorises a preservation-first, consent-second approach for uDCD. Programmes wishing to implement it require

Table 4.3 Controlled DCD (cDCD) versus uncontrolled DCD (uDCD): comparative pathway analysis

Feature	Controlled DCD (cDCD)—maastricht III/IV	Uncontrolled DCD (uDCD)—maastricht II/V
Trigger	Planned WLST following multidisciplinary futility determination	Refractory cardiac arrest after failed ACLS resuscitation
Event nature	Anticipated and elective; retrieval team pre-positioned before WLST	Sudden and unplanned; 'Code DCD' activated on futility declaration
Primary location	ICU/OR/ Recovery area	Emergency department / In-hospital ICU (Category V)
Operative ischaemia metric	fWIT: clock begins when SBP $\leq$ 50 mmHg or $SpO_2 \leq 70\%$	Total WIT: begins at the moment of witnessed cardiac arrest; to the start of organ preservation. Includes entire no-flow and low-flow period
Consent pathway	Obtained before WLST; separate additional consent for ante-mortem interventions (heparin, ante-mortem cannulation)	Obtained during NRP in international practice; preservation-first, consent-second model operates in a legislative gap in India
Organs retrievable	Heart, Lungs, Liver, Kidneys, Pancreas	Primarily Kidneys; Liver if NRP used and total WIT <45–60 min; Lungs if total WIT <90 min and TA-NRP feasible; Heart rarely viable
NRP configuration	TA-NRP (sternotomy, right atrial + aortic cannulation, surgical arch vessel clamping) OR peripheral/ abdominal NRP (femoral + EBOA)	Peripheral/abdominal NRP exclusively (femoral cannulation + EBOA); central sternotomy precluded by time constraints
Cerebral exclusion method	Surgical clamping of innominate artery, left common carotid artery, left subclavian artery (TA-NRP); EBOA in peripheral NRP	EBOA via contralateral femoral artery; position confirmed radiologically; absence of upper limb BP signal confirms exclusion
Primary logistical challenge	Predicting time to cardiac arrest; stand-down rate ~ 20%—primary driver of programme abandonment	Unknown or prolonged no-flow time; total WIT accumulation before team mobilisation; consent timing under legislative gap
Indian legal status	Operationally feasible under SC 2023 ruling; dual Medical Board WLST pathway established	Inclusion criteria feasible under THOTA; preservation-first consent model lacks explicit statutory authorisation and institutional ethics committee approval required

specific institutional ethics committee approval, documented legal counsel and a prospectively approved written protocol.

Competing Interests The author(s) has no competing interests to declare that are relevant to the content of this manuscript.

Ethics Approval The author(s) declares that this manuscript does not include primary research with human participants.

The author(s) declares that this manuscript does not include primary studies involving animals.

References

1. Supreme Court of India. Order modifying advance medical directive/withholding and withdrawing of life-sustaining treatment procedures (Common Cause case). Miscellaneous Application No. 1699 of 2019 in Writ Petition (Civil) No. 215 of 2005. Order dated 24 Jan 2023. New Delhi: Supreme Court of India; 2023.
2. Health and Family Welfare Department (Karnataka). Nomination of registered medical practitioners to the secondary medical board to certify withholding/withdrawing of life-sustaining treatment (WLST) [Internet]. Bengaluru: Health and Family Welfare Department; 2025. Available from: https://hfwcom.karnataka.gov.in/storage/pdf-files/NomineeofDHOonSecondaryBoard-1-1.pdf.
3. Seth AK, Mohanka R, Mani RK, et al. Organ donation after circulatory determination of death — consensus statement. Indian J Transplant. 2024;18(3):247–56. https://doi.org/10.4103/IJOT.IJOT_37_24.
4. Seth AK, Mohanka R, Haji J, Dhital K, Banker, et al. Consensus Statement of the National Consortium on Normothermic Regional Perfusion for Organ Donation after Circulatory Determination of Death in India. Indian J Transplant. 2026;20(1):23–35. https://doi.org/10.4103/ijot.ijot_81_25.
5. Lewis J, Peltier J, Nelson H, et al. Development of the University of Wisconsin donation after cardiac death evaluation tool. Prog Transplant. 2003;13(4):265–73. https://doi.org/10.1177/152692480301300405.
6. Seth AK, Mohanka R, Navin S, et al. Organ donation after circulatory determination of death in India: a joint position paper. Indian J Crit Care Med. 2022;26(4):421–38. https://doi.org/10.5005/jp-journals-10071-24198.

Normothermic Regional Perfusion in DCD

5

Jumana Yusuf Haji

Introduction

Donation after Circulatory Death (DCD) is rapidly becoming a global standard, largely due to its broad acceptance by donor families and its significant role in expanding the organ donor pool. In many Western nations, End-of-Life Care (EOLC) legislation permits the elective withdrawal of life-sustaining treatment when recovery to a functional life is no longer possible. These cases facilitate *controlled DCD*, specifically classified as *Maastricht Category III*.

The DCD process requires a mandatory *"no-touch" period* immediately following the cessation of life. This interval—confirmed by a flat-line ECG, absence of activity on echocardiography, and lack of palpable pulses—ensures the conclusive cessation of circulation and precludes any spontaneous return of brain viability. While the duration varies by country—ranging from 2 min in some jurisdictions to 20 min in Italy—the majority of nations adhere to a 5-min standard [1] (Table 5.1).

While DCD offers immense potential to increase organ availability, it presents significant physiological hurdles. As circulation fails during the dying process, organs transition to *anaerobic metabolism*, leading to a rapid loss of Adenosine Triphosphate (ATP). This metabolic decline accelerates during the *warm ischemia time (WIT)* of the no-touch period Fig. 5.1. Although subsequent cold perfusion slows this process, it does not halt it entirely. Consequently, any delay in procurement or transplantation can lead to irreversible damage, rendering the organs untransplantable. Ultimately, the success of a DCD transplant is dictated by the duration of warm ischemia the organs can endure.

J. Y. Haji (✉)
Fortis Hospital Mulund, Mumbai, Maharashtra, India
e-mail: ecmo@drjumana.in

S. P. Kolte et al. (eds.), *Organ Donation After Circulatory Death*,
https://doi.org/10.1007/978-981-92-6377-6_5

Table 5.1 Mandatory no-touch period after circulatory death country wise

Country	No-Touch Duration	Rationale/Notes
USA/Canada	2–5 min	Most common standard; focuses on permanent arrest.
UK/Australia	5 min	Standardized to ensure no spontaneous circulation (autoresuscitation).
France/Spain	5 min	Strictly regulated under Maastricht Category III protocols.
Switzerland	10 min	A more conservative approach to ensuring death.
Italy	20 min	The most stringent requirement globally to ensure total brain death.

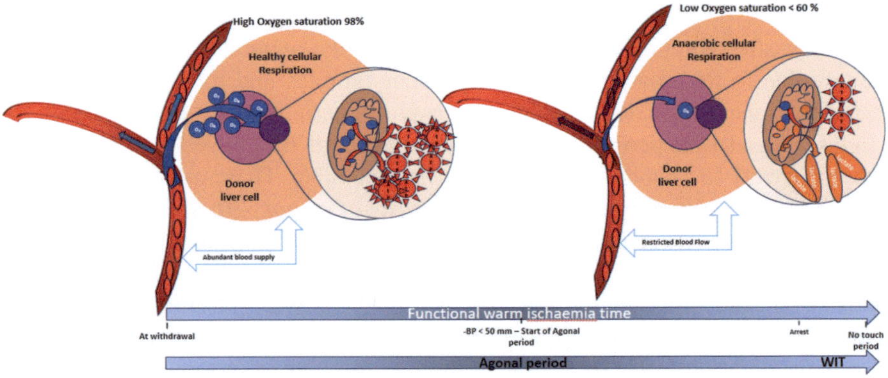

Fig. 5.1 Phases of cellular metabolism during functional warm ischemia time

There is immense variability in the methods of DCD donations internationally and each country needs to formulate pathways and Standard operating procedures from the outset to get good quality organs [2].

To this end there are currently 2 position statements describing the process of DCD donations in the Indian context [3, 4].

Comparison of Global "No-Touch" Periods

The "no-touch" period is the critical window between circulatory arrest and the start of organ procurement. As shown below, this duration varies significantly based on national legal and ethical frameworks.

Metabolic Impact: The ATP Depletion Pathway

When circulation stops, cells lose their primary fuel source (Oxygen). This triggers a cascade that determines whether an organ remains viable for transplant:

Phase 1: Ischemic Switch (Aerobic to Anaerobic)
With no oxygen, the mitochondria stop producing ATP via oxidative phosphorylation. Cells switch to *anaerobic glycolysis*, which is highly inefficient (producing 2 ATP vs. 36 ATP).
Phase 2: Lactic Acidosis
Anaerobic metabolism produces *lactic acid* as a byproduct. Intracellular pH drops (acidosis), damaging cell membranes and enzymes.
Phase 3: ATP Exhaustion and Structural Failure
As ATP stores hit zero, the cell can no longer power its "ion pumps." Sodium rushes into the cell, causing it to swell (*cellular edema*) and eventually burst, leading to irreversible tissue death.
Organs are thus susceptible to warm ischemic injury (WIT), leading to high rates of primary non-function (PNF) and ischemic cholangiopathy (IC). Normothermic Regional Perfusion (NRP) has emerged as a transformative technique that re-establishes circulation in situ restoring warm, oxygenated blood flow to organs following declaration of circulatory death. NRP mitigates warm ischemia, allows for metabolic recovery by ATP replenishment, and permits functional assessment prior to retrieval.
This is why *Normothermic Regional Perfusion (NRP)* is so effective—it restarts the oxygen supply *before* Phase 3 is reached, allowing the cell to "recharge" its ATP stores while still inside the donor.

Extracorporeal Membrane Oxygenation (ECMO) is a widely accepted form of cardiopulmonary support for critical care patients who are refractory to conventional treatment. Globally, the number of patients receiving ECMO in critical care settings has increased exponentially over the past 15 years [5]. Consequently, expanding organ donation eligibility to include patients on ECMO is essential.

The aim of using ECMO in donors declared dead—either by Brain Death (DBD) criteria or after Circulatory Death (DCD)—is to maintain organ viability. In these scenarios, the focus is on maintaining adequate oxygenated perfusion to preserve organs until they can be procured.

ECMO patients as brain-dead donors can expand the organ donor pool substantially in the years to come [6, 7]. Brain-dead donors on ECMO would need apnoea testing to be donors by DBD criteria. The process of apnoea testing on ECMO may be a bit tougher and many a times inconclusive [8–10]. In such cases withdrawal of life support and pursuing the DCD pathway would be convenient as the patient already has ECMO cannulations and consumables. The flow can be restarted after 5-min no-touch period with cerebral flow occlusion methods in place.

ECMO provides a vital bridge for families and medical teams to make decisions regarding organ donation. Studies have shown that using ECMO can improve transplant outcomes by reducing the ischemic damage that typically occurs between the time of death and organ retrieval. By enabling the use of organs from donors who might not otherwise have been considered, ECMO expands the donor pool and potentially reduces waiting times for recipients.

Normothermic Regional Perfusion

Normothermic Regional Perfusion is the preservation of in situ circulation in organs, using an extracorporeal oxygenator driven by a bypass or ECMO machine and temperature-controlled by a heater-cooler unit. The steps of DCD NRP are as shown in Fig. 5.2 [11].

The pathway additionally includes timing of cannulation and occlusion of circulation to the heart and brain to prevent reanimation of these organs, as it confuses the appearance of death.

The timing of cannulation varies according to the legislation of different countries. Italy has the longest warm ischemia time and hence permits insertion of cannulas before asystole. (Table 5.1) Most countries allow cannulation and heparization postmortem to prevent acceleration of the death process due to the risk of bleeding. A consent for the same is mandatory pre-mortem, but may not be needed postmortem. The occlusion of the circulation to the brain is done by either directly clamping the arch vessels or the abdominal aorta or inserting an Endovascular Balloon for Occlusion of the Aorta (EBOA) through a femoral artery and inflating it at the level of the abdominal aorta. The NRP circuit additionally needs a reservoir, as the native heart no longer acts as the reservoir. (Table 5.2).

The cannulation can be central through a thoracotomy, abdominal through a laparotomy or peripheral through cannulation of the femoral artery and vein in a VA ECMO configuration. The cannulation strategy depends on the type of DCD and the organs to be preserved.

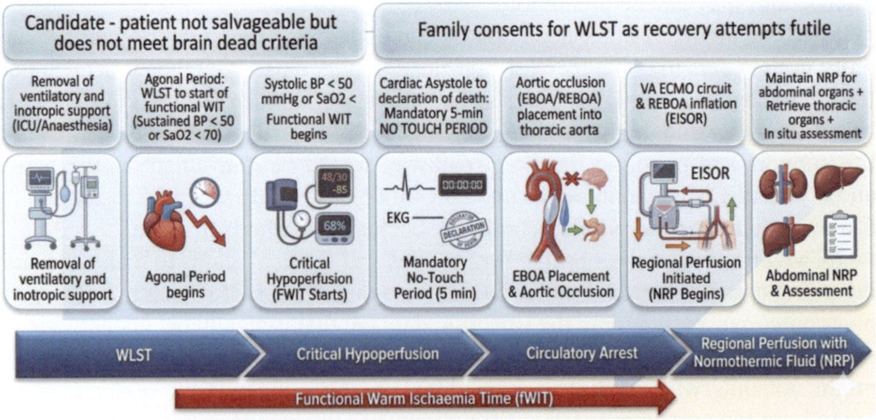

Fig. 5.2 Steps of DCD NRP and with the timelines to quantify ATP loss

Table 5.2 Types cannulation and cerebral circulation occlusion techniques related to various Maastricht Category donations

DCD type	Organs	Cannulation	Method of preventing reanimation of brain/ Brain + heart
II (uncontrolled)	Liver kidney pancreas and lungs	Femoral VA ECMO	EBOA
III (controlled)	Heart lung liver kidney pancreas intestines	Through sternotomy—RA to Aorta	Ligation of arch vessel to prevent brain circulation
		Through Laparotomy—internal iliac vessels/coeliac vessels	Clamp on the abdominal aorta
IV (uncontrolled)	Liver kidney pancreas and lungs	Femoral VA ECMO	EBOA
V (controlled)	All organs	Femoral VA ECMO	Not needed as patient certified brain dead

Management of DCD with NRP

DCD with NRP thus needs a multidepartment teamwork and coordination as shown in Fig. 5.3.

The critical care team decides the futility of continuation of care, then counsels the family for non-escalation of treatment or withdrawal of life support. It oversees the process till asystole, focusing on the comfort of the dying patient up to declaration of death while involving the organ transplant coordinators for keeping track of the ischaemia times and the ECMO team to plan logistics of cannulation and perfusion for NRP. In case of a type III donor, OT and cardiac and liver surgical teams are to be ready for either rapid retrieval or surgical cannulation while the ECMO team oversees the perfusion and monitors serial labs to ascertain organ viability.

NRP ECMO Hardware, Consumables and Circuit

Normothermic Regional Perfusion (NRP) utilizes a modified veno-arterial extracorporeal membrane oxygenation (VA ECMO) circuit to restore oxygenated blood flow to abdominal (A-NRP) or thoracoabdominal (TA-NRP) organs after death has been declared, allowing for in situ organ preservation and assessment. The hardware and consumables are similar to standard VA ECMO but tailored for rapid deployment and specific regional circulation control [11].

NRP Hardware Components (Fig. 5.4)

- *Centrifugal Pump*: Typically uses a magnetically levitated centrifugal to provide flow, which minimizes blood damage.
- *Console and Driver*: A portable console is usually chosen for rapid mobilization to the operating room.

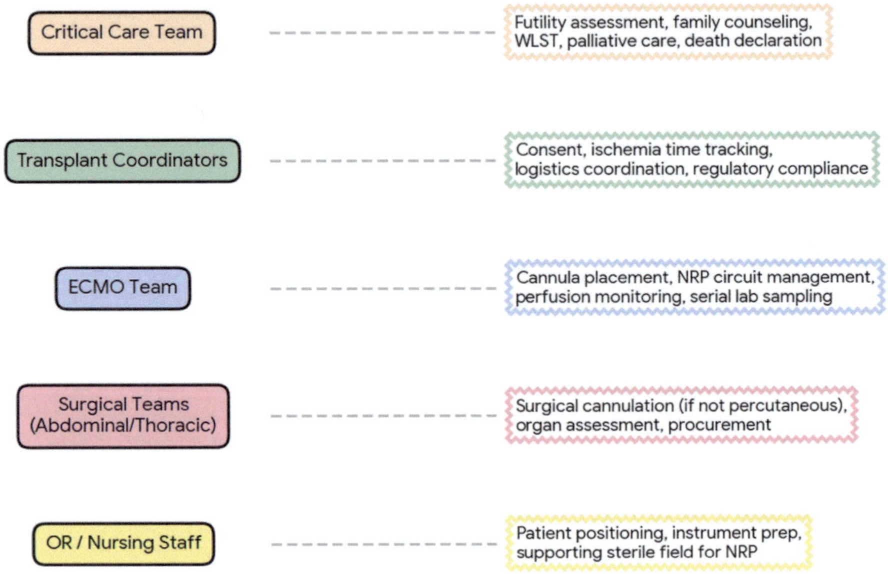

Fig. 5.3 Multidepartment teamwork in NRP-DCD Process

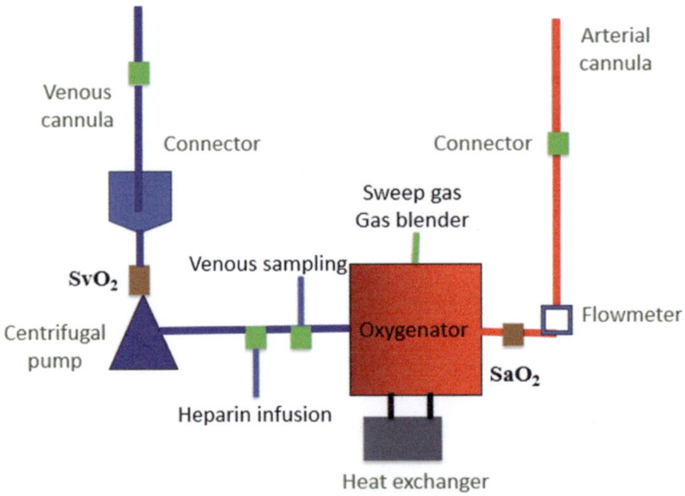

Fig. 5.4 NRP consumables and circuit setup

- *Heater-Cooler Unit*: A crucial unit (e.g., HICO or Sorin Stockert 3T) is used to maintain normothermia (37 °C) to reverse warm ischemic damage.
- *Gas Blender*: Connects to oxygen sources to manage sweep gas for the membrane oxygenator.

- *Flow/Pressure Sensors and Monitors*: Sensors integrated into the circuit monitor blood flow, pressure, and venous oxygen saturation ($SCVO_2$) to ensure adequate perfusion.

NRP Consumables and Circuit Setup

The circuit is designed as a closed loop that takes blood from the venous system, oxygenates it, and returns it to the arterial system.

- *Membrane Oxygenator*: Usually a PolyMethylPentene (PMP) oxygenator that includes an integrated heat exchanger.
- *Cannulae*:
  - *Venous Drainage*: Large bore (e.g.,21 F to 29 Fr), typically placed in the inferior vena cava (IVC) or right atrium.
  - *Arterial Return*: Smaller size (e.g., 17 to 21Fr), inserted into the abdominal aorta or femoral artery.
- *Tubing*: Polyvinylchloride (PVC) circuit tubing, often coated (e.g., heparin-coated) to reduce thrombosis, often with smaller (1/4)-inch or (3/8)-inch diameter to reduce priming volume.
- *Aortic Balloon Occlusion Catheter*: Specifically for TA-NRP, a Coda balloon catheter is used to isolate the abdominal organs and prevent perfusion of the brain.
- *Other Consumables*: Cardiotomy reservoir for blood collection, Y-connectors for bypass, blood gas sampling ports, and priming solution.

Key Differences in NRP Circuits

Unlike standard ECMO, NRP circuits are designed for short-term, high-efficiency use in a deceased donor.

- *Regionality*: Uses clamps or balloons to specifically limit perfusion to the liver, kidneys, and intestines.
- *Anticoagulation*: Because the donor is deceased, there is no need for systemic heparinization, although the circuit itself is typically biocompatible-coated.
- *Rapid Assembly*: Mobile NRP services use pre-assembled kits for rapid cannulation, often achieving flow within 2–3 min of cardiac arrest. A standard ECMO circuit consists of a mechanical blood pump, gas exchange device (membrane oxygenator), and a heat exchanger (Fig. 5.5).
- An *Endovascular Balloon Occlusion of the Aorta (EBOA)* is inserted via the contralateral femoral artery to restrict VA ECMO flow to the abdominal organs, preventing cerebral perfusion.

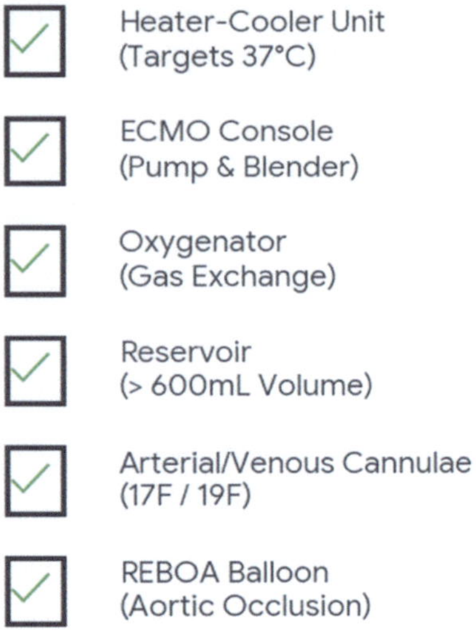

Fig. 5.5 NRP circuit and hardware checklist

Operational Parameters and Perfusate Management

Abdominal NRP can be maintained for *4–8 h* provided the following physiological targets are met:

- *Pump Flow*: NRP is aimed at maintaining oxygen delivery (DO2) by maintaining optimal Mean Arterial Pressure and optimal Hematocrit— [12].
  The protocols at each center varied slightly. Aim was to maintain a pump flow between 1.7 and 4 L/min, temperature 35.5–37.5 °C, pH 7.35–7.45, Hematocrit >20%.
  The optimal hematocrit during CPB appears to be above 23–24% in both adult and pediatric patients.
- *Volume Status*: Maintain a reservoir level using colloids or crystalloids to ensure adequate venous return.
- *Hematology*: Maintain a Hematocrit and add *Heparin* to keep the Activated Clotting Time (ACT) above 350 s.
- *Blood Gas Targets*: Maintain a pH between 7.35 and 7.45 and a between 100 and 150 mmHg. *Packed Red Blood Cells (PRBCs)* should be added to the perfusate to optimize oxygen-carrying capacity.

NRP Circuit and Hardware Checklist Fig. 5.5

NRP Circuit Priming and Anticoagulation Protocol

The success of the 4–8 h perfusion window depends on a meticulous "de-airing" of the circuit and aggressive anticoagulation to prevent clot formation within the donor organs.

1. *Priming Procedure*

   The goal of priming is to replace the air in the circuit with a biocompatible solution that mimics physiological conditions.

   - *Initial Flush*: The circuit is typically primed with *1–2 l of balanced crystalloid* (e.g., Plasmalyte or Ringer's Lactate). This ensures the oxygenator and pump head are free of air bubbles.
   - *Colloid/Blood Addition*: To maintain the required *reservoir volume (>600 mL)* and *Hematocrit (>20%)*, the crystalloid is partially replaced or supplemented with:
     - *5% Albumin*: To maintain oncotic pressure and prevent tissue edema.
     - *Packed Red Blood Cells (PRBCs)*: To ensure immediate oxygen delivery once NRP commences.
   - *De-airing*: The circuit is recirculated through the heater-cooler to reach *37 °C* and checked for microbubbles before the donor is cannulated.
2. *Anticoagulation Strategy (The Heparin Protocol)* (Table 5.3)
   In DCD, the cessation of circulation and subsequent stasis trigger a massive pro-thrombotic state. NRP must counteract this to ensure microvascular patency.
3. *Monitoring Organ Viability (Serial Labs)* [14]
   During Normothermic Regional Perfusion (NRP), the primary objective is to evaluate the metabolic recovery and functional capacity of the organs. This is achieved through a combination of half-hourly biochemical assessments—including *Arterial Blood Gases (ABG), Liver Function Tests (LFT), Hemoglobin (Hb), and Lactate kinetics*—alongside direct macroscopic inspection.

Organ-Specific Viability Criteria (Table 5.4)

- *Liver*:
  - *Metabolic Trends*: Assessment of lactate clearance (kinetic evolution) and normalization of blood pH.

Table 5.3 Heparin protocol for DCD

Parameter	Target value	Action/Rationale
Initial heparin dose	**300–400 units/kg**	Administered into the circuit or to the donor immediately upon NRP initiation
Target ACT	**> 350 s**	Monitored every 30–60 min to prevent fibrin deposition in the oxygenator and organ capillaries
Continuous infusion	**10–50 units/kg/h**	Adjusted based on serial ACT results during the 4–8 h perfusion

Table 5.4 Clinical viability dashboard

Organ	Marker	Ideal trend/Result
Global	**Lactate**	**Down-trending** (Clearance indicates mitochondrial recovery)
Global	**pH**	**7.35–7.45** (Resolution of metabolic acidosis)
Liver	**Bile**	**Golden/yellow** (Active production is a sign of health)
Liver	**ALT/AST**	**<3× baseline** (Minimal hepatocellular injury)
Kidney	**Urine**	**Present** (Indicates adequate glomerular filtration)
Pancreas	**Amylase**	**Stable** (Absence of sudden spikes)

  - *Enzymatic Stability*: Transaminases (SGOT/SGPT) should ideally remain less than three times the baseline or show a steady downward trend.
  - *Functional Output*: Observation of consistent bile production and assessment of the bleeding status at the biliary section.
  - *Visual & Histological*: Macroscopic "post-perfusion" appearance; if the visual assessment is non-convincing, a liver biopsy is performed while the NRP is ongoing.
- *Kidney*:
  - *Functional Output*: Monitoring of urine production (volume and consistency).
  - *Biochemical Assessment*: Analysis of urine chemistry and, if clinically indicated, a renal biopsy to assess chronic damage or acute tubular necrosis.
- *Pancreas*:
  - *Enzymatic Monitoring*: Serial measurement of Serum Amylase levels to screen for pancreatitis or significant ischemic injury.

Before formal procurement, the surgical team performs a final "bedside" assessment. A "convincing" liver should transition from a dark, congested appearance to a *bright, uniform pink/mahogany* color with soft turgor. Conversely, a "non-convincing" liver remains patchy, firm, or dusky, often requiring a frozen section biopsy to rule out macrosteatosis or irreversible ischemic necrosis.

Thoracoabdominal NRP (TA-NRP) Procedure (Fig. 5.6)

In Maastricht Category III DCD, the withdrawal of life-sustaining treatment (WLST) takes place directly within the operating theater (OT) to minimize the agonal phase and warm ischemia time. The TA-NRP technique allows for the simultaneous resuscitation of both thoracic and abdominal organs through a highly coordinated surgical approach.

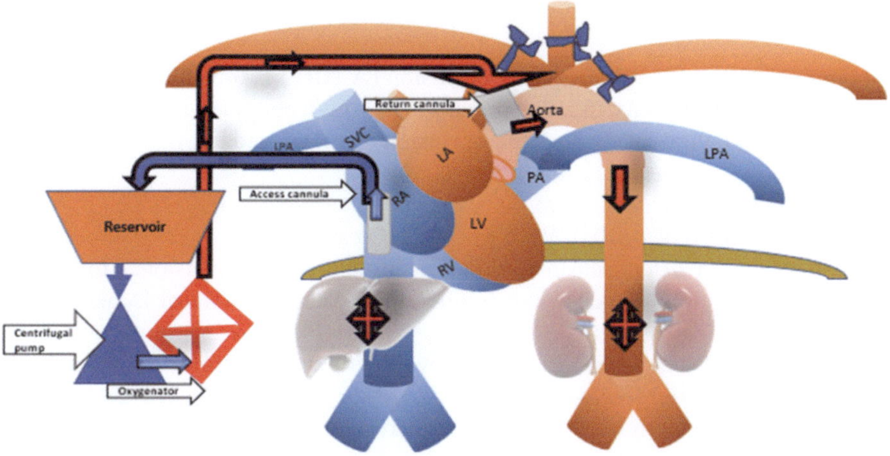

Fig. 5.6 Thoracoabdominal NRP using central cannulation and direct arch vessel ligation for prevention of cerebral circulation

Surgical Sequence and Vascular Control

1. Initiation: Following the declaration of death and the mandatory "no-touch" period, a rapid sternotomy and laparotomy are performed.
2. Cerebral Protection: To maintain ethical compliance and the "dead donor rule," the arch vessels (innominate, left carotid, and left subclavian arteries) are ligated. This prevents any restoration of blood flow to the brain once perfusion begins.
3. Thoracic Resuscitation: Central cannulation of the right atrium (RA) and the Aorta is established, and the ECMO circuit is initiated. As the heart is re-perfused with warm, oxygenated blood, it re-animates and resumes a functional beat.
4. Abdominal Transition: Once cardiac function is stabilized, iliac cannulation is performed to transition to abdominal NRP. The abdominal aorta is clamped to isolate the circuits as needed.
5. Simultaneous Retrieval: While abdominal NRP continues to optimize the liver and kidneys with warm perfusate, the thorax is flooded with sterile ice. The heart is then arrested with cold cardioplegia and retrieved for transplantation.

Key Advantages of TA-NRP

- Heart Transplantation: TA-NRP is the primary driver for the recent 15–30% expansion in the heart donor pool, as it allows the heart to be functionally assessed *inside* the donor before acceptance.
- Reduced "Stunned" Myocardium: Warm reperfusion allows the heart to recover ATP stores before being subjected to the second "hit" of cold storage and transport.

Abdominal NRP

Abdominal Normothermic Regional Perfusion (A-NRP) is broadly defined by isolating and perfusing only the abdominal cavity, the technique varies significantly based on cannulation location, aortic occlusion methods, and timing.

1. *By Cannulation Access Route*
   - *Peripheral (Femoral) A-NRP*: The ECMO catheters are inserted directly into the *femoral artery* and *femoral vein* through a groin incision. This allows rapid initiation of perfusion, minimizing postmortem warm ischemia time (Fig. 5.7).
   - *Central (Open) A-NRP*: Performed by directly opening the abdomen and cannulating the *infrarenal aorta* and *inferior vena cava (IVC)*. This technique is often used if peripheral vessels are atherosclerotic or inaccessible (Fig. 5.8).
2. *By Aortic Occlusion Mechanism (Isolating Cerebral Flow)*

   Ethical protocols dictate that blood must never flow back up to the brain after death declaration. This segregation splits A-NRP into two technique categories:
   - *Endovascular Balloon Occlusion*: An *intra-aortic balloon catheter* (often a Fogarty or EBOA balloon) is threaded up from the femoral artery and inflated in the descending thoracic aorta before starting the perfusion machine.
   - *Surgical Clamping*: Surgeons perform a rapid laparotomy or thoracotomy to place a physical *vascular clamp directly on the supraceliac aorta*.

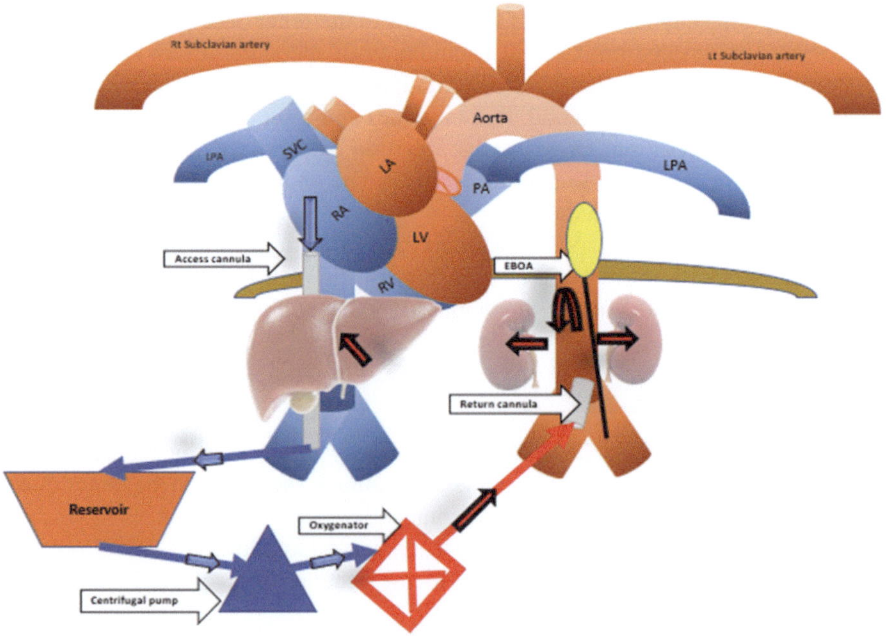

Fig. 5.7 Peripheral Veno-arterial ECMO with EBOA for NRP in ICU

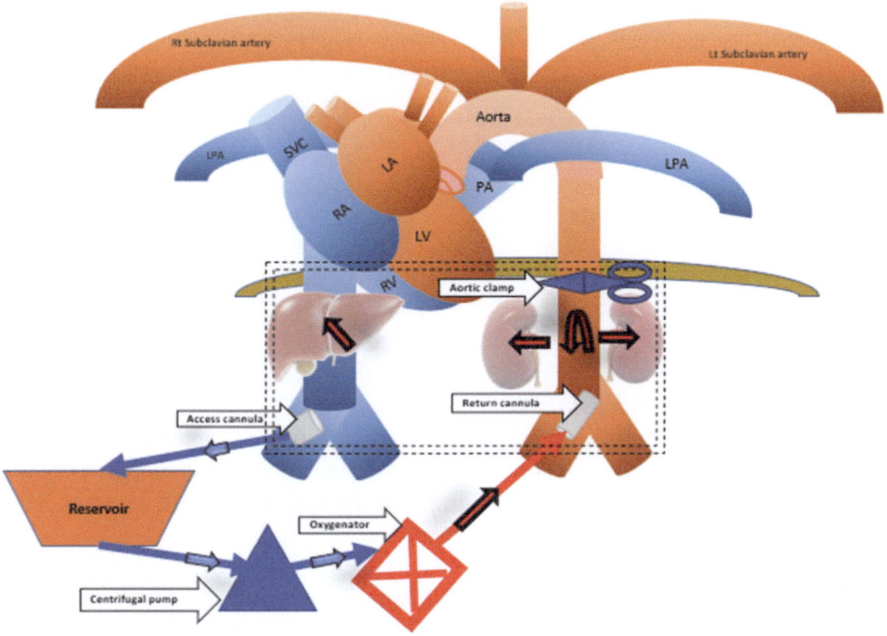

Fig. 5.8 Veno-arterial direct cannulation through laparotomy and direct clamping of abdominal aorta for abdominal NRP in OT

3. *By Cannulation Timing*
   - *Antemortem Cannulation (AMC)*: Cannulas are surgically placed in the donor's femoral vessels *before* the withdrawal of life-sustaining treatment (WLST). The circuit remains off until death is officially declared. This eliminates procedural delays, yielding the lowest possible warm ischemia times.
   - *Postmortem Cannulation (PMC)*: Vascular access and cannulation are strictly initiated *after* the donor's heart stops and the legally mandated "no-touch" waiting period ends.

Technical Direct Comparison (Table 5.5)

- *DCD and NRP Evidences Internationally*— [15, 16]
- International evidence indicates that controlled Normothermic Regional Perfusion (cNRP) and thoracoabdominal NRP (TA-NRP) in DCD donors yield liver and kidney graft outcomes comparable to DBD, with TA-NRP showing particularly high liver utilization. While early uncontrolled studies noted higher biliary complications, recent data confirms reduced graft loss and high 1-year survival rates for both liver and kidney transplants. Shapey et al. [15]: This systematic review published in Liver Transplantation analyzed early regional perfusion data (1997–2013). It found that while 1-year graft survival in uncontrolled DCD (uDCD) livers was initially lower than in DBD, patient survival remained

Table 5.5 Abdominal Normothermic Regional Perfusion (A-NRP) based on cannulation location, aortic occlusion methods, and timing

Feature variant	Peripheral access	Central access
Primary vessel used	Femoral Artery & Vein	Abdominal Aorta & IVC
Incision site	Groin area	Open midline abdomen
Speed to initiate	*Faster* if smaller conduit lines in place (Can begin immediately after death declaration)	*Slower* (Requires full surgical dissection first). Faster if patient ready on the OT table at time of WSLT

similar. It also noted that regional perfusion significantly reduced *delayed graft function (DGF)* in kidneys.

- Pelletier et al. [17]: Research from this team, often cited in summaries of controlled DCD (cDCD) outcomes, demonstrated that NRP-supported grafts achieved *91% 1-year patient and graft survival*, a risk profile comparable to DBD and superior to standard DCD methods.
- Bekki et al. [16]: Published in Transplantation Direct, this study used US registry data (2020–2021) to show that *TA-NRP* significantly increased liver utilization (70.6% vs. 39.0% in non-NRP-DCD) with excellent 1-year graft survival rates (91.3%).
- Schurink et al. (2023): A large-scale analysis of 1220 cDCD-NRP cases found a *1-year graft survival of 91%* and a remarkably low rate of *primary non-function (PNF)* at 3%.
- *Hessheimer et al./Spanish Protocols*: References to the established Spanish experience highlight that mandatory ligation and venting during TA-NRP effectively preclude brain perfusion, maintaining ethical standards while yielding outcomes similar to DBD.

In a systematic review on regional perfusion using ECMO for abdominal organ retrieval, Shapey et al. found raw data for RP-DCD liver transplantation. In all 3 uncontrolled RP-DCD studies, the rates of 1-year graft survival were lower than the rates with DBDs. However, no statistically significant difference was demonstrated for 1-year patient survival. Biliary complications were higher with NRP-DCD grafts, but the rates of operative mortality and HAT were similar for the RP-DCD and DBD groups in all these studies. Pelletier et al., in the only study of controlled Normothermic Regional Perfusion-supported donors after circulatory death (NRP-DCDs), reported a rate of 91% for 1-year patient and graft survival (10/11), and this resulted in a risk of graft loss comparable to that with DBDs and better than that with standard DCDs. For Kidneys, the 1-year patient and graft survival rates were better with RP-DCDs versus standard DCDs, and they were comparable to, if not better than, the rates with DBDs of all ages. Most studies reported PNF rates of 0%, with the remainder reporting rates comparable to those for DBDs older than 60 years [12].

In a more recent review Bekki et al. [13] showed that although the utilization rates of kidney and pancreas were comparable; that of liver in DCD with TA-NRP was significantly higher. Among 24 liver transplantations, 62 kidney transplantations, and 3 pancreas transplantations from DCD with TA-NRP, there were just 2 liver grafts and 1 kidney graft that failed within 1 year after transplantation.

The landscape of Donation after Circulatory Death (DCD) in India is currently at pivotal crossroads, shifting from established uncontrolled protocols to the emerging potential of controlled and perfusion-supported models.

The Status of DCD in India

- Legal Framework: DCD is legally recognized in India. The Indian Society of Critical Care Medicine (ISCCM) has recently published a position paper outlining the ethical and legal pathways, integrating organ donation into End-of-Life Care (EOLC) standards.
- Current Practice: Unlike Western nations, Maastricht Category III (Controlled DCD) is not yet standard practice in India. This is largely due to legal complexities and a lack of uniform guidelines regarding the Withdrawal of Life-Sustaining Treatment (WLST).
- Maastricht Categories in India: Current documented cases are predominantly Types II, IV, and V (Uncontrolled DCD). Consequently, kidney transplantation remains the primary successful outcome, as other organs are more sensitive to the warm ischemia common in uncontrolled scenarios.

In a recent position paper in the Indian Journal of Transplantation, a detailed account of implementing Normothermic Regional Perfusion (NRP), and discussion points have been addressed such as ethics of administration of Heparin and the timing of cannulation. The logistics of "Short Notice": Uncontrolled DCD (uDCD) requires a highly mobile and rapid-response team. Successful NRP in these cases requires 24/7 availability of skilled manpower: ECMO specialists and transplant surgeons ready for immediate deployment. On-hand stocks of expensive oxygenators, cannulae, and EBOA balloons must be available.

Financial Viability: The cost of NRP consumables and specialized labor is significant. Policies must be developed to determine how these costs are absorbed—whether by the transplant recipient, the hospital, or state-funded programs—to ensure equitable access.

Policy Recommendations for Indian Hospitals

To bridge the gap between current practice and the potential of *Controlled DCD (cDCD)* and *NRP*, the following institutional policies are recommended: [3, 4].

- *Establish "Conflict of Interest" Firewalls*: Protocols must strictly ensure that the treating intensive care team and the transplant team are separate. The team deciding on the futility of care must not be involved in the organ retrieval process.

- *Standardize WLST Procedures*: Hospitals should adopt clear internal guidelines for the *Withdrawal of Life-Sustaining Treatment* in line with the supreme court's simplified 2023 pathway for cDCD Category III.
- *Implement Integrated EOLC Pathways*: Organ donation should be presented as a standard option within the End-of-Life Care (EOLC) menu for terminal patients, ensuring families are counseled early but independently of the clinical prognosis.
- *NRP Readiness and Training*: Invest in the specialized consumables (e.g., EBOA balloons, high-flow oxygenators) and manpower training for *Normothermic Regional Perfusion* to move beyond kidney-only donation to include liver and thoracic organs.
- *NOTTO Registration*: Every hospital with an ICU should register as an organ retrieval center (ORC) with the National Organ and Tissue Transplant Organization to streamline logistics.

Conclusion: The Future of NRP-DCD in India

Normothermic Regional Perfusion (NRP) represents a paradigm shift in the management of Donation after Circulatory Death (DCD), offering a viable solution to India's chronic organ shortage. By transforming the "warm ischemia" period from a phase of inevitable damage into a window for active resuscitation and functional assessment, NRP-DCD has the potential to move India beyond the current "kidney-only" model toward a robust multi-organ recovery system.

The transition from uncontrolled (uDCD) to Controlled DCD (Maastricht Category III) is essential. This requires the integration of NRP into standard End-of-Life Care (EOLC) pathways, supported by the legal frameworks established by the ISCCM and the Supreme Court's guidelines on the withdrawal of life support.

The successful adoption of NRP in India hinges on investing in specialized ECMO hardware, REBOA technology, and the necessary consumables; training multidisciplinary "NRP Teams" capable of high-stakes coordination between the ICU, perfusion, and surgical departments and adopting serial lactate and enzyme monitoring as the gold standard for verifying organ viability in real-time.

While ethical debates regarding pre-mortem heparinization and the "dead donor rule" continue, the clinical evidence is undeniable: NRP-DCD yields graft survival rates comparable to those of brain-dead donors. For India, refining these methods is not merely a technical advancement but an ethical imperative to maximize the "gift of life" and honor the altruism of donor families.

Competing Interests The author(s) has no competing interests to declare that are relevant to the content of this manuscript.

Ethics Approval The author(s) declares that this manuscript does not include primary research with human participants.

The author(s) declares that this manuscript does not include primary studies involving animals.

References

1. Kootstra G, Daemen JH, Oomen AP. Categories of non-heart-beating donors. Transplant Proc. 1995;27(5):2893–4. PMID: 7482956.
2. Wind J, Faut M, van Smaalen TC, van Heurn EL. Variability in protocols on donation after circulatory death in Europe. Crit Care. 2013;17(5):R217. https://doi.org/10.1186/cc13034. PMID: 24090229; PMCID: PMC4057469.
3. Seth AK, Mohanka R, Navin S, Gokhale AGK, Sharma A, Kumar A, et al. Organ donation after circulatory determination of death in India: a joint position paper. Indian J Crit Care Med. 2022;26(4):423–40.
4. Seth AK, Mohanka R, Mani RK, Asthana S, Attawar S, Dhital KK, Gupta D, Gursahani R, Hote M, Kumar A, Kumar K, Kute VB, Mathur SK, Mehta D, Mirza DF, Modi P, Pandit RA, Sharma A, Shroff S. Organ donation after circulatory determination of death – consensus statement. Indian J Transplantat. 2024;18(3):247–56. https://doi.org/10.4103/ijot.ijot_37_24.
5. https://www.elso.org/registry.aspx
6. Soar J, Böttiger BW, Carli P, Couper K, Deakin CD, Djärv T, Lott C, Olasveengen T, Paal P, Pellis T, Perkins GD, Sandroni C, Nolan JP. European Resuscitation Council guidelines 2021: adult advanced life support, resuscitation. (n.d.). Available at: https://pubmed.ncbi.nlm.nih.gov/33773825/?dopt=Abstract. Accessed 27 June 2024.
7. Bronchard R, et al. Brain-dead donors on extracorporeal membrane oxygenation*. Crit Care Med. 2017;45(10):1734–41. https://doi.org/10.1097/ccm.0000000000002564.
8. Sady ERR, Junqueira L, Veiga VC, Rojas SSO. Apnea test for brain death diagnosis in adults on extracorporeal membrane oxygenation: a review. Rev Bras Ter Intensiva. 2020;32(2):312–8. https://doi.org/10.5935/0103-507x.20200048. Epub 2020 Jul 13. PMID: 32667442; PMCID: PMC7405745.
9. Kreitler KJ. et al. Declaring brain death on ECMO." Jefferson Digital Commons 2 May 2015. jdc.jefferson.edu/jhnj/vol12/iss1/7.
10. Greer DM, Shemie SD, Lewis A, et al. Determination of brain death/death by neurologic criteria: the world brain death project. JAMA. 2020;324(11):1078–97. https://doi.org/10.1001/jama.2020.11586.
11. Lequier L, Horton SB, McMullan DM, Bartlett RH. Extracorporeal membrane oxygenation circuitry. Pediatr Crit Care Med. 2013;14(5 Suppl 1):S7–12. https://doi.org/10.1097/PCC.0b013e318292dd10. PMID: 23735989; PMCID: PMC3742331.
12. Ranucci M, et al. Goal Directed Perfusion to reduce acute kidney injury: a randomized trial. J Thorac Cardiovasc Surg. 2018;156(5):1918–1927.e2.
13. Oniscu GC. Thoracoabdominal normothermic regional perfusion—it is not all about the heart. JAMA Netw Open. 2025;8(2):e2460039. https://doi.org/10.1001/jamanetworkopen.2024.60039.
14. Tanaka S, Umeda M, Ujike H, Ryuko T, Tomioka Y, Miyoshi K, Okazaki M, Sugimoto S, Toyooka S. Novel pulmonary abdominal normothermic regional perfusion circuit for simultaneous in-donor evaluation and preservation of lungs and abdominal organs in donation after circulatory death. Gen Thorac Cardiovasc Surg. 2025;73(9):700–8. https://doi.org/10.1007/s11748-025-02137-y. Epub 2025 Mar 16. PMID: 40089938; PMCID: PMC12378916.
15. Shapey IM, Muiesan P. Regional perfusion by extracorporeal membrane oxygenation of abdominal organs from donors after circulatory death: a systematic review. Liver Transpl. 2013;19(12):1292–303. https://doi.org/10.1002/lt.23771.
16. Bekki Y, Croome KP, Myers B, Sasaki K, Tomiyama K. Normothermic regional perfusion can improve both utilization and outcomes in DCD liver, kidney, and pancreas transplantation. Transplant Direct. 2023;9(3):e1450. https://doi.org/10.1097/TXD.0000000000001450. PMID: 36845854; PMCID: PMC9945290.
17. Pelletier SJ, Maraschio MA, Kingston H, et al. Donation after cardiac death as a strategy to increase deceased donor liver availability. Annals of Surgery. 2006;244(4):555–562. https://doi.org/10.1097/01.sla.0000239002.04603.

Machine Perfusion in DCD: Global Practices and Implications for Emerging Healthcare Systems

6

Devprakash Choudhary and Jasmine Sethi

Abbreviations

A-NRP	Abdominal Normothermic Regional Perfusion
D-HOPE	Dual Hypothermic Oxygenated Perfusion
DCD	Donation after Circulatory Death
DGF	Delayed Graft Function
EAD	Early Allograft Dysfunction
EVLP	Ex-Vivo Lung Perfusion
FMN	Flavin Mononucleotide
FWIT	Functional Warm Ischaemia Time
HMP	Hypothermic Machine Perfusion
HOPE	Hypothermic Oxygenated Perfusion
IFLT	Ischaemia-Free Liver Transplantation
IRI	Ischaemia-Reperfusion Injury
NAS	Non-anastomotic Strictures
NMP	Normothermic Machine Perfusion
NRP	Normothermic Regional Perfusion
SCS	Static Cold Storage

D. Choudhary (✉)
Department of Renal Transplant Surgery, PGIMER Chandigarh, Chandigarh, India

J. Sethi
PGIMER Chandigarh, Chandigarh, India

S. P. Kolte et al. (eds.), *Organ Donation After Circulatory Death*,
https://doi.org/10.1007/978-981-92-6377-6_6

The Decision That Changes Everything

'The kidneys appeared far from ideal, swollen, faintly mottled, and bearing the burden of more than sixty minutes of warm ischemia, compounded by stage III acute kidney injury in the donor. Under conventional criteria, these kidneys would likely have been discarded. Instead, they were placed on normothermic machine perfusion, where they received what they needed the most: warmth, oxygen, nutrients, and restored blood circulation. After six hours on the machine, renal blood flow had improved, urine was draining steadily, and kidneys once destined for waste were on their way to saving two lives'.

Case notes, Department of Renal Transplant Surgery, PGIMER, Chandigarh

There is a moment in every donation after circulatory determination of death (DCD) retrieval when a surgeon, often in the quiet hours of midnight, must decide whether an organ injured by warm ischaemia can still be rescued. For decades, that decision depended on the surgeon's eyes, hands and hard-earned intuition, refined over years at the operating table. The stakes could not have been higher: to accept the organs was to risk failure, and to decline them was to abandon the possibility of saving lives.

Machine perfusion has made that decision more hopeful by making it more informed and more objective. For the first time, the organ is no longer judged merely as a static object on ice, but observed as a living system in recovery. The surgeon can watch organ blood flow improve, vascular resistance fall, lactate clear, urine begin to drain, bile appear, enzymes stabilise and biomarkers emerge from the perfusate. The question is no longer simply, 'How damaged is this organ'? but something far more critical: 'Is it viable, and is the organ getting better on the machine'?

That shift from static preservation to dynamic assessment, from irreversible judgement to measurable recovery marks one of the most profound advances in the history of solid organ Transplantation.

The Organ Famine—A Public Health Emergency

The unmet need in solid organ transplantation extends far beyond statistics. In 2024, 173,727 solid organ transplants were performed worldwide, yet this represented less than 10% of the global need [1]. In India, the incidence of ESRD is estimated at 150–230 per million population, translating to approximately 200,000–300,000 new patients each year, while fewer than 5% receive a kidney transplant; the remaining die waiting for a kidney transplant on dialysis [2]. In the United States, more than 100,000 patients remain on the waiting list, and 17 die each day while waiting for a transplant [3]. These figures do not describe a niche medical problem but reflect a daily accumulation of preventable deaths and a structural public health emergency across the globe.

For decades, deceased organ donation has relied on a narrow biological window: the haemodynamically stable brain-dead donor whose organs remain oxygenated until retrieval. However, brain death accounts for only a small fraction of hospital deaths. Donation after circulatory determination of death (DCD) opens access to a much larger donor pool, including patients who die after failed resuscitation, withdrawal of life-sustaining treatment, or severe illness without meeting the standard neurological criteria for death. By transforming this previously underutilised donor pool into a viable source of grafts, DCD offers a critical pathway to expand access to transplantation to millions of people.

The impact of DCD is already evident. In the United Kingdom, it now accounts for more than 40% of deceased donor kidney transplants annually [4]. The Netherlands has sustained DCD kidney programmes since the 1980s, while Spain has demonstrated the feasibility of uncontrolled DCD when normothermic regional perfusion is deployed rapidly [5]. Despite this progress, DCD remains underused globally, with fewer than 25 countries reporting meaningful programme data to the Global Observatory on Donation and Transplantation [1].

With appropriate selection and preservation, long-term graft and patient survival after DCD kidney transplantation are comparable to DBD outcomes [6]. However, wider adoption of DCD remains limited by legal, logistical and biological barriers. Many systems lack clear frameworks for withdrawing life-sustaining treatment before donation, or the infrastructure needed for rapid retrieval. Even when these barriers are overcome, the central biological challenge remains warm ischaemia time, the cellular injury that begins when circulation stops.

This is where machine perfusion becomes transformative. Even in the mature UK system, the 2024/25 NHS Blood and Transplant report showed that 29.2% of retrieved DCD livers and 87.6% of offered DCD pancreases were not transplanted [4]. That's where the machine perfusion era transforms the central question of DCD from 'Should we discard this organ'? to 'Can we recover it enough to save a life?

The Biology of Warm Ischaemia—What Happens When the Heart Stops

To understand why machine perfusion works, we must first understand what warm ischaemia does to an organ and why cold storage is only a partial answer. When blood circulation stops, cellular injury begins almost immediately. ATP stores are rapidly depleted through anaerobic metabolism. Without ATP, cellular sodium-potassium pumps fail, calcium accumulates intracellularly and cells begin to swell [7]. Organ-specific vulnerability follows directly from this biology.

In the kidneys, this warm-ischaemic injury most often presents as delayed graft function (DGF) or primary non-function (PNF), reflecting tubular dysfunction and the need for post-transplant dialysis [8]. In livers, it appears as early allograft dysfunction, hepatocellular necrosis and, most characteristically, in DCD grafts as ischaemic cholangiopathy [9]. Hearts may develop primary graft dysfunction from myocardial stunning or microvascular injury, while lungs develop pulmonary graft dysfunction and oedema due to alveolar-capillary permeability changes [10, 11]. Each organ therefore carries a distinct DCD injury signature, which shapes both the clinical consequences of warm ischaemia and the preservation strategy required to mitigate it.

At the mitochondrial level, warm-ischaemic injury becomes even more precise. Complex I of the inner mitochondrial membrane, the first enzyme of the respiratory chain, is particularly vulnerable. During warm ischaemia, structural damage to Complex I leads to the release of its prosthetic group, flavin mononucleotide (FMN), into the perfusate. Over the past decade, FMN has emerged as one of the most specific biomarkers of ischaemic mitochondrial injury in transplantation, with its kinetics during machine perfusion predicting post-transplant biliary outcomes more accurately than conventional blood tests (9, 12). When circulation is restored in the recipient, these injured mitochondria may generate reactive oxygen species rather than produce efficient ATP. Neutrophils infiltrate, complement is activated, and the microcirculation becomes disrupted. This is ischaemia-reperfusion injury (IRI): an intrinsic feature of solid organ transplantation, and it is amplified in organs exposed to prolonged warm ischaemia time before preservation, like in DCD [7, 13].

Cold storage addresses this injury cascade in only one dimension: it slows the cellular engine. At 4 °C, metabolism falls sharply, decelerating injury but not reversing it. Waste products remain trapped within the cell, mitochondria remain primed to generate reactive oxygen species, and, crucially, there is no way to know whether the organ on ice is recovering or deteriorating. The organ is preserved, but so is the clinician's uncertainty until the moment of organ reperfusion.

Machine perfusion intervenes dynamically. At its simplest, circulating perfusate removes the metabolic waste that accumulates during static ice-cold storage. More importantly, normothermic perfusion restores near-physiological conditions, allowing cellular metabolism, mitochondrial recovery via vascular perfusion, urine or bile production and lactate clearance to be assessed in real time. The question is no longer merely whether the organ has survived preservation, but whether it is actively recovering.

The Maastricht Classification—A Taxonomy of Death and Its Clinical Significance

Not all DCD donors present the same clinical challenge. Therefore, preservation must be tailored to the circumstances of death. The revised Maastricht classification provides the operational framework, linking donor category to warm ischaemia exposure, retrieval logistics and the choice of perfusion strategy [14].

Categories I and II represent uncontrolled DCD. Category I refers to patients dead on arrival after out-of-hospital cardiac arrest without attempted resuscitation. Category II includes patients in whom cardiopulmonary resuscitation (CPR) has been attempted but is unsuccessful. In both, warm ischaemia is prolonged, unpredictable and often exceeds conventional organ-specific thresholds. Spain's pioneering uncontrolled DCD Programme was built largely around Category II donors, using mechanical CPR and rapid ECMO deployment to enable organ recovery [5]. Cat II also includes unexpected in-hospital cardiac arrest and, in some jurisdictions, donation following medically assisted dying (MAID) [15].

Category III refers to controlled DCD after planned withdrawal of life-sustaining therapy in the ICU. This is the dominant DCD pathway in the UK, the Netherlands, Belgium, Australia and, increasingly, the United States. Because the retrieval team is present and the agonal phase is monitored, functional warm ischaemia can be measured and often remains within acceptable limits.
Category IV describes cardiac arrest in a brain-dead donor during assessment or retrieval.

The key operational variable is functional warm ischaemia time (FWIT), commonly defined as the time from the point at which systolic blood pressure falls below 50 mmHg or oxygen saturation falls below 70% until the onset of cold perfusion. It is one of the strongest determinants of DCD organ quality. Most liver programmes use an upper FWIT threshold of approximately 30–45 min, whereas kidneys tolerate longer intervals (30–60 min), although risk increases with prolonged warm ischaemia [4, 14, 16].

Machine perfusion strategies follow this taxonomy. In controlled DCD with acceptable FWIT, end-ischemic hypothermic machine perfusion is established for kidneys and hypothermic oxygenated perfusion is increasingly used for livers [17]. In uncontrolled DCD, especially Categories I and II, in situ normothermic regional perfusion may be decisive. By restoring oxygenated circulation before retrieval, NRP limits ongoing warm-ischaemic injury and can convert otherwise unusable organs into clinically viable grafts [5].

The Machine Perfusion Arsenal—Modalities, Mechanisms and Devices

Machine perfusion is not a single technology but a family of approaches, differentiated primarily by temperature, oxygenation and whether perfusion occurs in situ (in the donor) or ex situ (in the retrieved organ). Understanding these differences is essential to interpreting the evidence base, selecting the right modality and planning implementation.

Static Cold Storage (SCS)—The Baseline Static cold storage remains the global reference standard because it is simple, inexpensive and available worldwide. An organ is flushed with cold preservation solution (typically University of Wisconsin, Custodial, or IGL-1), packed in ice and transported. It works by slowing metabolism, nothing more. Every machine perfusion modality earns its place by demonstrating improvement over this baseline in clinical outcomes, in discard rates, in health economics, or in the quality of the decision it enables [8, 10, 18, 19].

Hypothermic Machine Perfusion ***(HMP)*** Cold, pumped, non-oxygenated Hypothermic Machine Perfusion (HMP) is the oldest and most extensively validated of the dynamic preservation strategies. Where cold storage allows metabolic waste to accumulate around a static organ, HMP continuously washes those waste products away: lactate, adenosine and free radicals that prime the IRI response [20]. A second benefit is mechanical: pulsatile flow maintains microvascular patency, reducing the increased resistance associated with cellular swelling [8].

For kidneys, the original COMPARE RCT and 2024 Cochrane systematic review with twenty-two studies, 4007 participants, concluded with high certainty that HMP reduces DGF by roughly a fifth and improves graft survival compared to SCS [8, 20]. Belgium's national kidney HMP service translated that evidence into a health-system reality: DCD kidney volume doubled within a year of national roll-out, DGF rate reached 14.4% overall, and the projected saving in dialysis costs was €3.59 million per year [21]. Its cost-effectiveness has been demonstrated in several European healthcare systems, as well as in Brazil's public health system [8, 22].

Hypothermic Oxygenated Perfusion ***(HOPE)*** and its dual-vessel variant, D-HOPE, do something subtler and more ambitious: they allow injured mitochondria to recover. At four to twelve degrees Celsius, mitochondria remain metabolically active at a reduced rate. Supplying oxygen via the cold perfusate allows the respiratory chain to process its damaged components gradually, reducing the pool of primed complex I that would otherwise generate reactive oxygen species upon reperfusion [12]. A multicentre study from 10 centres confirmed that FMN kinetics during HOPE predict graft loss, biliary strictures and post-transplant kidney failure at the recipient level, enabling cross-centre use [23, 24]. In practical terms, HOPE allows clinicians to assess an organ's mitochondrial status within the first hour in a quantified and reproducible manner, something static cold storage never permitted [24].

In the DHOPE-DCD randomised trial of 160 patients, end-ischaemic D-HOPE reduced non-anastomotic biliary strictures at 6 months from 18% to 6%, while also lowering post-reperfusion syndrome and early allograft dysfunction [9]. Post-reperfusion syndrome fell from 27% to 12%, and early allograft dysfunction (EAD) from 40% to 26%. The five-year follow-up findings confirmed that these gains were durable: biliary stricture rates at 5 years were 14% versus 26%, and immune-mediated biliary complications, a measure of chronic bile duct injury, were zero in the HOPE group versus 32% in the SCS arm [18]. A separate multicentric randomised trial in extended-criteria DBD livers reached similar conclusions: HOPE reduced major liver-related complications 3.7-fold per patient and eliminated graft failures attributable to liver-specific causes [25].

The health-economic picture further strengthens the case. Embedded within the DHOPE-DCD trial, a full cost-effectiveness analysis found that D-HOPE saved an average of €15,427 per patient at 1 year, driven primarily by 28.4% lower intensive care costs [26]. For centres planning implementation, the lesson is direct: continuous HMP is ready for national service adoption and should not require further justification in policy frameworks. Oxygenation adds value in older and controlled DCD donors. The cost-effectiveness analysis embedded within DHOPE-DCD demonstrated a mean 12-month saving of €15,427 per patient (€110,794 vs €126,221), driven primarily by 28.4% lower ICU costs, with D-HOPE cost-effective from a single procedure in basic scenarios and from approximately 25 procedures per year when staffing and equipment depreciation are included [26].

One practical innovation deserves special mention here: the DHOPE-PRO study demonstrated that prolonged D-HOPE can be used as an overnight holding strategy; organs retrieved at night are preserved on oxygenated perfusion until morning, then transplanted in scheduled daytime sessions [27]. For centres without round-the-clock theatre capacity, this changes the logistics of DCD liver transplantation entirely.

Normothermic Regional Perfusion ***(NRP)*** takes a conceptually different approach. Rather than placing a retrieved organ on a machine, NRP uses an ECMO circuit to restore warm, oxygenated blood flow through the donor's own vasculature while the donor remains on the table, after the mandatory no-touch period following cardiac arrest. The surgeon can watch the organ change colour as it reperfuses, observe bile appearing in the gallbladder, and see the gut perfuse. The assessment is visual, immediate and happening in the organ's natural environment [28]. NRP works by re-establishing oxygenated perfusion and nutrient delivery after circulatory arrest, thereby attenuating warm-ischaemic injury before the onset of cold preservation. Conceptually, it shifts the DCD organ towards a more DBD-like physiological state.

This approach has produced some of the most compelling outcome data in DCD transplantation. Spain's national Programme demonstrated that abdominal NRP in controlled DCD significantly reduced biliary complications, ischaemic cholangiopathy and graft loss compared to super-rapid recovery [5]. The organisational achievements underpinning this programme, dedicated retrieval teams, 24/7 ECMO deployment, integration with emergency services, and the national ONT coordinating structure are at least as important as the technology itself. When abdominal NRP is followed by ex situ normothermic machine perfusion (NMP), the results are remarkable: zero cases of ischaemic cholangiopathy in the combined NRP-plus-NMP group versus 16.8% in those managed with SCS alone [29]. The combination appears synergistic: NRP enables in situ recovery before retrieval by mitigating warm-ischaemic injury, while NMP provides a platform for ex situ assessment and further reconditioning by limiting the consequences of cold ischaemia before implantation.

Thoracoabdominal NRP, which extends the perfusion circuit to include the thoracic organs, has made DCD heart and lung transplantation technically feasible at scale. It requires one additional safeguard: the cerebral circulation must be explicitly excluded via intra-aortic balloon and arch vessel management to satisfy the requirements of death determination [28]. A French study confirmed that with proper exclusion, transcranial Doppler monitoring shows no cerebral blood flow or electrical activity during TA-NRP [30, 59].

The American College of Physicians issued a position in 2021 calling for a pause on this practice pending further ethical clarification. The transplant community has responded substantively, and practice continues under national protocol frameworks in the UK, Spain, Italy, Belgium and France [30, 31].

Normothermic Machine Perfusion (NMP)—NMP is the most demanding of the current perfusion strategies, requiring a retrieved organ to be maintained for hours at physiological temperature on an oxygenated, blood-based perfusate, essentially keeping the organ alive and functioning outside the body. It is also the strategy with the most transformative clinical impact, for one reason above all others: it allows the clinician to watch the organ function before deciding whether to transplant it.

The two leading NMP platforms are the OrganOx metra (for livers; FDA-approved 2021) and the Organ Care System (OCS, TransMedics; FDA-approved for liver, heart and lung) [32–34]. The PILOT trial was the first randomised controlled trial of NMP in liver transplantation. In the SCS control, NMP halved peak transaminase levels, reduced discard rates from 25% to 11% and extended preservation time by 50% [36]. The PROTECT trial used the OCS Liver and demonstrated: EAD 18% vs 31%; 12-month ischaemic biliary complications 1.7% vs 8.5%; and DCD liver transplantation in 51% of the NMP arm versus 26% in SCS controls [19]. This expansion of the donor pool is not merely a consequence of preserving organs already destined for transplantation. It reflects the active recovery and rehabilitation of organs that would otherwise have been discarded. This is the central promise of NMP.

The VITTAL study addressed the livers formally declined by all UK centres [35]. After NMP, 22 of 31 (71%) met composite viability criteria (lactate clearance to ≤2.5 mmol/L within 4 h, plus biliary and metabolic criteria) and were transplanted. Ninety-day survival was 100%. This ‘rescue’ capacity for previously discarded organs is uniquely enabled by NMP and has no equivalent in any other preservation strategies. The ‘reconditioning effect’ during NMP is clinically important: organs that appear marginal at 60 min, with high lactate and limited bile flow, may recover substantially by 3–4 h. Premature discard decisions at 1 h are therefore potentially costly [35, 36].

The PILOT trial and PROTECT trial established NMP as the tool for pool expansion and logistics flexibility [19, 36]. The VITTAL study demonstrated NMP can rescue formally declined livers [35]. However, emerging U.S. real-world data show that the transition from trial success to routine clinical adoption is not seamless, with round-the-clock staffing and perfusate logistics becoming major operational bottlenecks [37]. The value of NMP lies especially in functional viability assessment and in enabling timed daytime transplantation.

Short-duration NMP in clinical kidney transplantation is supported by emerging clinical evidence, whereas prolonged perfusion remains an even earlier frontier [38–40]. The Oxford NKP1 phase I trial demonstrated the feasibility of 24-h ex situ kidney NMP, opening the possibility of scheduled daytime implantation and creating a platform for organ assessment, optimisation and therapeutic intervention before transplantation [41] (Table 6.1).

Table 6.1 Key machine perfusion platforms and clinical evidence by organ—what we know and how well we know it

Device/platform	Modality, regulatory status, key trial	Pivotal evidence and key outcome/finding	Evidence grade
Liver			
OrganOx metra	Liver · 35–37 °C NMP · FDA-approved 2021; PILOT trial (Nasralla 2018) [36]	Discard ↓50%; transplant pool +25%	**High**
OCS liver (TransMedics)	Liver · 37 °C NMP portable. FDA-approved 2021 (DCD indication) · PROTECT trial (Markmann 2022) [19]	EAD 18% vs 31%; organ discard rate reduced; DCD utilisation expanded	**High**
LifePort kidney transporter/ liver **assist**	Kidney, Liver · 4–12 °C HMP/HOPE · CE marked; EU clinical standard COMPARE [20]; DHOPE-DCD [9]	D-HOPE (DCD liver): NAS 6% vs 18% → 14% vs 26% at 5 yr.; cost-saving [12]. HOPE (DBD/ECD): Complications ↓3.7-fold; zero graft failures	**High**
NRP + NMP (sequential)	Liver · in situ NRP → ex situ NMP · emerging protocol · [29]	Ischemic cholangiopathy 0% vs 16.8% with SCS; DCD liver outcomes markedly improved	**Moderate**
Kidney			
LifePort kidney transporter	Kidney · 4–10 °C HMP portable · CE; FDA cleared; Belgium national standard [20, 21]	Cochrane 2024; DGF ↓20–25%; graft survival ↑; cost-saving vs SCS	**High**
Kidney assist transport (XVIVO)-HMP	Kidney · 4–12 °C oxygenated HMP · CE marked; EU clinical standard [42]	Fewer complications in DCD donors ≥50 years; eGFR difference NS overall	**Moderate**
(Research NMP platform)	Kidney · NMP 1 h end-ischemic [38] the first kidney NMP RCT	DGF 60.7% vs 58.5% (NS); NMP not superior to SCS (negative RCT)	**High (neg)**
(Research NMP platform)	Kidney · NMP NEXT-kidney study [39]	1–3 h of preimplantation NMP in DCD kidneys before implantation, DGF was lower than in contralateral cold-storage kidneys	**Low–mod**
Kidney assist (XVIVO)-NMP	Kidney · NMP, Stage III AKI donors PGIMER Chandigarh [40]	Feasibility of NMP in AKI kidneys and utilisation in resource-limited settings established	**Low–mod**
Heart			
OCS heart (TransMedics)	Heart · 37 °C NMP portable · FDA-approved 2021 [10]	6-month survival non-inferior to DBD heart transplant (94% vs 90%); enabled DCD heart utilisation accounts for more than 18% of US heart transplants by 2024	**High**

(continued)

Table 6.1 (continued)

Device/platform	Modality, regulatory status, key trial	Pivotal evidence and key outcome/finding	Evidence grade
TA-NRP (thoracoabdominal NRP)	Heart ·in situ NRP 37 °C · emerging technique [43]	1-yr survival 95.2% vs 90.1% (vs DPP); organ discard ↓; avoids ex situ perfusion cost approximately US$78,000 less per case than OCS-DPP	**Moderate**
Lung			
OCS lung (TransMedics)	Lung · 37 °C EVLP portable · FDA cleared (EXPAND trial) · INSPIRE trial [44, 45]	The EXPAND trial demonstrated 87% utilisation of extended-criteria lungs perfused with OCS lung, INSPIRE-non-inferiority to SCS for primary graft dysfunction grade 3 at 72 h; extended preservation time	**Moderate**
XPS + STEEN solution (XVIVO)	Lung · 37 °C EVLP · FDA cleared [11]	5-year survival comparable to non-EVLP lungs; transplant pool expanded with marginal donors	**Moderate**
TA-NRP	DCD lung transplantation using TA-NRP [46]	Confirming the feasibility of in situ lung perfusion before retrieval	**Low**
Pancreas			
NRP (multi-organ, in situ)	Pancreas · In situ NRP · Emerging technique (not a device) · UK registry; UNOS database [47, 48]	UK registry; UNOS Comparable graft survival for SPK transplantation; enables utilisation of higher-risk DCD pancreases	**Moderate**

Abbreviations: *NMP* normothermic machine perfusion, *HMP* hypothermic machine perfusion, *HOPE* hypothermic oxygenated perfusion, *O-HMP* oxygenated HMP, *EVLP* ex-vivo lung perfusion, *NRP* normothermic regional perfusion, *TA-NRP* thoracoabdominal NRP *DGF* delayed graft function, *EAD* early allograft dysfunction, *NAS* non-anastomotic biliary strictures, *eGFR* estimated glomerular filtration rate, *NS* not significant, *SPK* simultaneous pancreas-kidney, *AKI* acute kidney injury, *DBD* donation after brain death, *DCD* donation after circulatory death, *ECD* extended criteria donor, *SCS* static cold storage. Evidence grade: *HIGH* RCT or high-quality meta-analysis, *HIGH (neg)* high-quality RCT with negative result, *MODERATE* cohort/registry, *LOW–MOD* pilot/feasibility data only

Global Landscape—A Geography of Adoption

Machine perfusion adoption maps closely onto three factors: transplant system maturity, reimbursement and regulatory frameworks and organisational culture. The variation between and within countries is striking, and it is predominantly organisational rather than technological.

The Netherlands has the longest and most consistent record with HMP, dating to pioneering work by Rutger Ploeg in the 1980s. Dutch opt-out consent, centralised Euro transplant procurement and a culture of evidence-based practice created ideal conditions. HMP is universal for DCD kidneys, and D-HOPE for livers is increasingly routine. The Groningen and Leiden groups have shaped a remarkable proportion of the global kidney and liver machine perfusion literature to date.

United Kingdom—NHS Blood and Transplant established a national NMP Programme for livers, enabling the PILOT trial to run entirely within NHS infrastructure and to transition efficiently to routine practice [4]. DCD hearts using TA-NRP are now transplanted at Papworth, Royal Brompton and Newcastle. The UK's centralised structure, one procurement authority, standardised protocols and national auditing are the single most important factors enabling rapid, consistent adoption. UK discard rates for DCD livers remain high at 29.2% in 2024/25, suggesting that even in a leading system, realising the full potential of available technologies requires continued programmatic investment [4].

Spain's Organización Nacional de Trasplantes (ONT) model, repeatedly identified by the WHO as the gold standard for deceased donation coordination, has been exported to over 40 countries. Spain's unique contribution to machine perfusion is its uncontrolled DCD Programme. NRP across regional programmes demonstrates that organs from donors who died before reaching the hospital can produce transplantable results when logistical and technical infrastructure is properly designed [5]. The organisational achievement, including coordinated 24/7 ECMO deployment, is the primary innovation.

Belgium—Belgium's Eurotransplant membership and multi-institutional DCD experience have produced the most valuable economic evidence in kidney machine perfusion. The nationwide HMP analysis provided real-world proof that national HMP service roll-out is operationally feasible, clinically beneficial (DGF 14.4% overall; 9.5% in standard DCD; 19.6% in older DCD) and economically favourable (€3.59 million per year in dialysis savings) [21]. This single analysis is arguably the most policy-relevant evidence available to health ministries in middle-income countries considering HMP investment.

China—China's contribution to machine perfusion science comes primarily through the ischaemia-free liver transplantation (IFLT) Programme of the He Xiaoshun group at Sun Yat-sen University, which uses in-situ normothermic perfusion from procurement through back-table preparation and implantation, eliminating cold storage entirely, resulting in improved patient and graft survival when compared to conventional liver transplantation [49, 50]. New national regulations on organ donation and transplantation have strengthened donor consent and allocation standards, a prerequisite for Programme scale-up.

United States—The US landscape is fragmented: 56 organ procurement organisations, decentralised allocation, complex reimbursement and a regulatory pathway requiring FDA pre-market approval for perfusion devices have collectively slowed adoption relative to Europe. DCD kidneys represent approximately 20% of deceased donor kidneys compared to 40%+ in the UK [4, 51]. The OCS Liver received FDA approval in 2021, and multiple centres now have active NMP programmes. Since the 2021 DCD heart indication, economic modelling has suggested that NRP-based DCD heart transplantation may be approximately US$78,000 less expensive per case than OCS-DPP, a difference that could support broader adoption in cost-sensitive systems once regulatory and institutional barriers are resolved [52].

Japan faces structural barriers to DCD that go beyond technology. The legal framework for brain death determination was revised in 2009 but remains contentious, and DCD Programme development has been slow. A 2025 analysis identified cost, regulatory uncertainty and absence of consent frameworks as primary barriers. The first Japanese DCD heart transplant was attempted in 2024 [53]. Japan's well-developed living donor culture has reduced urgency around DCD, but demographic trends (ageing population, increasing ESRD) are driving renewed interest.

Brazil's most powerful contribution to evidence is economic analysis. A pharmacoeconomic Markov model projected that implementing HMP for expanded-criteria donor kidneys in Brazil's public SUS system would yield +1123 transplants, −815 patients on the waiting list and −120 deaths over 5 years, at a cost difference of US$4.49 million, cost-effective at accepted willingness-to-pay thresholds [22]. Brazil illustrates a broader principle: the political and budgetary case for machine perfusion in emerging systems should be built on dialysis avoidance and waiting-list outcomes, not on device cost alone.

PGIMER Chandigarh: Pioneering Machine Perfusion in South Asian Transplantation

Against the backdrop of high-income countries that have shaped most of the global evidence in machine perfusion, the experience of the Post Graduate Institute of Medical Education and Research (PGIMER) in Chandigarh occupies a special place in this chapter not for the scale of its cohort, but for what it demonstrates is achievable, and what it demands of the policy frameworks that surround it. It was a proof of concept for kidney transplantation across an entire continent.

In 2022, PGIMER reported Asia's first peer-reviewed clinical experience of ex-vivo NMP in kidney transplantation using the Kidney Assist device, with perfusion maintained for more than 2 h in AKI donor kidneys. This work was particularly significant because stage III AKI donor kidneys represent a high-risk graft category, with delayed graft function rates exceeding 75% and discard rates above 40%. In a country where deceased donor transplantation remains below one per million population, the near-routine abandonment of such organs is not only a clinical loss but also a public health failure [40]. The team hypothesised that NMP, by providing active metabolic support and enabling real-time viability assessment, could render these high-risk organs safely transplantable. A higher proportion of NMP kidneys demonstrated normal intrarenal resistive indices on Doppler ultrasound (0.5–0.7), while protocol biopsies showed milder acute tubular injury in the NMP group. Together, these findings provided functional and histological evidence that NMP was modifying ischaemia-reperfusion injury at the tissue level, rather than merely reflecting chance differences in donor quality.

The department is now conducting the SAFE-NMP trial—Safety Assessment for Extended Normothermic Machine Perfusion in Deceased Donor Kidney Transplantation: A Single-Centre Pilot Study, funded by The Transplantation

Society (TTS) Research Grant. At the time of writing, eight kidneys that would otherwise have been discarded have undergone prolonged ex-vivo NMP for 6–15.5 h and have been successfully transplanted, with publication in progress. This places PGIMER Chandigarh among the very few centres globally, after Oxford, to systematically explore prolonged NMP in clinical kidney transplantation.

The PGIMER experience demonstrates that NMP for high-risk donor kidneys is feasible even in a developing-country setting when supported by a committed multidisciplinary team. It provides a practical proof of concept that high-risk kidneys can be assessed, recovered and converted into clinically meaningful transplants rather than discarded (Fig. 6.1).

Lessons for the South Asian Region—Several aspects of the PGIMER experience are worth emphasising for institutions in South Asia and other emerging health systems considering machine perfusion adoption. The multidisciplinary team assembled at PGIMER, spanning renal transplant surgery, nephrology, pathology, immunopathology, biochemistry and anaesthesia, demonstrates that expertise can be built collaboratively within a single institution. The choice of high-risk donors as the focus was strategically correct: these are exactly the donors that a programme in a high-need, limited-resource setting should be trying hardest to use safely, and NMP is the tool best positioned to do so.

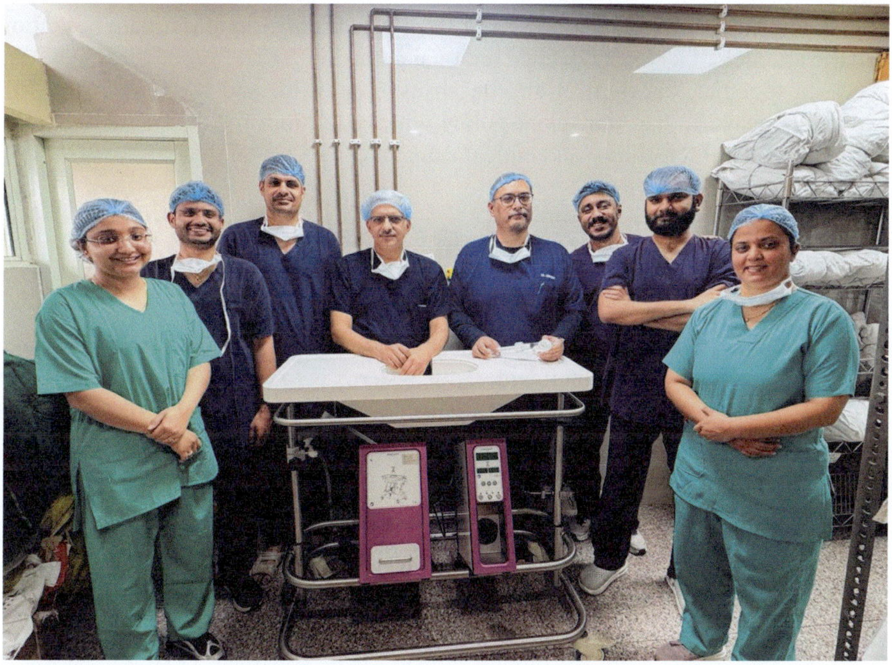

Fig. 6.1 Team of the department of renal transplant surgery at Postgraduate Institute of Medical Education and Research (PGIMER), Chandigarh, India

The Indian Policy and Regulatory Context

The clinical significance of the PGIMER work cannot be separated from the legislative and organisational context in which it was achieved. India's Transplantation of Human Organs Act (THOTA, 1994; amended 2011) does not explicitly provide for controlled DCD donation, nor does it define withdrawal of life-sustaining therapy as a precondition for organ donation. This legal ambiguity has constrained the development of DCD programmes nationally [54].

A joint position paper by the Indian Society of Critical Care Medicine, the Indian Society of Organ Transplantation and the Indian Network for Organ Sharing provides a comprehensive framework for DCD in India. It defines DCD categories I–V, specifies minimum no-touch intervals, supports the use of NRP and ex situ machine perfusion where available and outlines the necessary ethical safeguards. Importantly, this document represents the professional consensus on which future legislative reform can be built [54].

NOTTO's 2023–24 annual report documented continued growth in deceased donation, and 2025 data show India approaching 20,000 total organ transplants annually, quadruple the 2013 figure [55]. Yet India's deceased donor rate remains critically low, largely because donation after brain death continues to be the dominant pathway for organ donation. Despite the clear potential of DCD to expand the donor pool, this pathway remains severely underutilised in India, with only a few centres practising it consistently nationwide. This limited adoption reflects not a lack of clinical relevance, but persistent legal uncertainty, organisational hesitation and the absence of a clearly defined national pathway.

Taken together, the Seth et al. consensus framework and the PGIMER NMP experience leave Indian transplant policy with little room for delay: the scientific rationale, clinical feasibility and ethical safeguards are now in place.

Implications for Emerging Health Systems—Building A Programme Strategy, Economics, and Equity

The Correct Economic Frame—The most common error in the health-economic analysis of machine perfusion in emerging systems is to compare the device's cost to zero. The correct comparison is not perfusion versus no cost, but perfusion versus the full economic burden of organ discard and graft failure. In simplified terms:

> *Net value = (additional organs transplanted × mean QALYs gained per transplant × willingness-to-pay threshold per QALY) + avoided dialysis costs + avoided ICU costs from graft failure − programme fixed costs − variable perfusion costs.*

Under this whole-pathway model, kidney HMP and liver D-HOPE currently present the strongest health-economic case, with formal analyses demonstrating cost-saving or cost-effective outcomes in European and Latin American settings, as well as projected relevance to South Asian contexts [21, 22, 26]. The Belgian nationwide HMP data and the Brazilian pharmacoeconomic model are particularly relevant for health ministries in middle-income countries and should be cited in policy advocacy alongside clinical trial evidence [21, 22].

A Phased Implementation Roadmap Phase 1: *Organisational Foundation.* The first step is to establish or strengthen the organ procurement organisation or national coordinating body. This requires standardising donor identification, family approach, consent processes, retrieval logistics and reporting of deceased-donor activity. This organisational foundation is the non-negotiable prerequisite for any successful perfusion programme: Spain's success was built on the ONT model, not on technology alone.
Phase 2—Kidney HMP as Entry Point: The next step should be to implement a national or regional kidney HMP service, using the Belgian model as an operational template. Reimbursement must be structured at the procedure level to cover consumables, logistics and perfusion-related staffing. Training of dedicated perfusion teams should be developed in partnership with established European centres, allowing technical expertise, protocols and quality-assurance systems to be transferred safely into local practice [21].
Phase 3—HOPE at Regional Hubs: Controlled DCD programmes should next be developed at a small number of high-volume regional centres, supported by end-ischaemic HOPE. Lower-cost cold oxygenated perfusion platforms, such as VitaSmart and Kidney/Liver Assist, offer a feasible intermediate step with lower capital requirements than full NMP, while still providing mitochondrial protection and improved graft assessment in high-risk organs.
Phase 4—Selective NMP via Hub-and-Spoke: NMP should be introduced selectively through regional perfusion hubs rather than through device acquisition at every implanting centre. Because NMP requires round-the-clock support, reliable perfusate logistics and trained perfusionists, a hub-and-spoke model where one dedicated perfusion centre supports multiple retrieval and transplant hospitals is likely to be far more cost-effective in emerging systems. The PGIMER experience provides a practical South Asian template for this approach.
Phase 5—Regulatory and Reimbursement Reform: Sustainable expansion will require governance reform alongside technical adoption. This includes explicit legal frameworks for controlled DCD, pathway-level reimbursement that supports the entire donation-perfusion-transplant process rather than the device alone, and transparent adverse-event reporting systems to maintain public trust, clinical accountability and programme quality. (Table 6.2).

The Equity Imperative There is an uncomfortable truth at the heart of the global machine perfusion story: the technologies transforming transplant outcomes in Amsterdam, London and Cambridge remain, in their current commercial form, largely inaccessible to the populations with the greatest unmet need. A patient on dialysis in New Delhi has the same biological need as a patient on dialysis in Amsterdam, yet the technologies most capable of expanding access are being devel-

Table 6.2 Implementation tiers for machine perfusion in emerging health systems. Each tier requires both technology and governance infrastructure

Implementation tier	Entry modality	Prerequisites	Template/reference
Foundational	HMP	OPO/coordinator infrastructure; DCD legal framework; HMP devices (≤US$2-3K/case disposables); basic biochemistry	Belgium [21]; Netherlands; Brazil [22]
Intermediate	HOPE at hub	Moderate DCD volume; oxygen supply; outcome audit	DHOPE-DCD [9]; Endo 2025 [26]
Advanced	NMP; NRP	Round-the-clock perfusion teams; blood/Hb-carrier supply; logistics network; viability decision protocols	UK NHSBT NMP Programme [4]; Spain ONT [5], PGIMER [40]
Frontier	DCD heart; prolonged NMP	Full cardiac surgery + ECMO infrastructure; regulatory approval; cerebral exclusion validation; NRP legal framework	Schroder NEJM 2023 [10]; PGIMER [40]

oped, validated and manufactured far from the settings where the need is greatest. The WHO's 2024 World Health Assembly Resolution WHA77.4 explicitly calls for increased equitable access to transplantation and identifies technology transfer and differential pricing as essential mechanisms to achieve it [56].

Pathways to equity in machine perfusion must include technology-transfer agreements between device manufacturers and regional partners, differential pricing models calibrated to health-system expenditure, open-source perfusate formulations and public investment in lower-cost platforms designed specifically for LMIC contexts. The PGIMER experience demonstrates that clinical innovation is possible in these settings; however, individual institutional achievement cannot substitute for the systemic investment required to make such innovation scalable and equitable.

Health Economics: *The Evidence Behind the Investment Case*—Economic analysis of machine perfusion must extend beyond the immediate cost of the device or consumables and account for the full downstream consequences of transplantation or its absence. The avoided costs of long-term dialysis, repeat hospitalisation, graft failure, re-transplantation and premature death are all measurable, and each contributes substantially to the overall investment case for machine perfusion (Table 6.3).

Table 6.3 Health economic analyses in machine perfusion. All major analyses favour HMP and liver D-HOPE as cost-saving or cost-effective. DCD heart economics favours NRP over OCS-DPP on cost grounds when outcomes are comparable

Analysis	Setting	Modality	Key finding
Darius et al. [21]	Belgium (national)	Kidney HMP	€3.59 M/year dialysis savings; DCD volume 90 → 175/year; DGF 14.4%
Endo et al. [26]	Netherlands (DHOPE-DCD)	Liver D-HOPE	€110,794 vs €126,221 per patient (1 year); 28% ICU cost reduction; cost-effective ≥1 procedure
Tedesco-Silva et al. [22]	Brazil (Markov model)	Kidney HMP (ECD)	+1123 transplants; −120 deaths over 5 year; US$4.49 M incremental; cost-effective vs SUS threshold
Urban et al. [52]	United States	DCD heart NRP vs OCS-DPP	NRP ~US$78,000 less per case than OCS-DPP; comparable outcomes [57]
Guerre et al. [58]	France (tertiary centre)	Heart waitlist cost	Mean €21,324/patient waiting; type 4 patients €61,858 -denominator for device cost justification
Cochrane [8]	Multi-country (meta-analysis)	Kidney HMP	Cost-saving in the USA/Europe; cost-effective at ICER thresholds in Brazil, Canada

The Ethical Frontier

Machine perfusion has clarified several ethical issues in DCD transplantation but has also raised new ones. The central concern is NRP and its relationship to the dead donor rule. Under this rule, vital organs may be procured only after death has been declared, and procurement itself must not cause death. In DCD, death is declared after permanent cessation of circulation, confirmed by a mandatory no-touch interval. NRP subsequently restores warm oxygenated perfusion to the abdominal organs. For critics, this raises a difficult question: if circulation can be restored, even regionally, does the original declaration of circulatory death truly satisfy the requirement of permanence? [31].

The transplant community's response developed in the UK, and Canadian protocols, supported by French physiological data, is that the permanence requirement applies to the cerebral circulation: the flow that matters for death determination is flow to the brain, not flow to the gut [28]. With explicit exclusion of the cerebral circulation via intra-aortic balloon and arch vessel management, and confirmation that no transcranial blood flow occurs during NRP, the permanence criterion can be maintained while abdominal organ recovery proceeds [59]. The American College of Physicians called for a pause on this practice in 2021. The transplant community has responded substantively, and clinical practice continues under national frameworks across the UK, Spain, Italy, Belgium and France. This is a genuine ethical debate, not a solved problem and not one to be dismissed by clinical confidence. It requires national legal review and public transparency in every jurisdiction that introduces NRP.

Two other ethical dimensions of machine perfusion also deserve acknowledgement. The first is euthanasia-associated donation, practised in Belgium, the Netherlands, and increasingly Canada, where machine perfusion has enabled DCD heart donation following medically assisted dying [15]. The ethical defensibility of this pathway depends on strict separation between the assisted-dying decision and the donation process, with independent clinical teams, sequential consent and clear procedural safeguards. Although this model does not apply to jurisdictions where assisted dying is not legal, the rigour of its consent architecture offers broader lessons for donation governance.

The commercialisation of machine perfusion creates a structural tension that the field has not adequately addressed. The major platforms are manufactured by a small number of private companies with incentive structures that do not necessarily align with equitable access, transparent adverse event reporting, or the open publication of unfavourable data. As these technologies become standard of care, the reliance of transplant programmes on proprietary devices and consumables raises legitimate questions about sustainability, particularly in lower-income settings where import costs, currency fluctuations and supply chain fragility add systemic risk. WHO Resolution WHA77.4 frames access to technology as an obligation of the global medical community. Those framing matters need to shape how devices are priced, licenced and regulated.

Coda: The Organ That Was Going to Be Wasted

Return, finally, to the surgeon at two in the morning: an organ on the back table, a decision that cannot be deferred and a patient on a waiting list who does not know that this moment exists. That is where machine perfusion matters most. Not in the elegance of the circuit, not in the sophistication of the device, but in the narrow space between discard and transplantation.

For decades, transplantation has advanced through improvements in technique, immunosuppression, allocation and recipient care. Yet the central bottleneck remains unchanged: there are still too few usable organs. In that context, any technology that can recover a high-risk graft, reduce unnecessary discard and convert uncertainty into measurable viability is more than a technical advance. It changes the frontier of transplantation.

The PGIMER Chandigarh experience gives this argument particular force. It shows that machine perfusion is not the exclusive domain of high-income transplant systems. With institutional commitment, multidisciplinary collaboration and clinical courage, a South Asian public-sector centre used NMP to assess and transplant high-risk kidneys that might otherwise have been discarded elsewhere. These were not mere statistical gains; they were rescued organs converted into functioning transplants.

Machine perfusion will not solve the organ shortage. No single technology will. But it changes what transplant systems can do with the organs they already have. It transforms both controlled and uncontrolled DCD, as well as high-risk donation, from salvage procedures into structured pathways of assessment, recovery and optimisation.

The question now is no longer whether machine perfusion works. The evidence has answered that. The harder question is whether the benefits of this technology will remain concentrated in the health systems that least need expansion, or whether they will reach the regions where every recoverable organ carries the greatest human value.

That is the unfinished task. Machine perfusion has moved from innovation to evidence. It must now move from evidence to equitable implementation.

Competing Interests The author(s) has no competing interests to declare that are relevant to the content of this manuscript.

Ethics Approval The author(s) declares that informed consent to participate in the study and for the publication of the case report/data/ and/or photographs was obtained from all individual participants/legal guardians of participants.

The author(s) declares that this manuscript does not include primary studies involving animals.

References

1. Martin F, Carmona M, Mahillo B, Alvarez M, Luengo A, Chatzixiros E, et al. Organ donation and transplantation worldwide: the global observatory on donation and transplantation 2024 report. Transplantation. 2026;110(3):e655. https://doi.org/10.1097/TP.0000000000005657.
2. Modi GK, Jha V. The incidence of end-stage renal disease in India: a population-based study. Kidney Int. 2006;70(12):2131–3. https://doi.org/10.1038/sj.ki.5001958. PubMed PMID: 17063176.
3. Organ Donation Statistics | organdonor.gov [Internet]. [cited 2026 Jun 1]. Available from: https://www.organdonor.gov/learn/organ-donation-statistics?utm_source=chatgpt.com.
4. ODT Clinical – NHS Blood and Transplant [Internet]. [cited 2026 Jun 1]. Annual report on organ utilisation. Available from: https://www.odt.nhs.uk/statistics-and-reports/annual-report-on-organ-utilisation/.
5. Hessheimer AJ, de la Rosa G, Gastaca M, Ruíz P, Otero A, Gómez M, et al. Abdominal normothermic regional perfusion in controlled donation after circulatory determination of death liver transplantation: outcomes and risk factors for graft loss. Am J Transplant. 2022;22(4):1169–81. https://doi.org/10.1111/ajt.16899.
6. Rijkse E, Ceuppens S, Qi H, IJzermans JNM, Hesselink DA, Minnee RC. Implementation of donation after circulatory death kidney transplantation can safely enlarge the donor pool: a systematic review and meta-analysis. Int J Surg. 2021;92:106021. https://doi.org/10.1016/j.ijsu.2021.106021.
7. Eltzschig HK, Eckle T. Ischemia and reperfusion—from mechanism to translation. Nat Med. 2011;17(11):1391–401. https://doi.org/10.1038/nm.2507.
8. Tingle SJ, Thompson ER, Figueiredo RS, Moir JA, Goodfellow M, Talbot D, et al. Normothermic and hypothermic machine perfusion preservation versus static cold storage for deceased donor kidney transplantation. Cochrane Database Syst Rev. 2024;7 https://doi.org/10.1002/14651858.CD011671.pub3.
9. van Rijn R, Schurink IJ, de Vries Y, van den Berg AP, Cerisuelo MC, Murad SD, et al. Hypothermic machine perfusion in liver transplantation — a randomized trial. N Engl J Med. 2021;384(15):1391–401. https://doi.org/10.1056/NEJMoa2031532.

10. Schroder JN, Patel CB, DeVore AD, Bryner BS, Casalinova S, Shah A, et al. Transplantation outcomes with donor hearts after circulatory death. N Engl J Med. 2023;388(23):2121–31. https://doi.org/10.1056/NEJMoa2212438.
11. Divithotawela C, Cypel M, Martinu T, Singer LG, Binnie M, Chow CW, et al. Long-term outcomes of lung transplant with ex vivo lung perfusion. JAMA Surg. 2019;154(12):1143–50. https://doi.org/10.1001/jamasurg.2019.4079.
12. Schlegel A, Muller X, Mueller M, Stepanova A, Kron P, de Rougemont O, et al. Hypothermic oxygenated perfusion protects from mitochondrial injury before liver transplantation. EBioMedicine. 2020;60:103014. https://doi.org/10.1016/j.ebiom.2020.103014.
13. Dar WA, Sullivan E, Bynon JS, Eltzschig H, Ju C. Ischaemia reperfusion injury in liver transplantation: cellular and molecular mechanisms. Liver Int. 2019;39(5):788–801. https://doi.org/10.1111/liv.14091.
14. Thuong M, Ruiz A, Evrard P, Kuiper M, Boffa C, Akhtar MZ, et al. New classification of donation after circulatory death donors definitions and terminology. Transpl Int. 2016;29(7):749–59. https://doi.org/10.1111/tri.12776.
15. Bollen J, ten Hoopen R, Ysebaert D, van Mook W, van Heurn E. Legal and ethical aspects of organ donation after euthanasia in Belgium and The Netherlands. J Med Ethics. 2016;42(8):486–9. https://doi.org/10.1136/medethics-2015-102898. PubMed PMID: 27012736.
16. Heylen L, Jochmans I, Samuel U, Tieken I, Naesens M, Pirenne J, et al. The duration of asystolic ischemia determines the risk of graft failure after circulatory-dead donor kidney transplantation: a Eurotransplant cohort study. Am J Transplant. 2018;18(4):881–9. https://doi.org/10.1111/ajt.14526.
17. Patrono D, Zanierato M, Vergano M, Magaton C, Diale E, Rizza G, et al. Normothermic regional perfusion and hypothermic oxygenated machine perfusion for livers donated after controlled circulatory death with prolonged warm ischemia time: a matched comparison with livers from brain-dead donors. Transpl Int. 2022;35:10390. https://doi.org/10.3389/ti.2022.10390.
18. van Rijn R, Endo C, Küçükerbil EH, Blokzijl H, Blondeel J, Cortes Cerisuelo M, et al. Long-term follow-up after hypothermic oxygenated machine perfusion in DCD liver transplantation: results of a randomized controlled multicenter trial (DHOPE-DCD). Ann Surg. 2025;282(5):717. https://doi.org/10.1097/SLA.0000000000006876.
19. Markmann JF, Abouljoud MS, Ghobrial RM, Bhati CS, Pelletier SJ, Lu AD, et al. Impact of portable normothermic blood-based machine perfusion on outcomes of liver transplant: the OCS liver PROTECT randomized clinical trial. JAMA Surg. 2022;157(3):189–98. https://doi.org/10.1001/jamasurg.2021.6781.
20. Moers C, Smits JM, Maathuis MHJ, Treckmann J, van Gelder F, Napieralski BP, et al. Machine perfusion or cold storage in deceased-donor kidney transplantation. N Engl J Med. 2009;360(1):7–19. https://doi.org/10.1056/NEJMoa0802289.
21. Darius T, Jochmans I, Foguenne M, Hoste E, Randon C, Bracke B, et al. Nationwide hypothermic machine perfusion for ECD and DCD kidney transplantation in Belgium: one-year outcomes and impact on transplant rates and budget impact analysis. Transpl Int. 2025;38:15282. https://doi.org/10.3389/ti.2025.15282.
22. Tedesco Silva HJ, de Ramos TRM, de Carvalho DDBM, Ferreira GF, de Andrade JMM, de Andrade LGM, et al. Use of machine perfusion to increase the number of expanded criteria deceased donor kidney transplants: a pharmacoeconomic analysis. Transplant Direct. 2024;10(8):e1668. https://doi.org/10.1097/TXD.0000000000001668.
23. Eden J, Thorne AM, Bodewes SB, Patrono D, Roggio D, Breuer E, et al. Assessment of liver graft quality during hypothermic oxygenated perfusion: the first international validation study. J Hepatol. 2025;82(3):523–34. https://doi.org/10.1016/j.jhep.2024.08.030.
24. Sun K, Jiao C, Panconesi R, Satish S, Karakaya OF, Goeij FHCD, et al. Quantifying flavin mononucleotide: an internationally validated methodological approach for enhanced decision making in organ transplantation. EBioMedicine. 2025;116 https://doi.org/10.1016/j.ebiom.2025.105761. PubMed PMID: 40435722.
25. Schlegel A, Mueller M, Muller X, Eden J, Panconesi R, von Felten S, et al. A multicenter randomized-controlled trial of hypothermic oxygenated perfusion (HOPE) for human liver

grafts before transplantation. J Hepatol. 2023;78(4):783–93. https://doi.org/10.1016/j.jhep.2022.12.030.
26. Endo C, van Rijn R, Huurman V, Schurink I, van den Berg A, Murad SD, et al. Cost-effectiveness of dual hypothermic oxygenated machine perfusion versus static cold storage in DCD liver transplantation. Transplantation. 2025;109(2):e101. https://doi.org/10.1097/TP.0000000000005232.
27. Bodewes SB, Woltjes LC, Thorne AM, Eden J, Lantinga VA, Lascaris B, et al. Prolonged dual hypothermic oxygenated machine perfusion for daytime liver transplant. JAMA Netw Open. 2026;9(4):e265039. https://doi.org/10.1001/jamanetworkopen.2026.5039.
28. Manara A, Shemie SD, Large S, Healey A, Baker A, Badiwala M, et al. Maintaining the permanence principle for death during in situ normothermic regional perfusion for donation after circulatory death organ recovery: a United Kingdom and Canadian proposal. Am J Transplant. 2020;20(8):2017–25. https://doi.org/10.1111/ajt.15775.
29. Gaurav R, Paul S, Swift L, Martin J, Philipoff A, Webster R, et al. Sequential in situ normothermic regional perfusion and ex situ normothermic machine perfusion in controlled donation after circulatory death liver transplantation: a retrospective single-center experience. Transplantation. 2026;110(7):e1424–36. https://doi.org/10.1097/TP.0000000000005659.
30. Parent B, Caplan A, Moazami N, Montgomery RA. Response to American College of Physician's statement on the ethics of transplant after normothermic regional perfusion. Am J Transplant. 2022;22(5):1307–10. https://doi.org/10.1111/ajt.16947.
31. Glorion M, Briard JN, Roquebert L, Pizzi S, Menaouar A, Borie M, et al. Thoraco-abdominal normothermic regional perfusion does not restore cerebral blood flow or electrical activity despite collateral supra-aortic blood flow in a porcine model. JHLT Open. 2025;8:100221. https://doi.org/10.1016/j.jhlto.2025.100221.
32. OrganOx metra® Receives FDA Approval for Operation During Air Transport, Expanding Access to Life-Saving Liver Perfusion Technology | OrganOx [Internet]. [cited 2026 Jun 5]. Available from: https://www.organox.com/news/organox-metra-r-receives-fda-approval-for-operation-during-air-transport-expanding-access-to.
33. TransMedics Receives Full and Unconditional FDA IDE Approval for Next-Generation OCS Heart ENHANCE Trial | TransMedics [Internet]. [cited 2026 Jun 5]. Available from: https://investors.transmedics.com/news-releases/news-release-details/transmedics-receives-full-and-unconditional-fda-ide-approval/.
34. Ghinolfi D, Rreka E, De Tata V, Franzini M, Pezzati D, Fierabracci V, et al. Pilot, open, randomized, prospective trial for normothermic machine perfusion evaluation in liver transplantation from older donors. Liver Transpl. 2019;25(3):436. https://doi.org/10.1002/lt.25362.
35. Mergental H, Laing RW, Kirkham AJ, Perera MTPR, Boteon YL, Attard J, et al. Transplantation of discarded livers following viability testing with normothermic machine perfusion. Nat Commun. 2020;11(1):2939. https://doi.org/10.1038/s41467-020-16251-3.
36. Nasralla D, Coussios CC, Mergental H, Akhtar MZ, Butler AJ, Ceresa CDL, et al. A randomized trial of normothermic preservation in liver transplantation. Nature. 2018;557(7703):50–6. https://doi.org/10.1038/s41586-018-0047-9. PubMed PMID: 29670285.
37. van Leeuwen OB, Dutkowski P, Monbaliu D, de Meijer VE. Continuous normothermic machine perfusion of donor livers in the United States: the challenging road from the trial-world into the real-world. HepatoBiliary Surg Nutr. 2024;13(6):1022–6. https://doi.org/10.21037/hbsn-24-521.
38. Hosgood SA, Callaghan CJ, Wilson CH, Smith L, Mullings J, Mehew J, et al. Normothermic machine perfusion versus static cold storage in donation after circulatory death kidney transplantation: a randomized controlled trial. Nat Med. 2023;29(6):1511–9. https://doi.org/10.1038/s41591-023-02376-7. PubMed PMID: 37231075; PubMed Central PMCID: PMC10287561.
39. Hameed AM, Wang Z, Yoon P, Boroumand F, Singla A, Roberston P, et al. Normothermic ex vivo perfusion before transplantation of the kidney (NEXT-kidney): a single-center, non-randomized feasibility study. Transplantation. 2025;109(5):881. https://doi.org/10.1097/TP.0000000000005233.

40. Choudhary D, Sharma A, Singh S, Kenwar DB, Walker Minz R, Singh Kohli H, et al. Application of ex vivo normothermic machine perfusion in deceased donors with acute kidney injury with successful renal transplantation: a preliminary experience. Transplant Direct. 2022;8(11):e1391. https://doi.org/10.1097/TXD.0000000000001391. PubMed PMID: 36299442; PubMed Central PMCID: PMC9592475.
41. Dumbill R, Knight S, Hunter J, Fallon J, Voyce D, Barrett J, et al. Prolonged normothermic perfusion of the kidney prior to transplantation: a historically controlled, phase 1 cohort study. Nat Commun. 2025;16:4584. https://doi.org/10.1038/s41467-025-59829-5. PubMed PMID: 40382321; PubMed Central PMCID: PMC12085653.
42. Jochmans I, Brat A, Davies L, Hofker HS, van de Leemkolk FEM, Leuvenink HGD, et al. Oxygenated versus standard cold perfusion preservation in kidney transplantation (COMPARE): a randomised, double-blind, paired, phase 3 trial. Lancet. 2020;396(10263):1653–62. https://doi.org/10.1016/S0140-6736(20)32411-9.
43. Benkert AR, Keenan JE, Schroder JN, DeVore AD, Patel CB, Milano CA, et al. Early U.S. Heart transplant experience with normothermic regional perfusion following donation after circulatory death. JACC Heart Fail. 2024;12(12):2073–83. https://doi.org/10.1016/j.jchf.2024.06.007.
44. Warnecke G, Van Raemdonck D, Smith MA, Massard G, Kukreja J, Rea F, et al. Normothermic ex-vivo preservation with the portable organ care system lung device for bilateral lung transplantation (INSPIRE): a randomised, open-label, non-inferiority, phase 3 study. Lancet Respir Med. 2018;6(5):357–67. https://doi.org/10.1016/S2213-2600(18)30136-X.
45. Loor G, Warnecke G, Villavicencio MA, Smith MA, Kukreja J, Ardehali A, et al. Portable normothermic ex-vivo lung perfusion, ventilation, and functional assessment with the Organ Care System on donor lung use for transplantation from extended-criteria donors (EXPAND): a single-arm, pivotal trial. Lancet Respir Med. 2019;7(11):975–84. https://doi.org/10.1016/S2213-2600(19)30200-0.
46. Zhou AL, Ruck JM, Casillan AJ, Larson EL, Shou BL, Karius AK, et al. Early United States experience with lung donation after circulatory death using thoracoabdominal normothermic regional perfusion. J Heart Lung Transplant. 2023;42(6):693–6. https://doi.org/10.1016/j.healun.2023.03.001.
47. Callaghan CJ, Ibrahim M, Counter C, Casey J, Friend PJ, Watson CJE, et al. Outcomes after simultaneous pancreas–kidney transplantation from donation after circulatory death donors: a UK registry analysis. Am J Transplant. 2021;21(11):3673–83. https://doi.org/10.1111/ajt.16604.
48. Fischer RMJ, Muñoz N, Ong O, Abt PL, Gruessner AC, Parsons RF. Emerging national trends in normothermic regional perfusion for simultaneous pancreas–kidney transplantation. Clin Transpl. 2025;39(11):e70389. https://doi.org/10.1111/ctr.70389.
49. He X, Guo Z, Zhao Q, Ju W, Wang D, Wu L, et al. The first case of ischemia-free organ transplantation in humans: a proof of concept. Am J Transplant. 2018;18(3):737–44. https://doi.org/10.1111/ajt.14583.
50. Jia Z, Zhu J, Zhang J, Zhang J, Huang C, Zhang N, et al. Ischemia-free liver transplantation improves long-term outcomes in a 5-year follow-up study. JHEP Rep. 2025;7(7):101393. https://doi.org/10.1016/j.jhepr.2025.101393.
51. Israni AK, Zaun DA, Martinez A, Swanner K, Studenic E, Lozano C, et al. OPTN/SRTR 2024 annual data report: deceased organ donation. Am J Transplant. 2026;26:S551–84. https://doi.org/10.1016/j.ajt.2026.05.725.
52. Urban M, Ryan TR, Um JY, Siddique A, Castleberry AW, Lowes BD. Financial impact of donation after circulatory death heart transplantation: a single-center analysis. Clin Transpl. 2024;38(4):e15296. https://doi.org/10.1111/ctr.15296. PubMed PMID: 38545928.
53. Kotani Y. Barriers and solutions for introducing donation after circulatory death (DCD) in Japan. J Artif Organs. 2025;28(3):343–7. https://doi.org/10.1007/s10047-024-01491-7. PubMed PMID: 39812997; PubMed Central PMCID: PMC12373537.

54. Gupta S, Sahay M, Ramachandran B, Kumar A, Gursahani R, Sharma A, et al. Organ donation after circulatory determination of death in India: a joint position paper. Indian J Crit Care Med. 2022;26(4):423–40. https://doi.org/10.5005/jp-journals-10071-24198.
55. NOTTO : National Organ & Tissue Transplant Organisation [Internet]. [cited 2026 Jun 8]. Available from: https://notto.mohfw.gov.in/.
56. B158_12-en.pdf [Internet]. [cited 2026 Jun 8]. Available from: https://www.who.int/health-topics/transplantation#tab=tab_1.
57. Gouchoe DA, Satija D, Cui EY, Schroder JN, Milano CA, Bishawi M, et al. Rise of the machines: normothermic regional perfusion use in heart transplantation in the United States. J Thorac Cardiovasc Surg. 2025;170(1):268–276.e12. https://doi.org/10.1016/j.jtcvs.2024.12.001.
58. Atfeh J, Guerre P, Sebbag L, Pozzi M, Huot L. Economic burden and healthcare trajectories of patients awaiting heart transplantation in a French tertiary center. Transpl Int. 2025;38:13703. https://doi.org/10.3389/ti.2025.13703.
59. Frontera JA, Lewis A, James L, Melmed K, Parent B, Raz E, et al. Thoracoabdominal normothermic regional perfusion in donation after circulatory death does not restore brain blood flow. J Heart Lung Transplant. 2023;42(9):1161–5. https://doi.org/10.1016/j.healun.2023.05.010.

7 Surgical Retrieval of Abdominal Organs Following Donation After Circulatory Death: Controlled and Uncontrolled DCD Techniques

Ashish Sharma and Sarbpreet Singh

Learning Objectives

Upon completion of this chapter, the reader should be able to: (1) Distinguish between the Maastricht categories of DCD donation and understand their clinical and logistical implications; (2) Describe the anatomical and physiological basis for warm ischaemia in DCD retrieval; (3) Outline the operative steps for both rapid flush and normothermic regional perfusion (NRP) retrieval techniques; (4) Detail organ-specific retrieval considerations for the kidneys, liver, pancreas and intestine in the DCD context; (5) Appraise the role of machine perfusion technologies in mitigating ischaemia-reperfusion injury following DCD retrieval; and (6) Recognise the unique challenges of uncontrolled DCD retrieval and the ethical considerations surrounding abdominal normothermic regional perfusion.

Introduction

Donation after circulatory death (DCD) has emerged as an indispensable source of transplantable organs in an era defined by widening gaps between organ supply and demand. Historically sidelined in favour of donation after brain death (DBD), DCD programmes have undergone a renaissance since the late 1990s, driven by advances in surgical technique, organ preservation technology and a growing ethical acceptance of expanded donor criteria. Today, DCD accounts for a substantial and rising proportion of deceased donor activity in the United Kingdom, the Netherlands,

A. Sharma (✉) · S. Singh
Department of Renal Transplant Surgery, PGIMER, Chandigarh, India

S. P. Kolte et al. (eds.), *Organ Donation After Circulatory Death*,
https://doi.org/10.1007/978-981-92-6377-6_7

Australia, Spain and increasingly in North America. In India, several professional bodies, including the Indian Society of Organ Transplantation and the Indian Society of Critical Care Medicine, have issued consensus and position statements addressing the ethical, medical, legal, economic, procedural and logistical challenges associated with donation after circulatory determination of death (DCDD), while outlining a framework for the implementation of DCDD programmes in India [1, 2].

The central challenge of DCD retrieval—and the feature that distinguishes it categorically from DBD retrieval—is warm ischaemia. In DBD donation, the donor heart continues to circulate oxygenated blood until the moment of cross-clamping during retrieval. In DCD donation, circulatory arrest precedes organ retrieval and a period elapses during which organs are deprived of oxygenated perfusion at body temperature. This warm ischaemic period inflicts cumulative cellular injury that influences organ viability, post-transplant function and the risk of specific complications such as ischaemic cholangiopathy of the donor bile duct following liver transplantation.

This chapter provides a comprehensive account of the surgical techniques employed during DCD abdominal organ retrieval. It covers the anatomical, physiological and logistical foundations of both controlled DCD (cDCD) and uncontrolled DCD (uDCD) retrieval and addresses organ-specific considerations for the kidney, liver, pancreas and intestine. The role of normothermic regional perfusion (NRP) and machine perfusion technologies is discussed in the context of intraoperative decision-making. Ethical dimensions unique to uDCD retrieval, particularly abdominal NRP, are also considered. Other aspects of DCD transplantation—including recipient selection, post-transplant management and outcomes—are addressed in separate chapters of this volume.

Classification of DCD Donors: The Maastricht Categories

The internationally recognised framework for classifying DCD donors was established at the First International Workshop on Non-Heart-Beating Donors held in Maastricht in 1995 [2], subsequently modified in 2000 and expanded in 2013 [3, 4]. The Maastricht classification (Table 7.1) stratifies donors according to the circumstances of circulatory arrest, which has profound implications for the degree and duration of warm ischaemia and, therefore, for retrieval logistics and organ viability.

Categories I, II and V constitute uncontrolled DCD (uDCD), in which circulatory arrest is unexpected and resuscitation has either failed or been deemed futile. Category IV is generally considered controlled, but can resemble uncontrolled DCD when cardiac arrest occurs unexpectedly before brain death certification or organ recovery. The uncontrolled donors present the most extreme time pressures and organisational challenges: retrieval teams must respond rapidly, the duration of no-flow warm ischaemia is often poorly characterised and the legal and ethical frameworks governing uDCD vary considerably between jurisdictions. Opt-out systems, in which all citizens are presumed to have consented to organ donation after death unless they have formally registered an objection, help overcome many of the legal

Table 7.1 Modified Maastricht classification of donation after circulatory death

Category	Description	Subcategory	DCD Type
I	Dead on arrival to hospital	Ia: before arrival to hospital; Ib: after arrival to hospital	Uncontrolled
II	Unsuccessful resuscitation	IIa: out of hospital; IIb: in hospital	Uncontrolled
III	Awaiting circulatory arrest following withdrawal of life-sustaining treatment	–	Controlled
IV	Circulatory arrest in a brain-dead donor	–	Controlled or uncontrolled
V	Unexpected circulatory arrest in a critically ill hospitalised patient	–	Uncontrolled

Adapted from Thuong et al. [4]

and ethical challenges associated with utilisation of organs after uncontrolled circumstances surrounding death.

Category III—the planned withdrawal of life-sustaining treatment (WLST) with anticipated circulatory arrest—represents the dominant model in most active DCD programmes and is the paradigm for controlled DCD (cDCD). This setting permits preparation of the recipient, positioning of the surgical team and in many centres, the preoperative insertion of perfusion catheters or the commencement of NRP protocols at a defined moment of arrest. Category IV donors, in whom circulatory arrest occurs in an already brain-dead individual, occupy a hybrid position and their management may draw on elements of both DBD and cDCD protocols.

Warm Ischaemia in DCD Donation: Definitions and Thresholds

Physiologic Consequences Relevant to Retrieval

An understanding of warm ischaemia is fundamental to all aspects of DCD retrieval.

Warm ischaemia initiates multiple cellular and microvascular changes relevant to surgical retrieval.

(A) Endothelial Injury—Hypoxia results in endothelial dysfunction, leukocyte adhesion and impaired microvascular perfusion.
(B) ATP Depletion—Cellular energy stores decline rapidly during warm ischaemia, particularly within hepatocytes and cholangiocytes.
(C) Microvascular Thrombosis—Stagnant circulation promotes thrombosis within the splanchnic microvasculature, impairing subsequent flush quality.

(D) Hepatic Biliary Ischaemia—The biliary epithelium relies predominantly on hepatic arterial blood supply and is highly susceptible to ischemic injury. This vulnerability explains the increased incidence of ischemic cholangiopathy following DCD liver transplantation.
(E) Reperfusion Injury—Reoxygenation after transplantation activates inflammatory pathways, oxidative stress and mitochondrial dysfunction.

Understanding these processes underlies the technical emphasis on rapid perfusion, controlled reperfusion and preservation optimisation. The term ischaemia encompasses several distinct phases, each with differing implications for organ injury and precise definitions are essential for comparing outcomes across centres and studies.

Phases of Warm Ischaemia

The functional warm ischaemia time (fWIT) is the period during which haemodynamics are inadequate to sustain organ oxygenation and viability, conventionally defined as beginning when systolic blood pressure falls below 50 mmHg (or arterial oxygen saturation below 70%) and ending at cold perfusion during retrieval. This is widely regarded as the most clinically relevant measure of ischaemic injury.

The total warm ischaemia time (tWIT) is the interval from withdrawal of life-sustaining treatment to the commencement of cold perfusion. In controlled DCD, this includes the agonal phase, the mandatory no-touch period following the declaration of death (typically 2–5 minutes, depending on national guidelines) and the time required to initiate organ preservation. The asystolic warm ischaemia time (aWIT) refers specifically to the interval between circulatory arrest (asystole) and the start of organ preservation. This measure is particularly relevant in uncontrolled DCD, where prolonged no-flow periods after cardiac arrest may significantly affect organ viability..

Table 7.2 Approximate warm ischaemia thresholds and principal consequences for abdominal organs in DCD retrieval

Organ	Approximate fWIT threshold	Primary consequence of excess WIT	Adjustable by machine perfusion?
Kidney	≤60 min (typically)	Delayed graft function, primary non-function	Yes (HMP/NMP)
Liver	≤20–30 min (cDCD)	Ischaemic cholangiopathy, primary non-function	Yes (NMP strongly recommended)
Pancreas	≤20–30 min (cDCD)	Pancreatitis, thrombosis	Limited evidence (HMP)
Small intestine	≤60–90 min (cold)	Mucosal failure, graft enteritis	Experimental

fWIT functional warm ischaemia time, *HMP* hypothermic machine perfusion, *NMP* normothermic machine perfusion

Organ-Specific Ischaemic Thresholds

Organs differ substantially in their tolerance of warm ischaemia, reflecting differences in metabolic rate, energy substrate utilisation and susceptibility to ischaemia-reperfusion injury at the cellular level (Table 7.2). These thresholds inform retrieval decision-making and organ acceptance criteria (Fig. 7.1).

The liver is the most ischaemia-sensitive of the routinely retrieved abdominal organs, largely because of the vulnerability of the biliary epithelium (cholangiocytes) to ischaemic injury. Unlike hepatocytes, cholangiocytes rely primarily on the peribiliary capillary plexus—supplied by hepatic arterial flow rather than portal venous flow—making them disproportionately susceptible during periods of haemodynamic compromise preceding circulatory arrest. This explains why ischaemic cholangiopathy represents the signature complication of DCD liver transplantation and why the management of hepatic warm ischaemia has driven much of the innovation in DCD retrieval technique and machine perfusion technology.

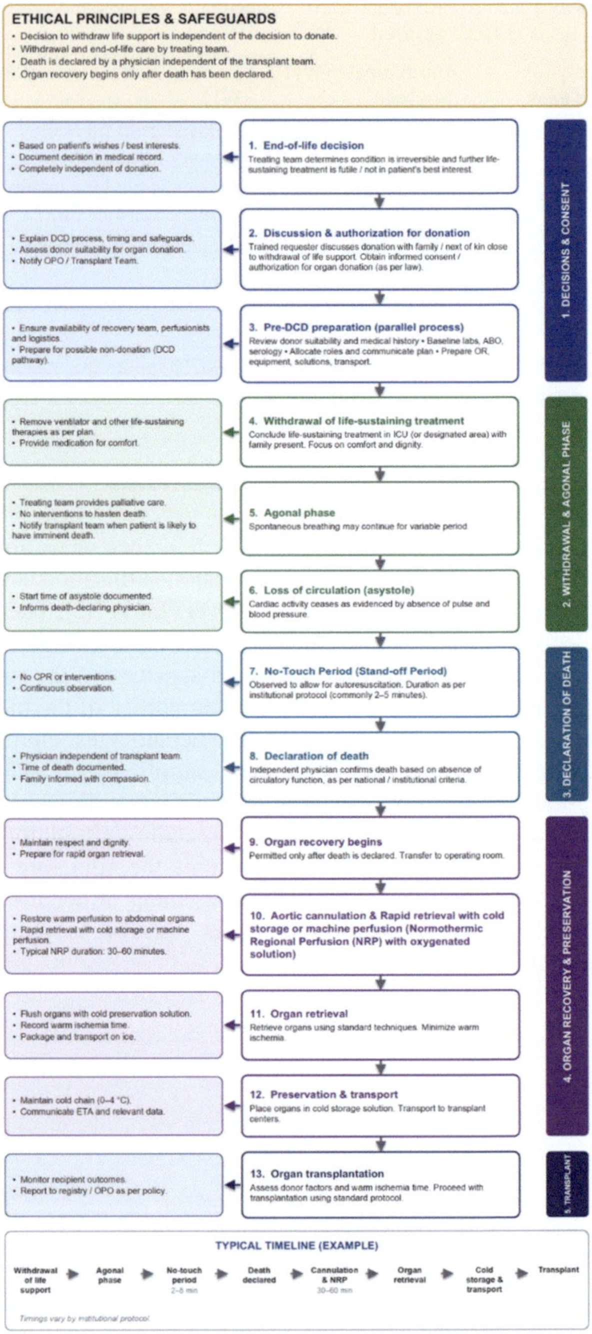

Fig. 7.1 Flow pathway for the determination of death by circulatory criteria III. WLST Withholding of life-sustaining treatments, nRP Normothermic regional perfusion

Preoperative Preparation and Theatre Setup for DCD Retrieval

Controlled DCD: Planning and Timing

The hallmark of controlled DCD retrieval is anticipation. Once WLST has been agreed upon and the family has consented to donation, the DCD process is coordinated between the intensive care unit, the operating theatre and recipient centres. Retrieval surgeons should communicate directly with recipient transplant teams to ensure that, wherever possible, recipients are selected, consented and admitted prior to the commencement of donor operation. However, no recipient preparation should be initiated until circulatory arrest has been confirmed and organ procurement is proceeding.

The retrieval team typically positions outside the room or in an anteroom during the WLST and dying process, entering the theatre—or a dedicated withdrawal room adjacent to the operating theatre suite—only after declaration of death. The interval between the decision to withdraw and actual circulatory arrest is variable and unpredictable; data from large cDCD series indicate that approximately 15–25% of potential donors fail to die within a timeframe that permits viable organ retrieval (conventionally within 60–90 min of WLST). These so-called "failed donors" represent a significant source of distress for families and teams alike, and the management of this possibility requires careful prospective counselling.

Surgical Team Composition and Roles

Abdominal DCD retrieval is typically performed by a two-surgeon team, with a senior retrieval surgeon and an assistant. For multi-organ retrieval involving thoracic organs—less common in DCD than in DBD—a cardiac surgeon needs to be present, though the additional warm ischaemia incurred by thoracic dissection in the DCD setting usually precludes heart retrieval in all but selected NRP programmes. The scrub nurse and anaesthetic team roles are modified in DCD retrieval: anaesthetic involvement ends at declaration of death, and the theatre team prepares the sterile field in advance.

Equipment and Preservation Solutions

Standard equipment for DCD abdominal retrieval includes:

- A major abdominal instrument set with vascular instruments (DeBakey forceps, bulldog clamps, vessel loops)
- Aortic and portal cannulae (typically 20–24 Fr for aortic cannulation)
- Ice slush bowls and sterile polystyrene containers for in situ topical cooling

- Preservation solution: University of Wisconsin (UW) solution, histidine-tryptophan-ketoglutarate (HTK), or Celsior for static cold storage; IGL-1 or proprietary solutions for machine perfusion
- Stapling devices (GIA, TA) for rapid bowel division if required
- NRP circuit if planned (roller pump, membrane oxygenator, heat exchanger, cannulae)

Preservation solutions differ in their ionic composition, oncotic properties and metabolic additives. UW solution remains the reference standard for hepatic and pancreatic preservation; HTK is preferred by some centres for its low viscosity, facilitating rapid and thorough organ flushing. For kidney preservation, both solutions are appropriate, though hypothermic machine perfusion (HMP) has largely superseded static cold storage for DCD kidneys at many institutions.

Surgical Technique: Controlled DCD (Maastricht Category III)

Overview of the Rapid Flush Technique

The rapid flush technique (also termed the in situ perfusion or super-rapid retrieval technique) was the original and remains a widely practised approach to cDCD abdominal retrieval. Its central principle is speed: the abdominal cavity is entered rapidly after declaration of death, the aorta and portal vein are cannulated, cold flush is initiated as swiftly as possible, and topical cooling is applied simultaneously to limit the continued accrual of warm ischaemic injury. The technique demands a disciplined, rehearsed team operating in a familiar environment.

Declaration of Death and Commencement of Surgery

In the United Kingdom, circulatory death is declared after a mandatory five-minute observation period following the loss of cardiac output, confirmed by continuous electrocardiographic monitoring. The precise duration of this no-touch period varies internationally (2 min in some jurisdictions; 5 min is standard in the UK and most European programmes). No surgical intervention may commence during this observation period. Once death is declared by a physician independent of the retrieval team, the surgical team may enter and proceed immediately.

The moment of declaration marks the start of the asystolic warm ischaemia time. Every minute from this point until cold perfusion is achieved represents continued ischaemic injury to donor organs. The target from declaration of death to aortic cannulation and cold flush is typically under 5 min, though this depends on whether preoperative preparation (e.g. laparotomy closure after pre-mortem cannulation) has been performed.

Laparotomy and Initial Exposure

A rapid midline laparotomy is performed from xiphisternum to pubis using a large knife blade or cutting diathermy. Self-retaining retractors (e.g. Omni-Tract or Bookwalter) are deployed immediately. The small bowel is eviscerated to the right to expose the posterior peritoneum and great vessels. An aortic "clamp site" is identified at the level of the infrarenal aorta, taking care to note the position of the inferior mesenteric artery and to preserve it if bowel retrieval is planned.

Aortic Cannulation and Cold Perfusion

The retroperitoneum overlying the infrarenal aorta is rapidly opened with scissors or diathermy. The aorta is mobilised circumferentially over a short segment and a purse-string suture (3/0 prolene) is placed, and a large-bore (18–24 Fr) aortic perfusion cannula is introduced through a small arteriotomy and secured. Some surgeons prefer to clamp the aorta proximally (infradiaphragmatically) using a digital or manual aortic clamp as the cannula is being positioned, to prevent retrograde perfusion and concentrate cold flush to the abdominal viscera.

Cold preservation solution is commenced immediately once the cannula is positioned and secured. Gravity-fed systems using two-litre bags elevated approximately one metre provide adequate perfusion pressure; some centres use pressurised bag systems or roller pumps to achieve 70–100 mmHg perfusion pressure. Adequate venous decompression is essential for effective perfusion. Therefore, an effluent drainage cannula is placed in the inferior vena cava (IVC) via the right iliac vein or infrarenal IVC, and venous blood and warm flush are vented to avoid venous hypertension and back-pressure in the organs. If thoracic organs are not being used, right atrial venting may also be performed. Topical cooling with ice slush (crushed surgical ice packed into the abdominal cavity around the viscera) is applied contemporaneously with cold flush. This in situ topical cooling arrests thermal injury at the organ surface and supplements the intravascular cold flush in achieving rapid core temperature reduction.

Portal Vein Flush

The liver receives its blood supply from both the hepatic artery (approximately 25% of total flow) and the portal vein (approximately 75%). Cold arterial flush alone is therefore insufficient to achieve uniform hepatic cooling and washout; portal venous flush is essential. In the rapid flush technique, portal perfusion is achieved either by cannulation of the inferior mesenteric vein (IMV)—which empties into the portal system just posterior to the transverse mesocolon—or by direct cannulation of the main portal vein after dividing the hepatoduodenal ligament. IMV cannulation is less disruptive and can be accomplished rapidly. A 14–16 Fr cannula is introduced via a small venotomy, secured with a tie, and connected to a separate preservation solution circuit.

Organ Dissection Following In Situ Cooling

Once cold perfusion has been established and the organs are visually inspected for perfusion (checked for pallor and temperature change). Organ dissection may then proceed at a somewhat less frantic pace. The liver, kidneys and pancreas are dissected in sequence according to the planned retrieval pattern. The hierarchy of organs—liver first, then pancreas, then kidneys—reflects the relative ischaemic sensitivity of each and is a broadly accepted convention, though the exact sequence may be modified based on individual donor anatomy and centre preference.

Normothermic Regional Perfusion (NRP) Technique in Controlled DCD

Normothermic regional perfusion has transformed cDCD retrieval at centres where it is available. Rather than accepting the inevitability of warm ischaemia during the rapid flush window, NRP restores oxygenated perfusion to the abdominal viscera at normothermia or near-normothermia within minutes of circulatory arrest, effectively resuscitating organs in situ before retrieval.

The abdominal NRP circuit is established by cannulating the aorta and IVC (Fig. 7.2)—most commonly via the femoral vessels, either percutaneously (using Seldinger technique with image guidance) before WLST or surgically after declaration of death—and connecting these to an extracorporeal membrane oxygenation (ECMO) circuit. The circuit consists of a centrifugal pump, membrane oxygenator, heat exchanger and reservoir. Blood is drained from the IVC, oxygenated and warmed and returned via the aorta. The descending thoracic aorta is clamped during abdominal NRP to prevent reperfusion of the thoracic organs and brain. When thoracic organs are also intended for retrieval, cerebral perfusion is excluded by occluding the supra-aortic (aortic arch) vessels, permitting regional reperfusion of the thoracic and abdominal organs while preventing restoration of cerebral blood flow. (In practice, the aorta is occluded at the level of the diaphragm to restrict perfusion to the abdominal compartment only, which carries important ethical implications discussed in section "Ethical Considerations Unique to DCD Retrieval").

Under abdominal NRP, the liver, kidneys and pancreas are perfused with warm oxygenated blood. Biochemical markers—lactate, pH, glucose, aminotransferases—are monitored and typically improve over the perfusion period (usually 60–240 min), providing a real-time assessment of organ viability that has no equivalent in the rapid flush technique. Lactate clearance and bile production from the liver are particularly informative. The NRP period also allows

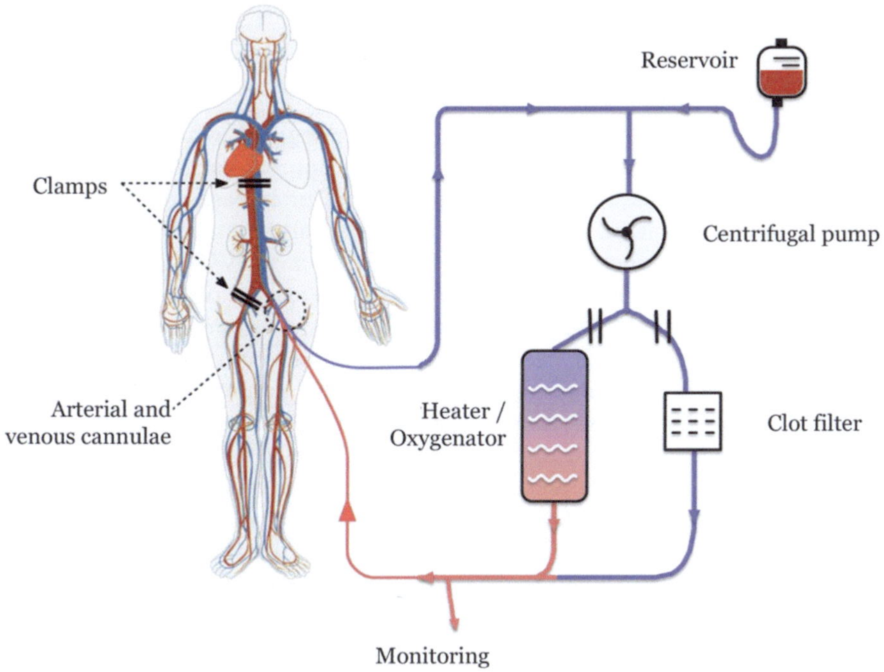

Fig. 7.2 Showing cardiac NRP circuit on the right and abdominal NRP circuit on the left

unhurried dissection of abdominal organs, reducing the technical risk associated with speed-driven retrieval.

Organ-Specific Retrieval Techniques

Kidneys

Anatomy and Dissection Principles

The kidneys are the most commonly retrieved organs in DCD donation and are the most tolerant of warm ischaemia among the abdominal viscera. Renal retrieval in cDCD follows the same anatomical principles as in DBD, but the imperative for speed during the interval before cold perfusion is achieved means that the sequence of steps is modified. Following establishment of cold perfusion and topical cooling, renal dissection proceeds from lateral to medial.

Gerota's fascia is incised along the lateral border of each kidney; the organ is rotated medially to expose the renal hilum. The ureter is identified in the retroperitoneum—taking a generous periureteral tissue cuff to preserve ureteric blood supply—and divided distally just above the bladder cuff or at the pelvic brim. An aortic patch (Carrel patch) incorporating all renal artery orifices is taken where possible, particularly in the presence of multiple renal arteries, to simplify the subsequent back-table vascular reconstruction.

En Bloc Versus Individual Kidney Retrieval

An en bloc retrieval of both kidneys on an aortic segment with the IVC allows the recipient centre to perform dissection under optimal back-table conditions which is especially required in paediatric donors or in cases of difficult hilar anatomy. In adult donors, individual kidney retrieval is standard. The left renal vein is divided at its junction with the inferior vena cava (IVC). The aorta is then opened longitudinally in the midline to expose the origins of the renal arteries. If multiple renal arteries are present—which occurs in approximately 20–25% of donors—all arterial ostia are removed together on a common Carrel patch of aortic wall to facilitate subsequent transplantation. To prevent damage to any accessory renal artery, dissection is limited between the great vessels and the kidneys. During upper-pole dissection, the surgeon should remain above the adrenal gland or through it and posterior to the lumbar fascia to minimise the risk of injury to the kidney and its vasculature. The kidneys are placed immediately in ice-cold preservation solution and transported to either a static cold storage container or, increasingly, onto a hypothermic machine perfusion (HMP) device.

Machine Perfusion for DCD Kidneys

Hypothermic machine perfusion with pulsatile flow (devices such as the LifePort, Kidney Assist, or NHBE machine) delivers cold preservation solution at controlled pressure through the renal artery while monitoring renal resistance and flow dynamics. Increasing evidence supports HMP over static cold storage for DCD kidneys including the landmark study by Moers and colleagues [5], demonstrating reductions in delayed graft function (DGF), primary non-function and 1-year graft loss. Perfusate biomarkers—including glutathione S-transferase (GST), lactate dehydrogenase (LDH) and fatty acid binding protein (FABP)—are emerging as tools for organ viability assessment during machine perfusion.

Liver

Anatomical Considerations in DCD Liver Retrieval

Liver retrieval in the DCD setting is anatomically identical to DBD retrieval but is profoundly affected by the preceding warm ischaemia. The hepatic artery is dissected from the coeliac axis, carefully preserving the replaced or accessory right hepatic artery (arising from the superior mesenteric artery in approximately 15–20% of individuals) and replaced or accessory left hepatic artery (from the left gastric artery in approximately 10%). These anatomical variants must be identified at the back table if not delineated during retrieval, as failure to recognise them risks hepatic artery insufficiency after transplantation.

Rapid Flush Liver Retrieval

After in situ cold perfusion via aortic and portal cannulae, the liver is mobilised by dividing the falciform ligament, triangular ligaments and gastrohepatic ligament. The hepatoduodenal ligament is dissected to expose the portal vein and hepatic artery; the common bile duct is divided and the gallbladder irrigated with cold saline to flush bile and prevent autolysis of the biliary mucosa. The suprahepatic IVC is divided either flush with the diaphragm or with a diaphragmatic cuff and the infrahepatic IVC is divided at the level of the renal veins. The portal vein is divided at the confluence with the splenic and superior mesenteric veins if pancreas retrieval is not planned or about 2 cm above the border of duodenum. The hepatic artery is divided at or near the coeliac origin, preserving as much length as possible.

NRP and the Liver: Clinical Evidence

Several large retrospective series and emerging prospective data indicate that abdominal NRP prior to liver retrieval is associated with substantially reduced rates of ischaemic cholangiopathy compared to rapid flush retrieval [6, 7]. The mechanism is both direct—NRP restores oxygen delivery to the biliary epithelium, ameliorating the ischaemic injury accumulated during the functional warm ischaemia period—and functional: lactate clearance during NRP identifies livers likely to recover adequate synthetic function post-transplantation. When NRP is not available, ex-vivo normothermic machine perfusion (NMP) of the retrieved liver using devices such as the OrganOx metra has demonstrated improved DCD liver outcomes by maintaining organ metabolism and permitting viability assessment prior to transplantation [8].

Bile Duct Injury and Ischaemic Cholangiopathy

Ischaemic cholangiopathy (IC) is the signature complication of DCD liver transplantation and its prevention is the principal driver of evolution of newer methods of preservation. IC manifests as non-anastomotic biliary strictures, typically affecting the intrahepatic and hilar ducts, and in severe cases may necessitate retransplantation. Warm ischaemia time is the dominant risk factor, but donor age, steatosis, cold ischaemia time and arterial reconstruction quality also contribute. The threshold beyond which IC risk becomes unacceptable is not fixed, but most programmes apply a functional WIT ceiling of 30 min for rapid flush DCD livers, with NRP permitting extension of these thresholds by effectively resetting the "ischaemic clock."

Pancreas

Retrieval Considerations

Pancreatic retrieval in the DCD setting is technically demanding and remains less common than renal or hepatic retrieval, reflecting concerns about the organ's sensitivity to ischaemia and the risk of post-transplant pancreatitis and graft thrombosis.

The pancreas receives its blood supply from the superior mesenteric artery (SMA) and coeliac axis via the gastroduodenal artery (GDA) and splenic artery, and its venous drainage is via the portal and splenic veins. The organ is anatomically inseparable from the duodenum—which provides the intrapancreatic component of the common bile duct and the site of drainage in pancreaticoduodenal transplantation—and the two are retrieved together as a composite block.

DCD pancreas retrieval follows the standard retrograde approach: the portal vein is transected approximately 1–2 cm proximal to the duodenal border, preserving an adequate portal vein length with the pancreas graft, the SMA is divided at its origin and the splenic artery is divided at its origin from coeliac axis, leaving a generous length for back-table reconstruction. The duodenum is stapled proximal to the pylorus and just beyond the ligament of Treitz. The spleen is left attached to the pancreatic tail to avoid traction injury to the splenic vessels and subsequently removed at the back table.

Functional Considerations in DCD Pancreas

Warm ischaemia inflicts injury to both the exocrine and endocrine pancreatic parenchyma. Acinar cell death contributes to post-reperfusion pancreatitis, elevation of serum amylase and lipase, and—in severe cases—peripancreatic necrosis. Islet cell injury from warm ischaemia is a determinant of islet yield if the organ is being processed for islet transplantation, and strict WIT thresholds (typically under 20–30 min) are applied by most islet isolation centres. Vascular thrombosis of the pancreatic graft remains a leading cause of early graft loss and appears to be potentiated by ischaemia-reperfusion injury.

Small Intestine

Overview and Indications

Intestinal retrieval in the DCD setting is rare, reflecting both the demanding recipient selection criteria for intestinal transplantation and the particular sensitivity of the intestinal mucosa to ischaemia-reperfusion injury. The gut is the most aerobically active of the abdominal viscera on a per-gram basis, and mucosal barrier disruption following warm ischaemia can lead to bacterial translocation, graft enteritis and rejection. Nevertheless, DCD intestinal transplantation has been reported from specialist centres, typically in the context of combined liver-intestinal retrieval from young donors with minimal comorbidity and short warm ischaemia times.

Retrieval Technique

Intestinal retrieval involves procurement of the small bowel from the ligament of Treitz to the terminal ileum with its mesenteric vascular pedicle. The SMA and SMV are the critical vascular structures; the SMA is taken with a Carrel patch from the aorta, and the SMV is divided at the portal confluence. Cold luminal irrigation via a nasojejunal tube or direct cannulation of the proximal jejunum is performed with balanced electrolyte solution to clear luminal content and limit mucosal bacterial load. In combined liver-intestinal retrieval, the hepatic portal vein and the intestinal SMV share the same venous outflow system; this requires careful coordination of the vascular division sequence to preserve adequate length for both organs.

Uncontrolled DCD (Maastricht Categories I, II and V)

Organisational and Logistical Framework

Uncontrolled DCD (uDCD) programmes operate in a fundamentally different environment from cDCD. The donor arrives at—or arrests within—a hospital setting after failed resuscitation, and the retrieval team must respond to an unpredictable event with a severely compressed time window. The warm ischaemia accumulated during the no-flow cardiac arrest phase, the resuscitation attempt, and the organisational response before preservation is initiated may be prolonged and is often incompletely documented.

Active uDCD programmes are concentrated in a small number of centres globally, with the most extensive published experience coming from Spain [9], France and Italy. These programmes depend on highly coordinated systems integrating prehospital emergency services, hospital emergency departments, organ procurement coordinators and surgical teams.

In-Hospital Resuscitation and Organ Preservation

When a potential uDCD donor is identified—typically a patient who has undergone out-of-hospital cardiac arrest (OHCA) with unsuccessful advanced cardiopulmonary resuscitation—a rapid decision-making process is initiated. If the patient meets broad criteria (appropriate age, no obvious contraindications to donation), the resuscitation effort is maintained or mechanical chest compression initiated (using devices such as the LUCAS or AutoPulse) to provide coronary and cerebral perfusion while the procurement team is mobilised.

Once the patient is in the emergency department and death is declared after failure of a defined resuscitation protocol, the transition to organ preservation must occur with minimal delay. Two main strategies are employed:

- Extracorporeal cardiopulmonary resuscitation (ECPR) with conversion to abdominal NRP: femoral cannulation is performed emergently and the ECMO circuit commenced to restore abdominal organ perfusion while the no-flow period from circulatory arrest to cannulation is minimised.
- In situ cold perfusion: femoral arterial cannulation and aortic balloon occlusion (using a Fogarty or dedicated intra-aortic balloon catheter) combined with cold flush via the iliac artery, employed when NRP infrastructure is not immediately available.

Abdominal NRP in Uncontrolled DCD

Abdominal NRP is the cornerstone of the most successful uDCD programmes. After femoral vessel cannulation—typically performed by the surgical team in the emergency department resuscitation bay—the ECMO circuit is established and abdominal organ perfusion is restored. The thoracic aorta is occluded (typically by an intra-aortic balloon inflated under fluoroscopic or ultrasound guidance, or by surgical clamping at laparotomy) to confine perfusion to the abdomen and prevent cerebral recirculation.

The perfusion period under abdominal NRP in uDCD serves several functions: it terminates ongoing ischaemia to the abdominal organs, provides a window during which consent for donation may be obtained from the family, allows logistical preparation of the retrieval team and enables viability assessment of individual organs. The monitoring of biochemical perfusate parameters—particularly lactate clearance, transaminase release and renal function markers—provides the most objective real-time viability data available in the retrieval setting.

Surgical Technique of uDCD Retrieval

Once abdominal NRP has been established, organ assessment has been satisfactory, and consent obtained, the retrieval proceeds as for cDCD. The aortic occlusion balloon or surgical clamp is removed, cold flush commenced via the established perfusion circuit and the abdomen opened for organ dissection. The technical sequence follows the same organ hierarchy as cDCD (liver, pancreas, kidneys), adjusted for anatomy and individual organ viability.

A notable difference in uDCD retrieval is the frequent need to assess and potentially exclude individual organs based on macroscopic appearance and perfusate biochemistry. Livers with evidence of significant fatty change, contusion, or inadequate perfusion are declined. Kidneys with evidence of cortical mottling or poor turgor may be biopsied and assessed on machine perfusion rather than accepted or declined at the time of retrieval. The decision-making framework in uDCD is necessarily more dynamic than in cDCD, and the retrieval surgeon must be empowered to make real-time organ acceptance decisions in conjunction with the recipient transplant surgeon.

Back-Table Preparation, Vascular Reconstruction, and Transplant

Back-table preparation is performed in a cold preservation bath and constitutes the final opportunity to assess organ quality, complete dissection and prepare vascular structures for recipient implantation. The back table is equally important in DCD and DBD retrieval, but in DCD the assessment of macroscopic ischaemic injury—areas of congestion, mottling, or inadequate flushing—takes on particular significance as a determinant of organ acceptance.

Kidney

Each kidney is inspected for cortical colour and perfusion uniformity. The renal artery and vein are trimmed to an appropriate length, and accessory renal arteries are prepared for reconstruction. If machine perfusion is planned, the renal artery is flushed with preservation solution and the organ mounted on either a hypothermic or normothermic perfusion device. Biopsies for histological assessment (to evaluate glomerulosclerosis, arteriosclerosis and acute tubular injury) may be obtained at this stage if indicated by donor history or macroscopic appearance. Normothermic machine perfusion can additionally facilitate functional assessment of the graft prior to transplantation and prevent unexpected primary non-function [10, 11] while hypothermic machine perfusion reduces delayed graft function and has become increasingly integrated into routine clinical practice [12].

Both increasing donor age and prolonged cold ischaemia time are independently associated with poorer graft survival. The adverse effect of cold storage is particularly pronounced in kidneys from older donors, indicating an interaction between donor age and preservation injury. Therefore, minimising cold ischaemia time is especially important when using kidneys from older DCD donors to optimise transplant outcomes [13].

Liver

The hepatic back table is the most technically demanding of the abdominal organs. The liver is inspected for homogeneity of cold flush and absence of congestion. The hepatic artery is inspected from coeliac to the bifurcation of the left and right hepatic arteries, with care taken to preserve any replaced or accessory vessels. If a replaced right hepatic artery has been identified, this is reconstructed. The portal vein is trimmed and any redundant soft tissue removed from the hilar plate. The bile duct is inspected and if NMP is planned, the bile duct is cannulated for bile collection during machine perfusion. The gallbladder is removed at this stage if retrieved along with the liver.

Livers from unexpected DCD donors have been successfully transplanted when preserved using NMP with strict selection and viability criteria [14]. Donors aged <55 years, with transaminase levels <4 times the upper limit of normal, good macroscopic liver appearance, satisfactory perfusion and consistency at procurement, absence of significant ischaemic injury, and exclusion of grafts with significant fibrosis or >30% macrovesicular steatosis on biopsy are associated with improved graft viability and more favourable post-transplant outcomes [15].

Pancreas

The spleen is removed from the pancreatic tail by careful ligation of the short gastric and splenic vessels at the splenic hilum, avoiding traction on the tail of the pancreas. Arterial reconstruction typically involves fashioning a "Y-graft" using the donor iliac vessels—the external iliac artery to the SMA and the internal iliac artery to the splenic artery—to create a single arterial inflow for the recipient anastomosis. This reconstruction is performed at the back table.

Hypothermic pulsatile machine perfusion of discarded human pancreases has been shown to be technically feasible and does not produce significant histological injury even up to 24-h preservation [16].

Ethical Considerations Unique to DCD Retrieval

The Dead Donor Rule and Determination of Death

All forms of DCD retrieval operate under the constraint of the dead donor rule (DDR), which requires that vital organs not be removed until the donor is dead and that the act of donation not itself cause death. The application of the DDR in DCD is straightforward in principle—circulatory arrest must be declared, and a no-touch observation period observed—but has generated sustained ethical debate in practice, particularly regarding the irreversibility of circulatory arrest.

The question of whether circulatory function is truly "permanently ceased" (the criterion in many jurisdictions) or merely "irreversibly ceased" (implying that restoration of function is impossible rather than merely not attempted) is of particular relevance when ECMO-based NRP is deployed. If NRP could, in principle, restore cardiac function, then the heart from a DCD donor on abdominal NRP has not necessarily met the criterion of irreversible cessation [17]. This interpretation does not invalidate DCD practices in most jurisdictions, but it underlines the importance of understanding the ethical basis of local standards.

Abdominal NRP and Cerebral Perfusion

The exclusion of cerebral perfusion during abdominal NRP is both a practical necessity—to prevent restoration of brain function in a donor who has been declared dead—and an ethically mandatory constraint. Failure to occlude thoracic aortic flow during abdominal NRP could result in restoration of cerebral perfusion and, theoretically, of consciousness in the donor. This is not merely hypothetical; it is a clinical risk that requires robust procedural safeguards, including mandatory verification of thoracic aortic occlusion (by imaging, transoesophageal echocardiography, or direct surgical inspection) before NRP flow is commenced.

Pre-mortem Interventions

In some cDCD programmes, interventions are performed before circulatory arrest—such as the pre-mortem insertion of femoral cannulae for NRP, heparin administration, or vasodilator infusion—with the purpose of improving organ preservation outcomes after death. These pre-mortem interventions are performed without direct benefit to the donor and carry a small risk of harm. They are ethically permissible in most frameworks only when: explicit donor consent exists (via advance directive or donor card indicating acceptance of such interventions), family agreement is obtained, the interventions do not hasten death, and institutional ethics approval has been secured. The regulatory and ethical landscape for pre-mortem interventions varies considerably internationally and continues to evolve.

Intraoperative Complications and Their Management

Vascular Injury

Vascular injury during DCD retrieval—particularly during the rapid flush phase when speed is prioritised—is an ever-present risk. Common injuries include inadvertent arteriotomy of the aorta or iliac vessels during cannula insertion, traction injury to the renal pedicle and damage to an unrecognised replaced hepatic artery during rapid dissection of the hepatoduodenal ligament. Immediate haemostasis with direct pressure and suture repair of the vessel, or in extreme cases, ligation and assessment of ischaemic injury, are required. Detailed back-table vascular reconstruction can usually salvage organs retrieved with minor vascular injuries.

Inadequate Cold Perfusion

Patchy or incomplete cold flushing—manifesting as areas of persisting congestion, or discolouration on the organ surface—may result from inadequate cannula positioning, unexpected vascular anatomy, severe atherosclerosis of the donor aorta, or hypotension-related stasis prior to death. Organs with demonstrably incomplete flush should be assessed by machine perfusion wherever available rather than accepted or declined based on macroscopic grounds alone.

NRP Circuit Failure

ECMO circuit failure during abdominal NRP—whether from cannula dislodgement, pump failure, oxygenator malfunction, or air embolism—risks abrupt termination of organ perfusion at normothermia. This scenario is managed by immediate transition to cold in situ flush via pre-positioned cannulae, with rapid correction of the circuit failure where possible. All NRP programmes should have a defined protocol for circuit failure, and back-up cold flush equipment must always be immediately available.

Summary

Key Points

1. DCD retrieval is classified by the Maastricht categories, with category III (controlled DCD following WLST) and categories I, II and V (uncontrolled DCD) representing the principal clinical contexts.
2. Warm ischaemia—Particularly functional warm ischaemia time—Is the defining challenge of DCD retrieval and drives organ-specific acceptance thresholds and technique selection.
3. The rapid flush technique prioritises speed to minimise warm ischaemia; abdominal NRP restores oxygenated perfusion after circulatory arrest and permits organ viability assessment, reducing ischaemic cholangiopathy risk in liver retrieval.
4. Kidney retrieval is the most common and most ischaemia-tolerant procedure; HMP is standard of care at most DCD centres.
5. Liver retrieval demands meticulous attention to warm ischaemia time and bile duct preservation; NRP and/or ex-vivo NMP have transformed DCD liver outcomes.
6. Pancreatic and intestinal retrieval in DCD are specialised procedures confined to centres with appropriate recipient programmes and strict WIT criteria.
7. Uncontrolled DCD requires an integrated emergency response system and is best supported by abdominal NRP with mandatory thoracic aortic exclusion.
8. Ethical safeguards—Including strict adherence to the dead donor rule, exclusion of cerebral perfusion during NRP, and transparent processes for pre-mortem interventions—Are non-negotiable features of every DCD programme.

Competing Interests The author(s) has no competing interests to declare that are relevant to the content of this manuscript.

Ethics Approval The author(s) declares that this manuscript does not include primary research with human participants.

The author(s) declares that this manuscript does not include primary studies involving animals.

References

1. Seth AK, Mohanka R, Mani RK, Asthana S, Attawar S, Dhital KK, et al. Organ donation after circulatory determination of death: consensus statement. Indian J Transplant. 2024;18(3):247–56.
2. Seth AK, Mohanka R, Navin S, Gokhale AG, Sharma A, Kumar A, et al. Organ donation after circulatory determination of death in India: a joint position paper. Indian J Crit Care Med. 2022;26(4):421–38. https://doi.org/10.5005/jp-journals-10071-24198.

3. Kootstra G, Daemen JHC, Oomen APA. Categories of non-heart-beating donors. Transplant Proc. 1995;27(5):2893–4.
4. Thuong M, Ruiz A, Evrard P, Kuiper M, Boffa C, Akhtar MZ, et al. New classification of donation after circulatory death donors: definitions and terminology. Transpl Int. 2016;29(7):749–59. https://doi.org/10.1111/tri.12776.
5. Moers C, Smits JM, Maathuis M-HJ, et al. Machine perfusion or cold storage in deceased-donor kidney transplantation. N Engl J Med. 2009;360(1):7–19. https://doi.org/10.1056/NEJMoa0802289.
6. van de Leemkolk FEM, Schurink IJ, Dekkers OM, Oniscu GC, Alwayn IPJ, Ploeg RJ, et al. Abdominal normothermic regional perfusion in donation after circulatory death: a systematic review and critical appraisal. Transplantation. 2020;104(9):1776–91. https://doi.org/10.1097/TP.0000000000003345.
7. Molina V, Mergental H, Hessheimer AJ, et al. Normothermic regional perfusion in controlled donation after circulatory death liver transplantation: a systematic review and meta-analysis. Transpl Int. 2024;37:13263. https://doi.org/10.3389/ti.2024.13263.
8. Mergental H, Laing RW, Kirkham AJ, Perera MTPR, Boteon YL, Attard J, et al. Transplantation of discarded livers following viability testing with normothermic machine perfusion. Nat Commun. 2020;11(1):2939. https://doi.org/10.1038/s41467-020-16251-3.
9. Mateos-Rodríguez AA, Navalpotro-Pascual JM, Del Rio Gallegos F, Andrés-Belmonte A. Out-of-hospital donors after cardiac death in Madrid, Spain: a 5-year review. Australas Emerg Nurs J. 2012;15(3):164–9. https://doi.org/10.1016/j.aenj.2012.05.002.
10. Choudhary D, Sharma A, Singh S, Kenwar DB, Walker Minz R, Singh Kohli H, et al. Application of ex vivo normothermic machine perfusion in deceased donors with acute kidney injury with successful renal transplantation: a preliminary experience. Transplant Direct. 2022;8(11):e1391. https://doi.org/10.1097/TXD.0000000000001391.
11. Hosgood SA, Nicholson ML. Normothermic machine perfusion in renal transplantation. Curr Transplant Rep. 2022;9:219–27. https://doi.org/10.1007/s40472-022-00378-x.
12. Markmann JF, Abouljoud MS, Ghobrial RM, et al. Hypothermic machine perfusion versus static cold storage in deceased donor kidney transplantation. N Engl J Med. 2022;387:2210–20. https://doi.org/10.1056/NEJMoa2118265.
13. Summers DM, Johnson RJ, Hudson A, Collett D, Watson CJE, Bradley JA. Effect of donor age and cold storage time on outcome in recipients of kidneys donated after circulatory death in the UK: a cohort study. Lancet. 2013;381(9868):727–34. https://doi.org/10.1016/S0140-6736(12)61685-7.
14. Fondevila C, Hessheimer AJ, Ruiz A, Calatayud D, Ferrer J, Charco R, et al. Liver transplantation using donors after unexpected cardiac death: novel preservation protocol and acceptance criteria. Am J Transplant. 2007;7(7):1849–55. https://doi.org/10.1111/j.1600-6143.2007.01846.x.
15. Nutu A, Justo I, Marcacuzco A, Caso Ó, Manrique A, Calvo J, et al. Liver transplantation for hepatocellular carcinoma using grafts from uncontrolled circulatory death donation. Sci Rep. 2021;11(1):13520. https://doi.org/10.1038/s41598-021-92976-5.
16. Prudhomme T, Kervella D, Le Bas-Bernardet S, Cantarovich D, Karam G, Blancho G, Branchereau J. Ex situ perfusion of pancreas for whole-organ transplantation: is it safe and feasible? a systematic review. Cell Transplant. 2020;29:963689720986931. https://doi.org/10.1177/0963689720986931.
17. Murphy NB, Slessarev M, Basmaji J, Blackstock L, Blaszak M, Brahmania M, et al. Ethical issues in normothermic regional perfusion in controlled organ donation after determination of death by circulatory criteria: a scoping review. Transplantation. 2025;109(4):597–606. https://doi.org/10.1097/TP.0000000000005161.

Donor Selection and Thoracic Organ Retrieval in Donation After Circulatory Death (DCD)

8

Prakash M. Ludhani and Kumud K. Dhital

Introduction

Heart and lung transplantation remain the definitive therapeutic options for selected patients with end-stage cardiopulmonary failure. The persistent shortage of suitable donor organs remains the principal limitation in serving the rising population of patients with advanced cardiopulmonary failure, and in limiting significant waitlist attrition. While patients with end-stage cardiac failure may be suitable for bridging or destination therapy with durable mechanical ventricular assist devices (VAD), no such alternative exists for those with advanced lung failure.

Excepting few initial historical heart transplants with donor and recipient co-location, both heart and lung transplants continued a necessary reliance on donation after brain death (DBD) donors. Over the past decade, a wider acceptance of the Maastricht definitions of categories relating non-heart beating donors, now referred to as donation after circulatory death (DCD), has resulted in a significant expansion of the donor pool that is available for conversion to clinical transplantation [1, 2]. While lung transplants were championed for both controlled and uncontrolled DCD donor organs with excellent outcomes [3, 4], concerns over the mandatory warm ischemic period associated with DCD donation left heart transplantation as being suitable only for donor hearts from the DBD pathway. Subsequent advances in organ preservation, machine perfusion technology, and refined procurement techniques have since enabled successful transplantation of DCD hearts also, with the first successful series reported from St Vincent's Hospital, Sydney, Australia in 2014 [5]. Since then, several centers across Australia, the United Kingdom, the United States, and Spain have established successful DCD thoracic programs [6–9].

P. M. Ludhani · K. K. Dhital (✉)
Institutes of Heart-Lung Transplantation and MCS, Apollo Hospital, Chennai, Tamil Nadu, India

S. P. Kolte et al. (eds.), *Organ Donation After Circulatory Death*,
https://doi.org/10.1007/978-981-92-6377-6_8

Functional warm ischemic time is an obligatory phase of the DCD pathway and significantly influences post-transplant graft dysfunction and survival. Therefore, donor selection, agonal phase assessment, retrieval technique, and optimized reperfusion strategies are central to ensuring a recipient-protective strategy for successful DCD transplantation [5, 7].

This chapter reviews donor selection and thoracic organ retrieval in DCD heart and lung transplantation, covering donor eligibility criteria, contraindications, evaluation protocols, ischemic time definitions, and preservation strategies. Detailed surgical retrieval techniques for DCD heart and lung procurement are described, including the techniques of direct procurement and perfusion (DPP), thoraco-abdominal normothermic regional perfusion (TA-NRP), abdominal NRP, adjunct ex situ lung perfusion (ESLP), together with logistical coordination, and emerging adaptations relevant to developing thoracic DCD transplant programs, particularly within the Indian context. Contemporary evidence demonstrates that DCD thoracic transplantation can safely expand the donor pool without compromising survival. With appropriate infrastructure, multidisciplinary clinical expertise and coordination, local legislation that permits donation after circulatory death, and protocol-driven retrieval strategies, the DCD donation pathway is emerging as an important approach to deliver significant and sustainable growth in heart and lung transplant activity. Controlled Maastricht category III DCD donors currently constitute the main source for thoracic DCD procurements globally because they permit planned retrieval logistics and controlled warm ischemic exposure.

Physiological Considerations in DCD Thoracic Donation

Unlike DBD donors, DCD donors undergo progressive hypoperfusion during withdrawal of life-sustaining therapy. The agonal phase is characterized by hypotension, hypoxia, metabolic acidosis, catecholamine surge, and inflammatory activation. Following circulatory arrest, complete cessation of organ perfusion occurs until reperfusion is re-established [10].

Critical ischemic intervals include the functional warm ischemic time (FWIT), the stand-off or no-touch period, the subsequent cold ischemic time, and the total ischemic time. For thoracic organs, FWIT is typically defined from the point at which systolic blood pressure falls below 50 mmHg and until the initiation of cold perfusion or reperfusion. Acceptable FWIT thresholds generally include less than 30 min for the heart and 60–90 min for the lungs [5, 11].

Donor Selection for DCD Heart and Lung Retrieval [8, 12–15]

See Tables 8.1 and 8.2.

Table 8.1 Inclusion and exclusion criteria for DCD heart donation

Parameter	Inclusion criteria	Exclusion criteria
Donor age	Preferably <50 years Coronary angiogram for >40 year	>50–60 years (relative)
Maastricht category	Controlled—III and IV	Uncontrolled (relative)
Cardiac function	Normal biventricular function	Moderate/severe LV or RV dysfunction
Coronary artery disease	No significant CAD	Significant CAD or prior MI
Structural heart disease	Normal cardiac anatomy	Cardiomyopathy or severe valvular disease
Hemodynamic stability	Stable with low vasoactive requirement	Refractory hypotension or high vasoactive cardiac support
Functional warm ischemic time (FWIT)	< 30 min	>30 min
Agonal phase prediction	Predicted rapid progression after WLST	Uncertain or prolonged agonal phase
Cardiac rhythm	Stable rhythm	Persistent ventricular arrhythmias
Troponin levels	Mildly elevated acceptable	Markedly elevated with dysfunction
Left ventricular hypertrophy	Mild/no LVH	Severe LVH (>1.4 cm)
Infection status	No uncontrolled sepsis	Active uncontrolled infection/ endocarditis
Metabolic profile	Acceptable lactate and acid-base status	Severe metabolic acidosis
Prior cardiac surgery	Preferably absent	Complex prior cardiac surgery
Substance abuse	Limited acceptable	Significant cocaine/ methamphetamine toxicity / current iv abuse
Malignancy	No transmissible malignancy	Active metastatic malignancy
Donor BMI	Acceptable BMI (adult weight ≥40 kg)	Severe obesity (relative)
Echocardiography	Normal EF with no structural abnormalities	Reduced EF, regional wall motion or structural abnormalities
Cardiac arrest duration	Short or absent	Prolonged downtime
Organ assessment	Acceptable OCS/NRP evaluation	Persistent lactate rise or poor recovery
Retrieval logistics	Predictable retrieval timing	Anticipated prolonged transport/ ischemia

Stand-Off Periods: A Comparative Perspective

Stand-off ("no-touch") period is the mandatory interval to confirm continued absence of circulation with no spontaneous auto-resuscitation, before death is certified. This interval varies substantially by jurisdiction and determines how much functional warm ischemic time a graft is exposed to before retrieval can

Table 8.2 Inclusion and exclusion criteria for DCD lung donation

Parameter	Inclusion criteria	Exclusion criteria
Donor age	Preferably <65 years	Advanced age with poor lung reserve
Maastricht category	Controlled—III and IV	Uncontrolled (relative)
Oxygenation	PaO_2/FiO_2 >300 mmHg	Severe refractory hypoxemia
Chest radiograph	Clear or minimal infiltrates	Diffuse bilateral infiltrates
Smoking history	<20 pack-years	Heavy smoking history
Bronchoscopy	Minimal secretions	Massive aspiration/purulent secretions
Pulmonary infection	No active pneumonia	Severe pneumonia or uncontrolled sepsis
Mechanical ventilation duration	Short/moderate acceptable	Prolonged ventilation with lung injury
Pulmonary compliance	Preserved compliance	Severe poor compliance
Lung trauma	Minimal contusions acceptable	Major pulmonary contusion/air leak
Aspiration	Minimal aspiration acceptable	Massive aspiration syndrome
Functional warm ischemic time	<90 min	>90 min
Ex situ organ perfusion assessment	Acceptable ex situ physiology	Progressive edema or oxygenation
Pulmonary edema	Mild acceptable	Severe pulmonary edema
Pulmonary hypertension	Mild acceptable	Severe donor pulmonary hypertension
Malignancy	No transmissible malignancy	Active transmissible malignancy
Airway anatomy	Normal anatomy	Severe airway injury
Viral/bacterial infection	Controlled/treated infection	Active uncontrolled infection
Donor BMI	Acceptable BMI	Severe obesity with poor mechanics
Thoracic surgery history	Minor acceptable	Complex thoracic surgical injury
Preservation logistics	Acceptable transport time	Excessive anticipated ischemic time

even begin. Excepting the Pittsburgh Protocol of a 2-min no-touch period, also practiced in New South Wales in Australia [16], most jurisdictions adhere to a more standard 5 min. Italy and Russia are outliers at 20 and 30 min, respectively marked outliers [17].

In India, under the Transplantation of Human Organs and Tissues Act, 1994, a 5-min no-touch period applies only where a do-not-attempt-resuscitation order has already been signed; donors without such an order require 30 min of cardiopulmonary resuscitation before death can be certified [12]. The protocol intended for use in a specific country therefore needs to state the applicable local stand-off requirement explicitly, rather than citing a single global figure, because the regulatory definition of death, not merely clinical practice, sets the ceiling on achievable FWIT.

DCD Heart Retrieval Techniques

Two principal strategies currently dominate DCD heart procurement: direct procurement and perfusion (DPP) and thoraco-abdominal normothermic regional perfusion (TA-NRP). More recently, the Vanderbilt University group in Nashville, USA, have described what may become a game changer with their REUP protocol [18].

Direct Procurement and Perfusion (DPP)

The principle of DPP is that the heart is rapidly retrieved after declaration of death, with primary cardioplegia, and following explant is re-perfused ex situ using a heart perfusion device (Heart OCS—TransMedics Inc., Andover, US). Required equipment includes sternotomy instruments, a cardioplegia setup, an ice preservation system, the Organ Care System (OCS), and cannulation equipment [5].

The surgical retrieval proceeds through seven steps. 1. Withdrawal of life-sustaining therapy (WLST) is performed in the ICU or operating room, with monitoring of arterial pressure and oxygen saturation. 2. Once circulatory arrest is confirmed, a mandatory no-touch period is observed, and certification of death declared. 3. The donor is then rapidly transferred to the operating room where the retrieval team is gowned and ready and transferred from the bed to the operating table. A rapid median sternotomy is then performed and the pericardium opened vertically. The aorta is cross-clamped and cold cardioplegia rapidly administered via the aortic root with additional topical cooling and venting of the left atrial appendage. Simultaneously, a two-stage venous cannula is inserted via the right atrial appendage in standard fashion and connected to a heparinized bag for collecting 1.5 l of blood for priming the OCS circuit. 4. Standard heart explant is performed respecting the need to leave adequate pulmonary artery, and left atrial tissue in the event the lungs are also being procured. 5. On the back table, the OCS cannula are attached to the aorta and the pulmonary artery. 6. The heart is then connected to the OCS platform for normothermic ex situ reperfusion. Following cardiac reanimation, the donor heart is transported back to the transplanting facility with interval check on hemodynamic parameters, ECG, lactate trends and assessment of contractility. Assuming the arteriovenous lactate levels downtrend and in favor of lactate consumption for cardiac metabolism, a final decision is made as to the suitability to proceed with the transplant. The heart then remains beating and non-ischemic until the recipient chest is prepared. 7. The final step is delivering cold cardioplegia to the donor heart on the device and then passing it on to the implanting team [5].

Thoraco-Abdominal Normothermic Regional Perfusion (TA-NRP)

The initial steps of TA-NRP are the same as that described above and differ only after median sternotomy. In this technique, the head and neck vessels are clamped just cephalad to the aortic arch, and circulation selectively restored to thoraco-abdominal organs with standard right atrial to ascending aortic cannulations and using either a heart-lung machine or a modified ECMO circuit. Ventilation is recommenced. This permits visual and functional assessment of the heart using transoesophageal echocardiography, hemodynamic measurements using a Swan-Ganz catheter. In situ reanimation terminates the ischemic insult and allows metabolic recovery. Standard procurement then proceeds, with cardioplegia administered and the heart retrieved in a manner similar to DBD procurement [7, 19].

The subsequent transport back to the recipient hospital follows two options. The typical modality has been to use the Heart OCS device as described above for the DPP method. Where the donor and recipient are collocated, then a brief period of static cold storage has been used in anecdotal cases.

See Table 8.3.

Table 8.3 Comparison between direct procurement and perfusion (DPP) versus thoraco-abdominal normothermic regional perfusion (TA-NRP)

Parameter	DPP	TA-NRP
Principle	Immediate organ retrieval followed by ex situ perfusion	In situ reperfusion and cardiac reanimation after death declaration
Reperfusion	Ex situ (OCS platform). Await more data from use of REUP and HOPE	In situ within donor body
Need for ex situ perfusion	Mandatory but await further data from REUP and HOPE	Optional/selective
Cerebral circulation	Not restored	Excluded by arch vessel clamping
Functional heart assessment	Limited ex situ assessment	Full physiologic assessment possible
Hemodynamic assessment	Limited	Comprehensive
Warm ischemia exposure	Higher	Lower
Lactate assessment	OCS-based monitoring	In situ physiologic recovery
Surgical complexity	Moderate	Higher
Retrieval speed requirement	Extremely rapid	Rapid but slightly more controlled
Perfusion technology dependence	High (may reduce with REUP)	Moderate
Cost	Higher due to OCS. HOPE is also expensive, but REUP will be economical	Potentially lower long-term
Resource utilization	Significant, except if future REUP data is compelling	Significant
Severe PGD rates	Slightly higher	Lower
ECMO requirement	Slightly more frequent	Reduced
Early survival	Excellent	Excellent

(continued)

Table 8.3 (continued)

Parameter	DPP	TA-NRP
Long-term survival	Comparable	Comparable
Rejection rates	Similar	Lower in some studies
Logistical complexity	Transport-focused. May be mitigated by REUP data	Cannulation and ECMO focused
Team expertise requirement	OCS expertise. Upskilling also for HOPE, but standard care with REUP	ECMO/NRP expertise
Organ recovery quality	Good	Superior metabolic recovery
Multi-organ procurement	More difficult coordination	Better abdominal-thoracic coordination
Increasing global adoption	Widely adopted initially	Rapidly expanding contemporary strategy
Major advantage	Simpler ethical framework	Better graft recovery and assessment
Major limitation	Cost	Ethical/legal complexity

The REUP Technique and Heart Preservation

The group at Vanderbilt University, Nashville, USA, have described their current DCD heart retrieval practice of a 10-min perfusion of the left and right vented heart using an extracorporeal circuit. The novel hyperoxygenated composition, perfused at 200 ml/min at 10–12 °C contains cross-matched packed red blood cells, del Nido cardioplegia, heparin, antibiotic, albumin, multivitamins, steroid, bicarbonate, valproic acid. The heart is then explanted in standard fashion and transported with static cold storage at 10 °C to the recipient hospital. In the initial cohort of 24 donors, the median age was 32 years, and the time from declaration of death to cardiac flush was less than 10 min, and survival was 92% at 90 days. That only 7 (29%) of the donors contributed lungs for transplantation is not dissimilar to the lung retrieval from TA-NRP [18].

This technique bypasses the high cost of mandatory ex situ perfusion with the standard DPP technique and avoids the ethical concerns with clamping of the arch vessels in the TA-NRP technique. It certainly aligns favorably in the Indian context largely from sparing very prohibitive costs of the ex situ perfusion device regardless of DPP or TA-NRP. It also dispenses with any post declaration due diligence of reanimating the heart for functional assessment, a factor that most practitioners have to date felt necessary given the uncertainly of what degree of myocardial injury is sustained with the variable warm ischemic time. We will have to wait for longer follow-up data to see if this truly represents a game changing strategy. One additional technique is that of post explant preservation using continuous Hypothermic Oxygenated Perfusion (HOPE). Its use in preserving DCD donor hearts has only been reported twice, so it will not be discussed further.

DCD Lung Retrieval Techniques

DCD lungs may be retrieved using rapid cold flush, TA-NRP-supported procurement, or ESLP assessment pathways [20, 21].

Following certification of death, lung retrieval proceeds through five steps. 1. Donor preparation involves endotracheal intubation and fiber-optic bronchoscopy, with aggressive recruitment maneuvres avoided. 2. A rapid median sternotomy is performed and the pleural cavities opened. 3. The main pulmonary artery is cannulated and prostaglandin E1 administered. 4. Antegrade flush follows, using low-potassium dextran solution (Perfadex Plus) infused while venting via the left atrial appendage. Topical cooling with ice slush is applied and the lungs inflated at low FiO_2. 5. A retrograde flush through the pulmonary veins clears clots and emboli. 6. Finally, the trachea is stapled, and both lungs are explanted en bloc [22].

The lungs can be safely transported with standard static cold storage.

Role of Ex Situ Lung Perfusion (ESLP)

ESLP has revolutionized DCD lung utilization. Its benefits include functional assessment, reconditioning of marginal lungs, extended preservation, and reduced turn-down rates [23–25]. Common ESLP systems include the Toronto protocol, the Lund protocol, and the Organ Care System Lung [26, 27]. Parameters assessed during EVLP include pulmonary vascular resistance, compliance, gas exchange, airway pressures, and ability to visualize radiographs for edema and other occult parenchymal pathology. Large cohort meta-analysis demonstrates that outcomes from DCD lung transplantation is similar with or without ESLP. Machine perfusion may not be necessary for standard DCD donor lungs, but may have value in the reconditioning of marginal organs by making them transplantable [3, 28].

See Table 8.4.

Table 8.4 Machine perfusion platforms in thoracic transplantation

Platform / strategy	Organ	Perfusion type	Temperature	Primary purpose	Key advantages	Major limitations
Organ care system (OCS) heart	Heart	Blood perfusion	Normothermic	DCD heart preservation and assessment	Functional assessment, lactate monitoring, prolonged preservation	Expensive, resource intensive
Thoraco-abdominal NRP	Heart ± lung and all abdominal organs	In situ ECMO reperfusion	Normothermic	Reanimation and organ recovery	Physiologic assessment, reduced PGD	Ethical/legal concerns
Abdominal NRP	Abdominal organs. Does permit heart and lung retrieval with rapid procurement	In situ ECMO reperfusion	Normothermic	Abdominal organ recovery	Improved organ quality	Does not assess heart
Ex situ lung perfusion (ESLP)	Lungs	Ex vivo perfusion/ ventilation	Normothermic	Lung assessment and reconditioning	Improves utilization of marginal lungs	Expensive, technically demanding
Toronto EVLP protocol	Lungs	Acellular perfusion	Normothermic	Extended assessment	Long evaluation periods	Expensive, and specialized expertise needed
Lund EVLP protocol	Lungs	Cellular perfusate	Normothermic	Functional reassessment	Good physiologic support	Increased complexity
Organ care system (OCS)lung	Lungs	Portable perfusion	Normothermic	Transport, reconditioning and preservation	Portable continuous assessment	High cost
Static cold storage (SCS)	Heart/lungs	No perfusion	4 °C	Conventional preservation	Simple, inexpensive	Limited ischemic tolerance
Hypothermic oxygenated perfusion (HOPE)	Heart	Oxygenated perfusion	Hypothermic	Ischemic protection	Reduced metabolic injury	Limited clinical experience
REUP transient blood-based cardioplegic perfusion	Heart	Hyperoxygenated static preservation	Hypothermic	Extended preservation	Potential prolonged transport capability	Lack of outcome data beyond short-term

Outcomes of DCD Heart and Lung Transplantation

Multiple studies demonstrate encouraging outcomes for DCD heart transplantation with comparable survival to transplants using DBD donor organs. The Sydney group has shown 1- and 5-year survival of 94% and 88% at 1 and 5 years, respectively. These are not statistically different from the DBD series with 87% and 81% survival of the DBD group at 1 and 5 years, respectively [8]. Reported benefits include significant donor pool expansion, comparable short to medium-term survival, and acceptable rates of primary graft dysfunction [7, 8, 28].

Outcomes of DCD Lung Transplantation

DCD lung transplantation has shown comparable survival to DBD lungs, similar chronic lung allograft dysfunction rates, and acceptable PGD incidence [22–33]. A major review and meta-analysis of five observational studies comprising 654 patients found survival to be 82.1% and 51.2%, respectively, at 1 and 5 years for DBD lung transplants, and 86.2% and 62.7% survival at 1 and 5 years, respectively, for the DCD cohort. While this shows a small but significant lower short-term survival with the DCD group at 1 year, the 5 year data suggest a similar advantage of DCD over DBD. Importantly, and despite these excellent outcomes, DCD lungs remain underutilized [28].

Comparative DCD Utilization Across Transplant Programs

The proportion of heart and lung transplant activity attributable to DCD donors varies widely by country, and this variation reflects differences in local legislation, procurement strategy, variations in the very definition of death, and on unit volume and experience.

In the United Kingdom, DCD heart transplants accounted for 28% of adult heart transplant activity in 2022/23, and the introduction of the DCD pathway in 2015 is estimated to have increased UK cardiac transplant activity by around 20% overall [34]. At St Vincent's Hospital in Sydney, Australia, home to the first modern adult DCD heart transplant in 2014, the DCD pathway accounted for 20% of the unit's total heart transplant activity across its first 8 years, using the DPP approach exclusively [8].

A 2023 multicenter study spanning 15 centers in the UK, Spain, the USA, and Belgium found that adopting thoraco-abdominal normothermic regional perfusion increased heart transplantation activity by 23% relative to DBD activity alone, with comparable 1-year survival between the two groups [9]. A decade since DCD heart transplants have become standard of care in numerous centers, the International Society for Heart and Lung Transplantation has reported that most programs adopting DCD heart transplantation are witnessing approximately 30% increase in their own transplant volume [35].

Ethical Controversy Specific to TA-NRP

TA-NRP raises an ethical question over the restoration of oxygenated circulation to the heart and abdominal organs after death has already been certified. With the heart reanimated in situ, critics argue it risks contradicting the dead donor rule. The central technical question is whether occluding or ligating the aortic arch vessels reliably and permanently excludes blood flow to the brain, or whether collateral circulation through intercostal and spinal vessels could theoretically permit some degree of cerebral reperfusion once systemic circulation is restored. The same critics also voice their unease at the prospect of converting a DCD donor into a DBD status by arch vessel occlusion.

A joint United Kingdom–Canadian proposal has argued that, provided arch-vessel occlusion is performed correctly and its adequacy confirmed, TA-NRP maintains the permanence standard required for a valid declaration of circulatory death rather than reversing it [36]. This position has been directly challenged by an ethical and logistical analysis, aligned with concerns later raised by the American College of Physicians, which viewed the in situ reanimation of the heart and restoration of circulation to major organs after death has been declared, as being difficult to reconcile with a genuine, irreversible cessation of circulatory function, and called for caution before wider adoption of TA-NRP in the United States pending further evidence and public deliberation [37].

The International Society for Heart and Lung Transplantation, in its 2022 position paper on controlled DCD thoracic transplantation, acknowledges this unresolved tension and recommends that individual programs adopt explicit, auditable safeguards, with confirmed arch-vessel occlusion, absence of arterial pressure or flow above the clamp, and family consent specific to the NRP technique, rather than treating the ethical question as settled [38]. Any center considering TA-NRP therefore needs a documented institutional position on the dead-donor-rule question before adopting the technique, not merely a technical description of the perfusion circuit and surgical procedure.

Challenges in Emerging Nations and the Indian Perspective

Implementation of DCD transplantation in emerging nations faces multiple barriers, including legislation permitting the withdrawal of life support as part of end-of-life care, legal uncertainty over the definition and certification of circulatory death, limited access to machine perfusion technology, critical care and retrieval infrastructure limitations, financial constraints, organ transport logistics, and limited public awareness of DCD as distinct from the more familiar brain-death pathway [12].

India's regulatory framework already permits DCD donation under the Transplantation of Human Organs and Tissues Act, 1994, but deceased donation in India remains overwhelmingly brain-death-based: fewer than 10 deceased-donor transplants per million population are performed nationally, compared with more than 100 per million population in the United States, and reported DCD experience to date has been almost entirely limited to a small number of kidney cases rather than thoracic organs [12].

A 2022 joint position paper by Indian transplant and critical care societies set out a DCD framework specific to Indian practice: where brain death has been formally certified through both necessary brain-stem death tests, that cardiopulmonary resuscitation and a stand-off period are not required for category IV donation, where only one test set has been completed. The 30 min of CPR remains a requirement unless a do-not-attempt-resuscitation order is in place, in which case a 5-min stand-off period applies instead [12]. The same position paper identifies the prohibitive cost of ex situ perfusion systems as the principal barrier to thoracic DCD specifically and calls for development of indigenous organ care systems and preservation solutions, alongside structured data submission and outcome audit, to build clinical confidence and gain public trust [12].

This has since progressed with a clear understanding that the highlighted shortcomings do not permit a wholesale adoption of the European, North American, Australian, and British practices. An additional national consensus statement has been specifically published to inform about normothermic regional perfusion and how best it may be modified and applied in an Indian DCDD practice [39].

Potential advantages for India include expansion of the donor pool, reduction in waitlist mortality, and better utilization of existing tertiary-care ECMO and cardiac surgical infrastructure. The principal open challenges remain the cost of perfusion technology, the absence of a thoracic-specific DCD track record, and the need for retrieval-team training specific to time-critical DCD logistics rather than the brain-death pathway India's transplant coordinators are already familiar with.

Conclusion

Heart and lung transplantation following donation after circulatory death represent one of the most important advances in contemporary thoracic transplantation. Careful donor selection, minimization of warm ischemic injury, meticulous surgical retrieval, and modern perfusion technologies have enabled successful utilization of DCD hearts and lungs with outcomes comparable to DBD transplantation.

Normothermic regional perfusion and ex vivo organ preservation platforms are rapidly redefining the boundaries of acceptable donor utilization, of the ability to resuscitate marginal organs ex situ, and likely to offer far more in future with ex situ therapies for immune modulation and to mitigate the currently inevitable onslaught of chronic rejection. As global transplant demand continues to rise, DCD thoracic transplantation will likely become an essential component of future heart and lung transplant programs as already evidenced in many the western nations.

The development of structured DCD pathways, upskilling healthcare staff, informing the communities, building locally affordable devises, are all necessary, and offer a unique opportunity to significantly expand thoracic transplant capacity while reducing waitlist mortality and saving more lives.

Competing Interests The author(s) has no competing interests to declare that are relevant to the content of this manuscript.

Ethics Approval The author(s) declares that this manuscript does not include primary research with human participants.

The author(s) declares that this manuscript does not include primary studies involving animals.

References

1. Kootstra G, Daemen JH, Oomen AP. Categories of non-heart-beating donors. Transplant Proc. 1995;27(5):2893–4.
2. Thuong M, Ruiz A, Evrard P, et al. New classification for donation after circulatory death donors definitions and terminology. Transpl Int. 2016;29(7):749–59.
3. Levvey B, Harkness M, Chambers D, et al. Are DCD lungs superior? excellent intermediate results from a donation after cardiac death lung transplant national collaborative. J Heart Lung Transplant. 2020;29(2 Suppl):S117–8.
4. Suberviola B, Mons R, Ballesteros M, et al. Excellent long-term outcome with lungs obtained from uncontrolled donation after circulatory death. Am J Transplant. 2019;19(4):1195–201.
5. Dhital KK, Iyer A, Connellan M, et al. Adult heart transplantation with distant procurement and ex-vivo preservation of donor hearts after circulatory death: a case series. Lancet. 2015;385:2585–91.
6. Chew HC, Macdonald PS, Dhital KK. The donor heart and donation after circulatory death. Heart Lung Circ. 2019;28:316–22.
7. Messer S, Cernic S, Page A, et al. A 5-year single-centre early experience of heart transplantation from donation after circulatory -determined death donors. J Heart Lung Transplant. 2020;39(12):1463–75.
8. Joshi Y, Scheuer S, Chew H, et al. Heart transplantation from DCD donors in Australia: lessons learned from the first 74 cases. Transplantation. 2023;107(2):361–71.
9. Louca J, Ochsner M, Shah A, et al. The international experience of in-situ recovery of the DCD heart: a multicentre retrospective observational study. EClinMedicine. 2023;58:101887. https://doi.org/10.1016/j.eclinm.2023.101887.
10. Iyer A, Chew HC, Gao L, et al. Pathophysiological trends during withdrawal of life support. Circulation. 2016;134:1562–74.
11. Bello I, Palleschi A, Cypel M, et al. Unlocking the potential of uncontrolled DCD in lung transplantation: a review of 2 decades of experience. J Heart Lung Transplant Open. 2025;10:100374. https://doi.org/10.1016/j.hlto.2025.100374.
12. Seth A, Mohanka R, Navin S, et al. Organ donations after circulatory determination of death in India: a joint position paper. Indian J Crit Care Med. 2022;26(4):423–40.
13. British Transplantation Society. UK Guidelines on Transplantation from deceased donors after circulatory death. 2023.; https://bts.org.uk/transplantation-from-deceased-donors-after-circulatory-death/.
14. Belousova N, Cheng NA, Matelski J, et al. Effects of donor smoking history on early post-transplant lung function measured by oscillometry. Fron Med. 2024;11 https://doi.org/10.3389/fmed.2024.1328395.

15. Van Raemdonck D, Neyrinck A, Verleden GM, et al. Lung donor selection and management. Proc Am Thorac Soc. 2009;6:28–38.
16. DeVita M, Snyder J. Development of the University of Pittsburgh Medical Centre policy for the care of terminally ill patients who may become organ donors after death following the removal of life support. Kennedy Inst Ethics J. 1993;3(2):131–43.
17. Lomero M, Gardiner D, Coll E, et al. Donation after circulatory death today: an updated overview of the European landscape. Transpl Int. 2020;33:76–88.
18. Williams A, Trahanas J, Bommareddi S, et al. Donation after circulatory death heart transplant without preimplant reanimation using rapid ultra oxygenated recovery. JAMA. 2026;335(10):885–93.
19. D'Alessandro DA, Hoffman JR, Knecht KR, et al. Heart transplantation from controlled DCD donors using normothermic regional perfusion. Ann Thorac Surg. 2019;108:1450–6.
20. Van Raemdonck D, Keshavjee S, Levvey B, et al. Donation after circulatory death in lung transplantation. J Thorac Dis. 2015;7:1471–6.
21. Keshavjee S, Cypel M. Human lung transplantation from donation after circulatory determination of death donors. Am J Transplant. 2011;11:2001–2.
22. Cypel M, Levvey B, Van Raemdonck D. Donation after circulatory death lung transplantation. Semin Thorac Cardiovasc Surg. 2015;27:112–8.
23. Cypel M, Keshavjee S. Extracorporeal lung perfusion (EVLP). Curr Transplant Rep. 2015;2:161–70.
24. Valenza F, Rosso L, Coppola S, et al. Ex vivo lung perfusion to improve donor lung function and increase the number of organs available for transplantation. Transpl Int. 2014;27:553–61.
25. Cypel M, Rubacha M, Yeung J, et al. Normothermic ex vivo perfusion prevents lung injury compared to extended cold preservation. J Thorac Cardiovasc Surg. 2009;138:783–9.
26. Cypel M, Yeung JC, Hirayama S, et al. Technique for prolonged normothermic ex vivo lung perfusion. J Heart Lung Transplant. 2008;27:1319–25.
27. Warnecke G, Moradiellos J, Tudorache I, et al. Normothermic perfusion of donor lungs for preservation and assessment. Lancet. 2012;380:1851–8.
28. Costa B, Coelho B, Grillo I, et al. Ex vivo lung perfusion in donation after circulatory death lung transplantation: a systematic review and meta-analysis. J Heart Lung Transplant Open. 2026;11:100480. https://doi.org/10.1016/j.hlto.2026.1000480.
29. Cypel M, Levvey B, Van Raemdonck D, et al. International Society for Heart and Lung Transplantation donation after circulatory death registry report. J Heart Lung Transplant. 2015;34:1278–82.
30. Snell GI, Levvey BJ, Oto T, et al. Early lung transplantation success utilizing controlled DCD donors. Am J Transplant. 2008;8:1282–9.
31. Levvey BJ, Harkess M, Hopkins P, et al. Excellent clinical outcomes from a national donation-after-determination-of-cardiac-death lung transplant collaborative. Am J Transplant. 2012;12:2406–13.
32. Osaki S, Anderson JE, Johnson MR, et al. Donation after cardiac death in lung transplantation. Ann Thorac Surg. 2010;89:1735–41.
33. Spadaccio C, Salsano A, Altarabsheh S, et al. Short and long-term outcomes of lung transplantation from brain dead vs circulatory death donors: a meta-analysis of comparative studies. J Heart Lung Transplant Open. 2025;44(5):708–18.
34. NHS Blood and Transplant. Annual report on heart transplantation: report for 2022/2023. NHSBT; 2023.
35. International Society for Heart and Lung Transplantation. DCD heart transplantation reaches 10-year mark, now up to 30% of transplant volumes. ISHLT News; 2025.
36. Manara A, Shemie SD, Large S, et al. Maintaining the permanence principle for death during in situ normothermic regional perfusion for donation after circulatory death organ recovery: a United Kingdom and Canadian proposal. Am J Transplant. 2020;20:2017–25.

37. Parent B, Moazami N, Wall S, et al. Ethical and logistical concerns for establishing NRP-cDCD heart transplantation in the United States. Am J Transplant. 2020;20(6):1508–12.
38. Holm AM, Courtwright A, Olland A, Zuckermann A, Van Raemdonck D. ISHLT position paper on thoracic organ transplantation in controlled donation after circulatory determination of death (cDCD). J Heart Lung Transplant. 2022;41:671–7.
39. Seth AK, Mohanka RM, Mani RK, Asthana S, Attawar S, Dhital KK, et al. Consensus statement of the national consortium on normothermic regional perfusion for organ donation after circulatory determination of death in India. Indian J Transplant. 2026;20(1):23–35.

Part III

Organ Allocation, Logistics and Policy Framework in DCD

Logistics in DCD Transplantation

9

Shrikanth Srinivasan, Jumana Yusuf Haji,
and Aravinth Srinivas

Introduction and Historical Context

Donation after Circulatory Death (DCD), also historically referred to as Non-Heart Beating Organ Donation (NHBD), has become a cornerstone of modern transplantation, now accounting for approximately half of all organ donors in some nationwide registries [1]. However, the practise of DCD is not a modern invention; in fact, it represents the historical origins of organ transplantation [2, 3].

Before the widespread clinical and legal adoption of Brainstem Death (BSD) criteria in the 1970s, DCD was the standard procedure and only mechanism for organ procurement [2, 3]. Despite its early use, DCD was largely abandoned as the medical community transitioned to BSD donors, primarily because early DCD grafts suffered from the damaging effects of unmitigated warm ischaemic time (WIT) [2].

In recent decades, however, the incidence of BSD has steadily declined due to improvements in road and workplace safety, alongside advancements in neurological critical care [2]. This decline, juxtaposed against an ever-growing international demand for donor organs, created a significant shortage that necessitated expanding the donor pool [4]. Advancements in immunosuppression, organ storage, and novel machine perfusion technologies have mitigated historical concerns regarding ischaemia, allowing DCD outcomes to approach equivalence with DBD (Donation after

S. Srinivasan (✉)
Manipal Institute of Critical Care Medicine, Manipal Hospitals, New Delhi, Delhi, India

J. Y. Haji
Fortis Hospital Mulund, Mumbai, Maharashtra, India
e-mail: ecmo@drjumana.in

A. Srinivas
Manipal Hospital, Delhi, India

S. P. Kolte et al. (eds.), *Organ Donation After Circulatory Death*,
https://doi.org/10.1007/978-981-92-6377-6_9

Brain Death) outcomes for several organs, sparking a global resurgence in DCD programmes [2].

Classification of DCD Donors: The Maastricht Categories

To standardise the logistical and ethical protocols surrounding DCD, donors are classified using the Maastricht Categories, originally described in 1995 and subsequently updated in Paris in 2013. These categories distinguish whether the permanence and irreversibility of circulatory death are based on a "cannot resuscitate" scenario (uncontrolled) or a "will not resuscitate" scenario (controlled) [2].

Uncontrolled DCD (uDCD) refers to permanent and irreversible circulatory death following failed resuscitation. Due to the unpredictable nature of these deaths, uDCD presents immense logistical challenges and narrow windows for intervention before irreversible organ damage occurs [5]. The categories include:

- *Category Ia*: Found dead, unwitnessed cardiac arrest out-of-hospital.
- *Category Ib*: Found dead, unwitnessed cardiac arrest in-hospital.
- *Category IIa*: Witnessed cardiac arrest out-of-hospital.
- *Category IIb*: Witnessed cardiac arrest in-hospital.

Controlled DCD (cDCD) occurs when circulatory death is determined after a planned "Do Not Attempt Resuscitation" order is executed, allowing for carefully coordinated logistical planning.

- *Category III*: Death follows the elective withdrawal of life-sustaining therapy (WLST) in-hospital. This is the most common DCD pathway, typically involving patients with devastating, non-recoverable neurological injuries, end-stage respiratory failure, or those being withdrawn from Extra-Corporeal Life Support (ECMO).
- *Category IV*: Cardiac arrest occurring in a patient who has already met (or is undergoing evaluation for) Brainstem Death criteria. This can be either a controlled or uncontrolled event depending on the circumstances [2].

Definitions of Ischaemia Time (Warm, Functional Warm, Cold)

The central logistical constraint in any DCD procurement is the management of ischaemic times. In DCD, organs are subjected to a period of hypoperfusion that inevitably occurs during the dying process, distinct from the immediate cold preservation seen in brain-dead donors [2]. Standardising these definitions is critical for assessing organ viability:

- *Warm Ischaemia Time (WIT)*: Broadly, WIT is the total period of hypoperfusion and anoxia. It begins when the donor's systolic blood pressure (SBP) or oxygen saturation (SaO_2) falls below a critical threshold (often SBP <50 mmHg or SaO_2 <70%) and ends when the organs are flushed with cold perfusion fluid [2, 6].

- *Functional Warm Ischaemia Time (fWIT)*: This metric specifically tracks the phase where end-organ ischaemia actively causes damage. While definitions can vary internationally and by institution, fWIT is most commonly defined as starting when the donor's SBP drops below 50 mmHg (or SaO_2 <70%) and ending with the administration of cold cardioplegia or the initiation of normothermic regional perfusion (NRP) [4, 6]. Depending on the organ, maximum tolerable fWIT limits are strict: generally 20–30 min for the liver, 30–60 min for the pancreas, 60–90 min for lungs, and up to 120 min for kidneys [6].
- *Asystolic Warm Ischaemia Time (aWIT)*: This tracks the time specifically from circulatory arrest (asystole) to the delivery of cold flush. Prolonged aWIT has been significantly associated with severe primary graft dysfunction and post-operative complications [4, 7, 8].
- *Cold Ischaemia Time (CIT)*: This is the period of cold static preservation. With the advent of ex vivo machine perfusion (EVLP), CIT is now frequently split into two phases: CIT1 (from cross-clamp/cold flush to the start of machine perfusion) and CIT2 (from the end of machine perfusion to implantation in the recipient) [9].

Pre-procurement Logistics: OPO Coordination, and Donor Identification

Prior to any surgical recovery, the logistical coordination of a potential DCD donor requires meticulous collaboration between the Organ Procurement Organization (OPO) and the hospital's patient care team. Because death has not yet occurred during the pre-procurement phase, the primary physician or their clinical designee remains fully responsible for the medical management of the patient [5].

Once authorisation for donation is obtained, the OPO clinical coordinator conducts a thorough evaluation of the potential donor. This includes reviewing the patient's medical and behavioural history, performing a physical examination, and ordering necessary diagnostic tests to assess organ viability. The OPO is required to obtain specific donor testing, which ranges from standard arterial blood gases and infectious disease screening to more advanced organ-specific diagnostics like echocardiograms, cardiac catheterisations, and bronchoscopies.

Active critical care management and adherence to standard Donor Management Goals (DMGs) have been shown to increase the number of transplantable organs and improve post-transplant graft survival [10]. These goals focus on maintaining physiological stability, such as a mean arterial pressure of 60–110 mmHg and adequate oxygenation. In some systems, to ensure standardised and dedicated care, haemodynamically stable donors with prior authorisation may be transferred to a specialised hospital-based Donor Care Unit (DCU) prior to the withdrawal of life support [5]. Effective communication throughout this phase is critical; OPO personnel must clearly explain to the Legal Next of Kin that donation will only proceed after life-sustaining therapies are withdrawn and a qualified healthcare professional formally declares death [5].

Withdrawal of Life-Sustaining Therapy: Process and Separation of Roles

A fundamental ethical and logistical tenet of DCD is the strict separation between end-of-life care and the organ donation process. The decision to execute the Withdrawal of Life-Sustaining Therapy (WLST) must be made exclusively by the patient's healthcare team and their family, completely independent of the OPO's goals [11]. Under no circumstances may the OPO, transplant surgeons, or organ recovery teams guide palliative care, participate in the WLST process, or declare the patient's death. WLST and the verification of death must be performed by a physician or group of physicians who are completely separate from the organ recovery teams [2].

The WLST process typically involves the discontinuation of mechanical ventilation and inotropic support, while the primary intensive care team manages comfort-focussed medications to relieve distress and maintain the patient's dignity. While the ideal location for WLST is often the Critical Care Unit to allow the patient to remain in a familiar environment with their family, it can also take place in the Operating Room (OR) to minimise ischemic time, provided the family and healthcare teams agree. If WLST occurs in the OR, prepping and draping the patient prior to the declaration of death is highly discouraged to preserve donor dignity, unless specifically agreed upon by the family and clinical staff [12].

Before WLST, certain premortem interventions may be administered to optimise the viability of the organs. The most notable intervention is the systemic administration of heparin to prevent microthrombi formation in the small vessels of the transplanted organs. The use of antemortem heparin or the insertion of specific cannula is strictly dictated by local legislation and hospital protocols, and it must be clearly discussed with the family during the authorisation process [5, 12, 13].

Declaration of Death: The No-Touch Interval and Autoresuscitation

Following WLST, the patient's vital signs are continuously monitored via indwelling arterial catheters, pulse oximetry, and electrocardiography [2]. Death must be determined independently by the attending physician based on the permanent cessation of circulation and respiration. This is clinically characterised by unresponsiveness, apnoea, and the absence of an arterial pulse or heart sounds. In the context of DCD, "permanent" indicates that no resuscitative efforts will be made and the physiological ability to autoresuscitate has been lost [5].

To clinically confirm this permanence, a mandatory "no-touch" observation period is required immediately following circulatory arrest before any organ recovery activity or perfusion can begin [14]. Most international and institutional protocols mandate a strict 5-min continuous observation period of asystole or absent pulsatile flow. Some jurisdictions require a longer observational period; for instance, certain countries legally mandate up to 20 min of electrical asystole before death can be declared [15].

During this no-touch interval, the patient is carefully monitored for "autoresuscitation," which is defined as the unassisted return of spontaneous circulation, such as the spontaneous return of an arterial waveform, a pulse, or respiratory effort [15, 16]. While autoresuscitation has never been documented in controlled DCD scenarios, protocols dictate that if any persistent circulation is observed, the donation process must be paused immediately. If this occurs, end-of-life care continues in the best interest of the patient, and a new observation period must be completed once the circulatory activity ceases [2, 15].

Furthermore, if the patient does not die within a predefined timeframe following WLST—often between 60 and 90 min depending on the targeted organs and local criteria—the ischemic damage to the organs is considered too severe. In these cases, the organ donation process is "stood-down," and the patient receives ongoing routine palliative care [17, 18].

Operating Room Preparation and Team Coordination

The preparation and coordination of the Operating Room (OR) in a DCD procedure begins well before the patient is transported. Prior to the withdrawal of life-sustaining therapy (WLST), the OR must be fully set up with all anticipated equipment, surgical instrumentation, and cold preservation fluids to eliminate any delays once death is declared.

A formal "time-out" process is critical, involving the intensive care physician or anaesthetist, ICU and theatre nursing staff, the OPO coordinator, and the transplant retrieval teams. Close collaboration ensures that all expectations and potential clinical outcomes are explicitly understood by all parties before WLST. This includes confirming the exact duration of the mandatory no-touch period and establishing a clear plan for a "stand-down" if the patient does not die within the acceptable ischaemic timeframe [5].

If WLST takes place in the OR rather than the ICU, pre-prepping and draping the patient prior to the declaration of death is highly discouraged to preserve donor dignity, unless strictly agreed upon by the family and clinical staff for logistical necessity. Furthermore, if advanced perfusion techniques like Normothermic Regional Perfusion (NRP) are planned, the OR staffing must be scaled accordingly. An Abdominal-NRP (A-NRP) protocol requires a dedicated team that includes at least two surgeons, a scrub nurse, a circulating nurse, and a perfusionist to manage the extracorporeal circuit [3, 5].

Surgical Procurement: Minimising Warm Ischaemia Time

Once death is declared and the mandatory no-touch observation period elapses, the surgical teams initiate recovery with extreme urgency. The primary objective is to minimise the asystolic Warm Ischaemia Time (aWIT)—the specific duration from circulatory arrest to the delivery of cold flush [4]. Prolonged aWIT is significantly associated with primary graft dysfunction (PGD) and a higher likelihood that the recipient will require post-operative mechanical support, such as ECMO [4, 7, 8].

To mitigate ischaemic damage, the surgical team performs a rapid laparotomy (and sternotomy, if thoracic organs are being recovered). In standard rapid flush procedures, the aorta is immediately cross-clamped, and cold preservation fluids are rapidly infused to arrest cellular metabolism and flush out micro-thrombi. Colloid-containing solutions—such as University of Wisconsin (UW) solution or IGL-1 for abdominal organs, and Perfadex for lungs—are the standard of care. Following the onset of the cold flush, the organs must be extracted as swiftly as possible, either sequentially or en bloc, to limit any further warm ischaemic damage [2, 6, 19].

Controlled DCD Procurement: Rapid Flush vs. Normothermic Regional Perfusion

Organ recovery in controlled DCD primarily utilises two distinct logistical strategies: Direct Procurement and Perfusion (DPP/Rapid Flush) and Normothermic Regional Perfusion (NRP).

Direct Procurement and Perfusion (DPP) involves rapid in situ cold flushing immediately after the declaration of death, followed by prompt extraction and cold static storage. While historically the standard approach, DPP subjects the organs to unmitigated warm ischaemia during the dying process and does not allow for in vivo physiological assessment of the organs prior to procurement [3, 5].

Normothermic Regional Perfusion (NRP) represents a major advancement in DCD practice. It utilises an extracorporeal membrane oxygenation (ECMO) circuit to restore warm, oxygenated blood flow to targeted organs after circulatory death is permanently confirmed. By temporarily re-establishing perfusion, NRP replenishes depleted cellular energy substrates, clears toxic by-products of anaerobic metabolism, and limits further ischaemic injury. Crucially, NRP allows transplant surgeons to assess the real-time viability and physiological function of the organs before deciding to procure them [3, 5].

Because NRP restores regional circulation, strict cerebral isolation strategies are an absolute ethical and technical mandate to ensure compliance with the dead donor rule. To prevent any return of cerebral perfusion following the declaration of death, procedural safeguards are required:

- In Abdominal-NRP (A-NRP), the descending thoracic aorta must be clamped and vented.

- In Thoraco-abdominal NRP (TA-NRP), the aortic arch vessels must be clamped and vented [20].

Current guidelines strongly recommend A-NRP over rapid flush for controlled DCD abdominal procurement, as high-certainty evidence shows it significantly reduces the rates of ischaemic cholangiopathy and early allograft dysfunction in livers [6]. Furthermore, clinical meta-analyses comparing NRP and DPP suggest that while 30-day mortality is comparable (96.9% for NRP vs. 97.0% for DPP), NRP may lower the incidence of Primary Graft Dysfunction (PGD), dropping from 21% in DPP recipients to 14% in NRP recipients, largely due to the shorter functional warm ischaemic times afforded by immediate in situ reperfusion [4].

Uncontrolled DCD: Emergency Logistics and ECMO/eCPR Integration

Uncontrolled DCD (uDCD) procedures present an immensely challenging and unpredictable logistical environment, characterised by a very narrow window for intervention before irreversible organ damage occurs. Solid organ transplantation from uDCD donors without some form of regional perfusion is highly uncommon, and current guidelines strongly recommend the use of Abdominal Normothermic Regional Perfusion (A-NRP) over standard in situ rapid flush [5, 21].

Even with the implementation of NRP, utilising solid organ grafts from uDCD donors requires extreme caution; clinical teams must continuously weigh the risk of the recipient's continued time on the waiting list against the risk of primary non-function and adverse graft outcomes [22]. Because of the unplanned nature of uDCD, emergency logistics are governed by strict time limits. Protocols typically mandate that the maximal accepted time between the initial cardiac arrest and the start of basic life support must fall between 15 and 90 min. Following this, the maximum accepted interval between the initiation of basic life support and the start of the NRP circuit is strictly limited, varying between 30 and 150 min depending on specific institutional criteria [5].

Simultaneous Thoracoabdominal Procurement: Challenges and Team Dynamics

In controlled DCD settings, the implementation of Thoraco-abdominal NRP (TA-NRP) allows the heart to be reperfused alongside the abdominal organs, providing a platform for robust physiological functional assessment and enabling DCD heart transplantation. However, this simultaneous procurement introduces complex logistical and technical challenges. If the heart functions poorly after reperfusion or requires high-dose inotropic support, adequate perfusion to the abdominal organs is immediately put at risk. Consequently, surgical teams must establish clear, pre-agreed contingency plans to rapidly convert the procedure to A-NRP or an in situ rapid flush should cardiac complications arise during the perfusion phase [23].

In a TA-NRP procurement, the team dynamics and choreography within the Operating Room are paramount. Continuous, clear communication between the abdominal surgical team, the thoracic surgical team, and the perfusionist is critical to ensuring favourable outcomes for all recovered organs. The thoracic team must practise meticulous surgical haemostasis to control caval tributaries in the chest and prevent severe blood loss from the circuit. Furthermore, to maintain strict adherence to the dead donor rule during TA-NRP, the aortic arch vessels must be securely clamped and vented to ensure there is absolutely no cerebral reperfusion while the heart is circulating blood [20, 23].

Ex Vivo Machine Perfusion: Hypothermic and Normothermic Strategies

While NRP optimises the donor organs in situ, ex vivo machine perfusion isolates the organ for physiological assessment, reconditioning, and preservation outside of the body. There is increasing evidence that utilising ex vivo organ perfusion improves overall outcomes for DCD livers and kidneys, specifically by allowing for additional viability testing before transplantation [24].

In lung transplantation, Ex Vivo Lung Perfusion (EVLP) has become a transformative logistical tool. Two widely used protocols demonstrate different logistical strategies: the Toronto EVLP method utilises an acellular perfusate within a closed circuit in a static setting, while the Organ Care System (OCS) Lung uses a portable system with a blood-based perfusate and an open left atrium [9]. EVLP not only allows teams to evaluate the metabolic activity of the lung graft, but it also provides a unique platform for targeted therapies. Because the lung is isolated from the systemic circulation, high-dose antibiotics, fibrinolytic drugs (like alteplase for pulmonary emboli), and even gene or cell-based therapies can be administered directly into the circuit without the risk of systemic toxicity to the donor or recipient [9].

For abdominal organs, hypothermic machine perfusion is frequently utilised for DCD kidneys—particularly—those recovered from uDCD settings—to—improve preservation and mitigate the high rates of delayed graft function associated with prolonged ischaemia [24].

Organ Transport: Cold Storage, Portable Perfusion, and Distance Constraints

Following procurement or perfusion, transporting the organ to the recipient hospital introduces the final logistical constraint. Traditionally, organs have been transported via static cold storage on ice. While cold storage is less logistically complex and facilitates transport across large geographical distances, it subjects the organ to ongoing cold ischaemia and prevents physiological assessment during transit [6, 9].

Portable normothermic perfusion devices (such as the OCS for hearts and lungs) mitigate ischaemic damage by maintaining the organ in a metabolically active state during transportation. However, the substantial cost and logistical complexity of deploying these specialised devices and trained personnel to distant donor hospitals limit their universal application and equitable distribution [9, 25].

To address these constraints, a "centralised organ repair hub" model is emerging. In this logistical model, donor organs are recovered at the donor hospital using standard cold preservation and then transported to a dedicated, high-volume facility equipped with EVLP and machine perfusion technology. The organs are actively reconditioned and assessed at the hub, and if accepted, are subsequently transported to the recipient hospital. By significantly extending the overall safe preservation time (splitting the cold ischaemia into two shorter periods), this centralised model allows transplant programmes to proactively optimise operating room availability, clinical staffing, and the transportation of the recipient [9, 25].

Organ-Specific Logistical Considerations (Heart, Liver, Kidney, Lung, Pancreas)

Because different organs have varying tolerances to hypoxia and hypoperfusion, DCD logistics must be tailored to the specific organs being procured. The maximum tolerable warm ischaemic time (WIT) strictly dictates the viability of the grafts.

- *Liver*: The liver is highly sensitive to warm ischaemia, and most protocols strictly limit the acceptable WIT to 20–30 min [6]. When evaluated during Normothermic Regional Perfusion (NRP), liver acceptance is ideally based on the evolution of hepatic transaminases (targeting <4x the upper limit of normal), a declining lactate trend in the perfusate, active bile production, and a macroscopic assessment showing <30% macrosteatosis [26, 27].
- *Kidneys*: Kidneys are the most resilient to ischaemic injury, tolerating a maximum WIT of up to 120 min [6]. While kidneys from uncontrolled DCD (uDCD) settings have higher rates of primary non-function, viability assessment is often based on macroscopic appearance, renal resistance on pump, and urine production—though guidelines caution against discarding a kidney solely due to the absence of urine output during perfusion [6, 24].
- *Heart*: Logistical evaluation of the heart during Thoraco-abdominal NRP (TA-NRP) involves assessing the left ventricular ejection fraction (LVEF), cardiac index, flow-volume curves, and crucially, the heart's ability to support the thoraco-abdominal circulation after the NRP circuit is weaned [23, 28].
- *Lungs*: Lungs can tolerate a WIT of approximately 60–90 min. Donor lungs are frequently subjected to aspiration injuries during the dying process. Acceptance criteria during procurement or ex vivo evaluation typically require a PaO_2/FiO_2 ratio of >300 mmHg [9, 19].
- *Pancreas*: The pancreas is generally assessed based on its macroscopic appearance, with a maximum tolerable WIT of 30–60 min [6].

Donor Selection Criteria and Organ Assessment

Standardising the identification and medical management of potential DCD donors is critical to expanding the donor pool and optimising graft survival. In addition to basic inclusion criteria—such as age limits, witnessed cardiac arrest (in uDCD cases), and low anticipated risk of transmissible diseases or cancer—clinical teams focus heavily on Donor Management Goals (DMGs) prior to the withdrawal of life-sustaining therapy (WLST) [10].

Active critical care management aims to achieve specific physiological benchmarks, such as maintaining a Mean Arterial Pressure (MAP) of 60–110 mmHg, a Central Venous Pressure (CVP) of 4–12 mmHg, a left ventricular ejection fraction ≥50%, serum sodium ≤155 mEq/L, and blood glucose ≤180 mg/dL. Achieving these goals increases the number of transplantable organs yielded per donor [10].

A major logistical hurdle in controlled DCD is accurately predicting the time of death following WLST. If the donor does not die within the acceptable ischaemic window (typically 60–90 min), the donation must be stood-down To mitigate operating room delays and resource waste, predictive models such as the DCD-N Score and the Wisconsin DCD Evaluation Tool are used. These tools evaluate independent variables such as the aetiology of neurological injury, Glasgow Coma Scale, absent reflexes, oxygenation index, and inotropic requirements to estimate the probability that a patient will expire within the necessary timeframe [29].

Ethical and Legal Framework Governing DCD Logistics

The logistics of DCD are fundamentally anchored in public trust and rigorous ethical safeguards, primarily the Dead Donor Rule, which dictates that organs can only be recovered after death is determined and that organ recovery must never cause death [11, 30].

To ensure an ethical process, there must be a strict legislative separation between the patient's end-of-life care and the organ recovery process. The decision to withdraw life support and the subsequent declaration of death must be performed by the primary healthcare team, completely independent of the Organ Procurement Organization (OPO) or transplant surgeons. To confirm the permanence of circulatory arrest and rule out autoresuscitation, a mandatory "no-touch" observation period—most commonly a continuous 5-min interval—is legally required prior to any surgical incision [14, 15].

If advanced techniques like NRP are utilised, cerebral isolation strategies are an absolute ethical mandate to prevent the reanimation of the brain once circulation is temporarily restored to the organs. For TA-NRP, the aortic arch vessels must be confirmed clamped and vented; for Abdominal-NRP, the descending thoracic aorta must be clamped and vented [5, 20, 30].

Another significant ethical debate surrounds antemortem interventions, such as the administration of systemic heparin prior to WLST to prevent micro-thrombi in the grafts. While evidence shows that premortem heparin is associated with lower rates of primary non-function and graft thrombosis—particularly in livers and pancreases—without hastening the patient's death, its use is heavily governed by localised legislation [31].

International Variation in DCD Programmes and Practices

While the Maastricht Classification provides a universal language for DCD, logistical and legal protocols vary drastically on an international scale [32, 33].

- *The No-Touch Period*: While the United States, United Kingdom, and Australia generally adhere to a 5-min observation period to confirm death, legislation in other jurisdictions, such as Italy, mandates a prolonged 20-min period of electrical asystole before death can be formally declared [15, 33].
- *Antemortem Interventions*: The permissibility of placing surgical cannula, guidewires, or administering heparin before the declaration of death differs widely. The UK and the Netherlands strictly prohibit any antemortem interventions. Conversely, Spain permits antemortem surgical cannulation. Belgium, France, Italy, and Norway allow the antemortem insertion of guidewires or catheters, and varying degrees of heparin administration. In Italy, heparin is only permitted after functional warm ischaemia begins, defined as systolic blood pressure dropping below 50 mmHg [18, 32].

Future Directions and Emerging Technologies

As DCD transplantation evolves, new logistical models and perfusion technologies are reshaping the landscape to maximise organ utilisation and alleviate hospital constraints.

Donor Care Units (DCUs) and Centralised Hubs: To reduce the logistical burden on smaller or non-specialised hospitals, "Donor Care Units" are emerging. In this model, haemodynamically stable, authorised donors are transferred to a dedicated, hospital-based ICU/OR setup specifically designed to standardise donor management and WLST [34]. Furthermore, a Centralised Organ Repair Hub model is being trialled for ex vivo lung perfusion (EVLP). Organs are procured at regional hospitals and transported to a high-volume hub where dedicated specialists perform advanced physiological assessment and reconditioning before the organs are dispatched to the final recipient hospital [9, 25].

EVLP as an Advanced Therapeutic Platform: Normothermic machine perfusion is no longer just a preservation tool; it is evolving into a platform for targeted interventions. Because the organ is isolated outside the body, localised therapies can be administered at doses that would be systemically toxic to a living patient. Current clinical and pre-clinical applications on the EVLP circuit include:

- *Fibrinolysis*: Administering alteplase or urokinase directly into the circuit to dissolve pulmonary emboli in DCD lungs.
- *High-Dose Antimicrobials*: Administering high-dose broad-spectrum antibiotics to clear bacterial loads [9].
- *Light Therapy*: Using Ultraviolet C (UVC) irradiation integrated into the EVLP circuit to safely reduce viral loads, which has been shown to prevent the transmission of Hepatitis C from an HCV-positive donor to a recipient [35].
- *Surfactant and Gene Therapy*: Utilising intra-airway lavage and surfactant replacement to repair aspiration injuries, or utilising adenoviral vectors for anti-inflammatory IL-10 gene therapy [9].

Conclusion

Donation after Circulatory Death is a highly complex but an established and effective pathway. That has successfully expanded the global organ donor pool. Unlike Donation after Brain Death, DCD requires surgical teams and Organ Procurement Organizations to operate within strict ischaemic time constraints, while adhering strictly to the ethical boundaries of the dead donor rule and the separation of end-of-life care. Through the integration of standardised donor management goals, predictive end-of-life scoring tools, and emerging technologies like Normothermic Regional Perfusion and Ex Vivo Machine Perfusion, the historical limitations of DCD are progressively being overcome.. As international frameworks continue to adapt to these advances, DCD grafts are increasingly achieving outcomes that rival standard criteria brain-dead donors, offering viable alternatives for patients on transplant waiting lists worldwide.

Competing Interests The author(s) has no competing interests to declare that are relevant to the content of this manuscript.

Ethics Approval The author(s) declares that this manuscript does not include primary research with human participants.

The author(s) declares that this manuscript does not include primary studies involving animals.

References

1. Husain SA, Motter JD, Stewart D, et al. Changes in organ donation after circulatory death in the United States. JAMA. 2026;335(12):1087–9. https://doi.org/10.1001/jama.2026.0976.
2. Finotti M, Wall A, D'Alessandro A, et al. The Dallas Donation after Circulatory Death Transplantation Summit: expanding donation after circulatory death procedures through process improvement, broader utilization, and innovation. HepatoBiliary Surg Nutr. 2024;13(5):82436–836. https://doi.org/10.21037/hbsn-23-503.
3. Thuong M, Ruiz A, Evrard P, et al. New classification of donation after circulatory death donors definitions and terminology. Transpl Int. 2016;29(7):749–59. https://doi.org/10.1111/tri.12776.

4. Jolliffe J, Brookes J, Williams M, et al. Donation after circulatory death transplantation: a systematic review and meta-analysis of outcomes and methods of donation. Ann Cardiothorac Surg. 2025;14(1):117–27. https://doi.org/10.21037/acs-2024-dcd-0132.
5. Jochmans I, Hessheimer AJ, Neyrinck AP, et al. Consensus statement on normothermic regional perfusion in donation after circulatory death: report from the European Society for Organ Transplantation's Transplant Learning Journey. Transpl Int. 2021;34(11):2019–30. https://doi.org/10.1111/tri.13951.
6. UK guidelines on transplantation from deceased donors after circulatory death. British Transplantation Society. August 1, 2023. https://bts.org.uk/transplantation-from-deceased-donors-after-circulatory-death/. Accessed 15 May 2026.
7. Williams AM, Ahmad A, Trahanas J, et al. Ten-minute asystolic warm ischemic time (AWIT) predicts mortality and severe primary graft dysfunction in donation after circulatory death hearts recovered with thoracoabdominal normothermic regional perfusion. J Heart Lung Transplant. 2026;45(4):555–65. https://doi.org/10.1016/j.healun.2025.07.015.
8. Wang CC, Petrovic M, Ahmad A, et al. The effect of warm ischemic intervals on primary graft dysfunction in normothermic regional perfusion for donation after circulatory death heart transplant. J Thorac Cardiovasc Surg. 2025;170(4):1109–1116.e3. https://doi.org/10.1016/j.jtcvs.2025.03.037.
9. Watanabe T, Cypel M, Keshavjee S. Ex vivo lung perfusion. J Thorac Dis. 2021;13(11):6602–17. https://doi.org/10.21037/jtd-2021-23.
10. Franklin GA, Santos AP, Smith JW, Galbraith S, Harbrecht BG, Garrison RN. Optimization of donor management goals yields increased organ use. Am Surg. 2010;76(6):587–94. https://doi.org/10.1177/000313481007600621.
11. Vergano M, Metaxa V, Citerio G. Ten ethical challenges in donation after circulatory death (DCD): a practical guide for intensivists. Intensive Care Med. 2026;52(1):170–2. https://doi.org/10.1007/s00134-025-08229-w.
12. DCD-ICSI-Guideline.pdf. https://jficmi.anaesthesia.ie/wp-content/uploads/2017/05/DCD-ICSI-Guideline.pdf. Accessed 15 May 2026.
13. ASA Statement on Controlled Organ Donation after Circulatory Death. American Society of Anesthesiologists. Available at: asahq.org.
14. AST-ASTS Statement on DCD. American Society of Transplantation. https://www.myast.org/ast-asts-statement-on-dcd. Accessed 15 May 2026.
15. Zorko DJ, Shemie J, Hornby L, et al. Autoresuscitation after circulatory arrest: an updated systematic review. Can J Anaesth. 2023;70(4):699–712. https://doi.org/10.1007/s12630-023-02411-8.
16. Sheth KN, Nutter T, Stein DM, Scalea TM, Bernat JL. Autoresuscitation after asystole in patients being considered for organ donation. Crit Care Med. 2012;40(1):158–61. https://doi.org/10.1097/CCM.0b013e31822f0b2a.
17. Kelso CM, Lyckholm LJ, Coyne PJ, Smith TJ. Palliative care consultation in the process of organ donation after cardiac death. J Palliat Med. 2007;10(1):118–26. https://doi.org/10.1089/jpm.2006.0118.
18. O'Rourke J, Crowe G, Turner R, Gaffney A. Donation after circulatory death: a narrative review of current controversies, attitudes, and the evolving role of regional perfusion technology. AME Med J. 2024;9(0) https://doi.org/10.21037/amj-23-65.
19. Van Raemdonck D, Van Slambrouck J, Ceulemans LJ. Donor lung preservation for transplantation—where do we go from here? J Thorac Dis. 2022;14(9):3125–30. https://doi.org/10.21037/jtd-22-949.
20. ASTS Statement on Thoracoabdominal Normothermic Regional Perfusion Donation after Circulatory Determination of Death (TA-NRP DCD).
21. Pionnier Y, Darius T, Penaloza A, et al. Solid organ transplantation originating from uncontrolled donation after circulatory death in Europe: a narrative review. Scand J Trauma Resusc Emerg Med. 2024;32:130. https://doi.org/10.1186/s13049-024-01305-y.

22. Pinho A, Sampaio S, Alencastre I, et al. Kidney transplantation from uncontrolled donation after circulatory death maintained by normothermic regional perfusion: an 8-year Portuguese single-centre experience. Transpl Int. 2025;38:14651. https://doi.org/10.3389/ti.2025.14651.
23. Hoffman JRH, Hartwig MG, Cain MT, et al. Consensus statement: technical standards for thoracoabdominal normothermic regional perfusion. Transplantation. 2024;108(8):1669–80. https://doi.org/10.1097/TP.0000000000005101.
24. Kang M, Kim S, Choi JY, et al. Ex vivo kidney machine perfusion: meta-analysis of randomized clinical trials. Br J Surg. 2024;111(4):znae102. https://doi.org/10.1093/bjs/znae102.
25. Ragheb K, et al. A narrative review on ex vivo lung perfusion: up-to-date role in lung transplantation. Current Challenges in Thoracic Surgery 2025. Available at: ccts.amegroups.org/article/view/96957/html.
26. Steinberg I, Patrono D, De Cesaris E, et al. Viability assessment of livers donated after circulatory determination of death during normothermic regional perfusion. Artif Organs. 2023;47(10):1592–603. https://doi.org/10.1111/aor.14622.
27. Schurink IJ, van de Leemkolk FEM, Fondevila C, et al. Donor eligibility criteria and liver graft acceptance criteria during normothermic regional perfusion: A systematic review. Liver Transplant. 2022;28(10):1563–75. https://doi.org/10.1002/lt.26512.
28. Bona M, Wyss RK, Arnold M, et al. Cardiac graft assessment in the era of machine perfusion: current and future biomarkers. J Am Heart Assoc Cardiovasc Cerebrovasc Dis. 2021;10(4):e018966. https://doi.org/10.1161/JAHA.120.018966.
29. Nijhoff MF, Pol RA, Volbeda M, et al. External validation of the DCD-N score and a linear prediction model to identify potential candidates for organ donation after circulatory death: a nationwide multicenter cohort study. Transplantation. 2021;105(6):1311–6. https://doi.org/10.1097/TP.0000000000003430.
30. Wall AE, Fiedler A, Karp S, Shah A, Testa G. Applying the ethical framework for donation after circulatory death to thoracic normothermic regional perfusion procedures. Am J Transplant. 2022;22(5):1311–5. https://doi.org/10.1111/ajt.16959.
31. Honarmand K, Alshamsi F, Foroutan F, et al. Antemortem heparin in organ donation after circulatory death determination: a systematic review of the literature. Transplantation. 2021;105(12):e337–46. https://doi.org/10.1097/TP.0000000000003793.
32. Domínguez-Gil B, Ascher N, Capron AM, et al. Expanding controlled donation after the circulatory determination of death: statement from an international collaborative. Intensive Care Med. 2021;47(3):265–81. https://doi.org/10.1007/s00134-020-06341-7.
33. Wind J, Faut M, van Smaalen TC, van Heurn EL. Variability in protocols on donation after circulatory death in Europe. Crit Care. 2013;17(5):R217. https://doi.org/10.1186/cc13034.
34. Emily A, Vail MD, Varun K, Goyal MD, Ashley C, McGinity MD, et al. Best practices for hospital-based donor care unit operations. Chest Crit Care. 2025;3(2):100144. https://doi.org/10.1016/j.chstcc.2025.100144.
35. Cypel M, Feld JJ, Galasso M, et al. Prevention of viral transmission during lung transplantation with hepatitis C-viraemic donors: an open-label, single-centre, pilot trial. Lancet Respir Med. 2020;8(2):192–201. https://doi.org/10.1016/S2213-2600(19)30268-1.

National Framework for DCD Organ Allocation: Indian Context

10

Anil Kumar and Vivek B. Kute

Abbreviations

ALT	Alanine Aminotransferase
AMI	Antemortem Interventions
AST	Aspartate Aminotransferase
ASTS	American Society of Transplant Surgeons
BSD	Brain-Stem Death
cDCD	Controlled Donation after Circulatory Death
CRRT	Continuous Renal Replacement Therapy
DCD	Donation after Circulatory Death
DDR	Dead Donor Rule
DGF	Delayed Graft Function
ECMO	Extracorporeal Membrane Oxygenation
fWIT	functional warm ischaemia time
HMP	Hypothermic Machine Perfusion
ICU	Intensive care unit
IT	Information Technology
MELD	Model for End-stage Liver Disease
NMP	Normothermic Machine Perfusion
NOTTO	National Organ and Tissue Transplant Organization

A. Kumar
National Organ and Tissue Transplant Organization (NOTTO), Directorate General of Health Services, Ministry of Health & Family Welfare, Government of India, New Delhi, Delhi, India
e-mail: dr.anilkumar@nic.in; dir@notto.nic.in

V. B. Kute (✉)
Department of Nephrology, Institute of Kidney Diseases and Research Center-Institute of Transplantation Sciences, Ahmedabad, India

S. P. Kolte et al. (eds.), *Organ Donation After Circulatory Death*,
https://doi.org/10.1007/978-981-92-6377-6_10

NRP	Normothermic Regional Perfusion
OPTN	Organ Procurement and Transplantation Network
OT	Operation Theater
PIO	Persons of Indian Origin
ROTTO	Regional Organ and Tissue Transplant Organizations
SOPs	Standard Operating Procedures
SOTTO	State Organ and Tissue Transplant Organization
THOTA	Transplantation of Human Organs and Tissues Act
TTS-ISODP	The Transplantation Society–International Society for Organ Donation and Procurement
WLST	Withdrawal of Life-Sustaining Treatment

Overview of Organ Transplantation in India and the Case for Donation After Circulatory Death (DCD)

India's organ transplantation program has grown substantially since the enforcement of the Transplantation of Human Organs and Tissues Act (THOTA) in 1994. India is ranked as third worldwide in volume considering the substantial rise in the total number of transplants from 4990 in 2013 to 18,911 in 2024 [1]. However, this accomplishment is shadowed by a profound imbalance: India simultaneously leads the world in living donor transplants. The deceased organ donor rate in India (approximately 0.81 per million population in 2024) remains comparable to the Southeast Asian average of 0.76 per million population, but well below from the global average of 8.67 per million population [2]. A large population of patients still constitutes a large cohort for renal waitlist; many of them spend years on dialysis before a transplant becomes available. Road accidents, cerebrovascular accidents, and head injuries generate a substantial pool of patients who suffer catastrophic, non-survivable brain injuries yet do not progress to meet strict brain-stem death (BSD) criteria. These individuals are potential controlled DCD (cDCD) candidates, and represent the most immediate addressable structural gap in India's deceased donation system.

DCD accounted for approximately 28% of total 47,180 deceased donors worldwide in 2024, while in many Western countries, cDCD now exceeds 50% of all deceased donors [3]. In India, the pathway is legally permissible as THOTA 1994 explicitly defines a deceased person in both neurological and cardiopulmonary terms [4], but it remains largely unclaimed in practice due to ethical ambiguity around Withdrawal of Life-Sustaining Treatment (WLST), and limited infrastructure for time-critical organ preservation. There is a felt need for having standardized national guidelines. This chapter outlines the framework within which addresses the gap.

Legal and Ethical Framework

Is DCD Permissible Under Indian Law?

This question is settled affirmatively by the statute itself. THOTA 1994 defines a "Deceased person" as a person in whom permanent disappearance of all evidence of life occurs, by reason of brain-stem death or in a cardiopulmonary sense at any time after live birth has taken place [4]. This dual definition (neurological or cardiopulmonary) explicitly recognizes circulatory death as a valid basis for the deceased donor pathway. However, there has been a lack of the standardized practice, nationally, including uniform protocols for WLST, death determination, no-touch periods, and organ procurement that are fully consistent with the statute and with the ethical obligations of the clinical community.

The 2023 Supreme Court judgment [5] in "Common Cause vs. Union of India" has provided the procedural architecture for WLST that was previously missing. The judgment mandates: (a) evaluation of futility of care by a Primary Medical Board; (b) review by a Secondary Medical Board comprising a nominee of the district Chief Medical Officer and two independent experts; (c) informed consent of the next of kin; and (d) intimation to a judicial magistrate prior to initiating WLST. While this process is more time-consuming compared to WLST frameworks prevailing in Europe or North America, it provides the clear medico-legal path within which cDCD category III becomes feasible in India.

The Dead Donor Rule (DDR) and Its Application to DCD

DDR, which defines that organ procurement must occur after death and must not itself cause death, underscores all ethical frameworks for deceased donation worldwide. In DCD, the DDR is satisfied by two requirements: First, death must be accurately declared by cardiorespiratory criteria before any incision for organ recovery; and second, the stand-off (no-touch) period must be observed to exclude autoresuscitation [6]. The determination of circulatory death in DCD is based on the irreversible or, in some frameworks, the permanent cessation of circulatory and respiratory functions. There is an ongoing international philosophical debate about whether "5 minutes of asystole" truly constitutes irreversibility or merely permanence at that point in time—a distinction that matters because the heart could theoretically be restarted if resuscitation were attempted [6]. The prevailing consensus, endorsed by the Transplantation Society–International Society for Organ Donation and Procurement (TTS-ISODP), and the UK Academy of Medical Royal Colleges, is that permanence (confirmed by the formal decision not to attempt resuscitation) is sufficient to satisfy the DDR, provided that the stand-off period is scrupulously observed [7].

The Modified Maastricht Classification

The Modified Maastricht Classification [8] provides a standardized international framework for categorizing DCD donors based on the circumstances of cardiac arrest (Table 10.1). The Indian transplant community's 2022 joint position paper and the 2024 consensus statements recommend category III as India's primary DCD pathway [9].

Ethical Boundaries

Several ethical issues are associated with DCD and must be explicitly addressed in a national framework.

- *Separation of Care from Donation*: The decision to withdraw life support must be made entirely independently of any consideration of organ donation. The treating team (intensivists, neurologists, neurosurgeons) must not include members of the transplant team, and the transplant coordinator may approach the family only after the WLST decision has been finalized and documented.
- *Antemortem Interventions (AMI)*: Procedures performed before death (heparinization, femoral cannulation, etc.) benefit the potential recipient. They are ethically permissible only with specific, explicit written informed consent from the family/legal representative, obtained after the WLST decision and entirely separate from the consent for donation.
- *Conflicts of Interest*: The perpetual risk that a treating team's clinical decisions might be influenced by the transplant team's desire for organs requires structural safeguards: formal firewalls, audit mechanisms, and independent ethics committee review.
- *Socio-cultural Context*: India's multi-religious and cultural landscape generates additional sensitivities around end-of-life decision-making, withdrawal of support, and body handling after cardiac death. Effective DCD programs include

Table 10.1 Modified Maastricht classification

Category	Name	Description
I	Found dead	Cardiac arrest outside (IA) or inside (IB) hospital with no attempt at resuscitation. Uncontrolled DCD
II	Witnessed cardiac arrest	Sudden cardiac arrest with unsuccessful resuscitation—out-of-hospital (IIA) or in-hospital (IIB). Uncontrolled
III	Controlled DCD	Anticipated cardiac arrest following planned WLST in a patient with irreversible brain injury who does not meet full brain-stem death criteria. Most common pathway
IV	Controlled	Cardiac arrest occurs after brain death is diagnosed but before organ recovery begins
V	Unexpected arrest	Unexpected cardiac arrest in a hospitalized patient

DCD Donation after Circulatory Death, *WLST* Withdrawal of Life-Sustaining Treatment community engagement, culturally sensitive communication, and religious leader involvement in awareness campaigns.

Clinical Framework: WLST, Stand-Off (No-Touch) Period, and Stepwise Protocol

WLST

In the context of cDCD (category III), WLST refers to a carefully planned and intentional decision to stop all medical interventions that are maintaining body's circulation and respiration in a patient whose continued treatment has been determined to be ineffective. The components of WLST include stopping mechanical ventilation, extubation, discontinuation of vasopressors and inotropes, cessation of Continuous Renal Replacement Therapy (CRRT), and removal of Extracorporeal Membrane Oxygenation (ECMO) support, if any [8, 9] (Fig. 10.1).

A fundamental principle—mentioned in all national DCD protocols and consistent with the 2023 Supreme Court framework [5]—is that medical staff involved in organ procurement or transplantation surgery are strictly excluded from participating in the WLST process. This separation is not merely procedural but purely ethical: the dying patient's care must remain the uncompromised responsibility of the treating team alone. In India, the current reality is that most terminally ill patients with catastrophic brain injuries who do not meet BSD criteria are discharged against medical advice or leave the ICU informally, dying shortly thereafter at home or in transit [8]. This approach—while understandable in light of financial constraints and cultural norms—forecloses the DCD opportunity entirely. A national DCD program requires a shift: patients and families must be offered an option of a planned and dignified end-of-life care pathway within the hospital, with the knowledge that their decision for WLST may also enable life-saving organ donation for needy patients.

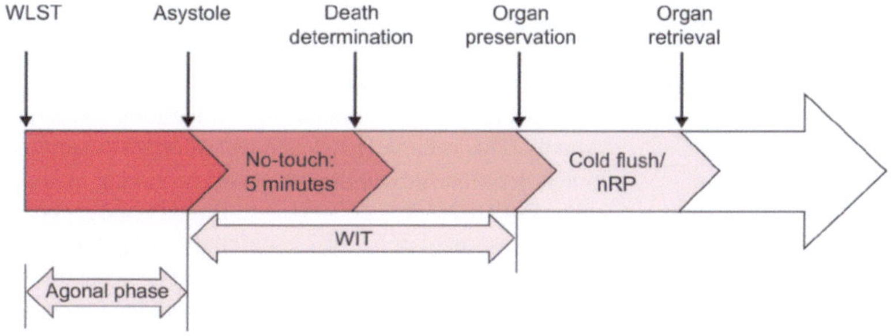

Fig. 10.1 Pathway for cDCD category III. cDCD Controlled Donation after Circulatory Death, nRP Normothermic Regional Perfusion, WIT Warm Ischaemia Time, WLST Withdrawal of Life-Sustaining Treatment

The Stand-Off (No-Touch) Period

Following asystole, a mandatory waiting period (typically 5 min) is observed by the medical team before death is declared. This stand-off period exists to ensure that autoresuscitation (spontaneous return of circulation, the Lazarus phenomenon) does not occur [10]. The 5-min standard is endorsed by the UK, USA, Australia, and the 2024 consensus paper [8]. No interventions whatsoever, including organ preservation, may be initiated during this period. The procurement team may not be allowed to enter the room. The declaration of death is made by the treating physician; then after only the retrieval team takes over.

It bears emphasis that the stand-off period is not the only determinant of DCD feasibility. The functional warm ischemia time (fWIT), defined as the period from the point when systolic blood pressure falls below 50 mmHg (or SpO^2 <70%) to the onset of organ cooling or Normothermic Regional Perfusion (NRP), is the clinically critical interval. Previous research (2024) demonstrated that fWIT is a significant predictor of DCD kidney transplant outcomes [11]. The Organ Procurement and Transplantation Network (OPTN) recommendation is to allow waiting up to 4 h for DCD kidney donation as long as fWIT remains below 30 min [11]. For liver, fWIT limits are stricter: most programs specify a maximum of 20–30 min [12].

Stepwise cDCD Protocol for India

Table 10.2 presents the proposed stepwise cDCD protocol for India, prepared from the National Organ and Tissue Transplant Organization (NOTTO) operational framework, 2022 joint position paper and 2024 consensus paper, and the 2023 Supreme Court WLST guidelines.

Table 10.2 Stepwise protocol for controlled DCD (category III) in India

Step	Stage	Action/details
1	Patient identification	Patient with catastrophic, non-recoverable brain injury dependent on life-sustaining treatment but not meeting brain-stem death criteria—potential cDCD category III candidate
2	Futility decision	Treating team (intensivists, neurosurgeons) determines in consultation with the family that continued support is futile. Decision documented formally. This is entirely independent of organ donation consideration
3	WLST documentation	Formal decision for withdrawal of life-sustaining treatment (WLST) and/or DNR/DNAR is documented. Primary and secondary medical boards constituted as per 2023 supreme court guidelines
4	Referral firewall	Only after the WLST decision is finalized does the transplant coordinator receive notification to approach the family separately for donation counseling
5	Consent	Separate, specific informed consents obtained for: (a) withdrawal of support; (b) organ donation; (c) antemortem interventions (heparinization, femoral cannulation) where applicable

(continued)

Table 10.2 (continued)

Step	Stage	Action/details
6	WLST execution	Controlled withdrawal—stopping ventilation, extubation, cessation of inotropes, vasoconstrictors, CRRT, ECMO—performed by treating physician, not the transplant team
7	Asystole	Onset of cardiac arrest is noted and timed precisely
8	Stand-off period	Mandatory 5-min (minimum) no-touch observation period to confirm irreversibility of circulatory cessation—satisfying the Dead Donor Rule
9	Death declaration	Treating physician—not the transplant team—declares death based on cardiorespiratory criteria
10	Organ preservation	Immediately after declaration, retrieval team initiates rapid cannulation, cold flush (in situ cooling) or NRP. Final procurement decision after surgeon visually assesses organ condition
11	Recovery	Standard surgical organ retrieval proceeds. Recipient team activated in parallel from step 4 onwards

cDCD Controlled Donation after Circulatory Death, *CRRT* Continuous Renal Replacement Therapy, *DNAR* Do Not Attempt Resuscitation, *DNR* Do Not Resuscitate, *ECMO* Extracorporeal Membrane Oxygenation, *NRP* Normothermic Regional Perfusion, *WLST* Withdrawal of Life-Sustaining Treatment

Organizational Framework and Organ Allocation Architecture

India's Three-Tier Network

India's deceased donation and organ allocation program operates through a hierarchical three-tier structure under THOTA 1994 and the 2014 Rules [4]. At the apex is NOTTO—the National Organ and Tissue Transplant Organization under the Ministry of Health and Family Welfare—which maintains the national waitlist, issues Unique IDs to all registered patients, and oversees the policy and coordination across the country. Below NOTTO are five Regional Organ and Tissue Transplant Organizations (ROTTOs) and 26 State Organ and Tissue Transplant Organizations (SOTTOs), with more than 1000 registered hospitals (transplant/retrieval hospitals) as the operational units at the ground level [1, 13]. Organ allocation follows a tiered geographic priority: organs are first offered to registered recipients on the Hospital List (the donor hospital's in-house waitlist), followed by the State List (SOTTO), Regional List (ROTTO), and finally the National List (NOTTO). Special provisions apply to Persons of Indian Origin (PIO) and foreigners too. This structure, though designed for BSD donation, provides the foundational framework within which DCD allocation can be put into operation—with critical modifications to account for time sensitivity.

Why DCD Allocation Demands a Different Algorithm

DCD allocation is fundamentally more time-pressured than BSD allocation. Table 10.3 presents the key algorithmic differences between the two pathways. The most significant operational difference is the starting point of allocation planning. In

Table 10.3 Allocation algorithm differences—DCD vs DBD/BSD

Feature	Donation after brain death (DBD/BSD)	Donation after circulatory death (DCD)
Time sensitivity	Moderate—Donor is stable in ICU; adequate time for logistics and recipient workup	Critical—Organs undergo progressive warm ischemia; every minute from WLST to procurement counts
Allocation priority	National/regional waitlist based on medical urgency (MELD/SOFA) and waiting time	Local or regional priority to minimize cold ischemia and transport time; fast-track protocol mandatory
Fast-tracking	Less common; standard offer–accept workflow	Routinely employed; backup recipient lists activated simultaneously
Organ types routinely transplanted	Heart, lungs, liver, kidneys, pancreas, intestine—full complement	Primarily kidneys and liver; heart and lungs only with advanced NRP; pancreas selectively
Allocation start point	After BSD declaration, allocation begins sequentially	Allocation planning starts before WLST—recipient matching, blood group/HLA sampling, transport booking, OR scheduling [9, 10]
Role of machine perfusion	Optional; used to extend viability or assess marginal organs	Near mandatory for liver/heart; NRP and HMP substantially improve DCD organ utilization and outcomes
Key coordinator role	Sequential communication—NOTTO → ROTTO/SOTTO → transplant centers	Parallel, real-time communication—All stakeholders simultaneously looped in from the outset

BSD Brain-Stem Death, *DBD* Donation after Brain Death, *DCD* Donation after Circulatory Death, *HLA* Human Leukocyte Antigen, *HMP* Hypothermic Machine Perfusion, *MELD* Model for End-stage Liver Disease, *NOTTO* National Organ and Tissue Transplant Organization, *NRP* Normothermic Regional Perfusion, *ROTTO* Regional Organ and Tissue Transplant Organization, *SOFA* Sequential Organ Failure Assessment, *SOTTO* State Organ and Tissue Transplant Organization, *WLST* Withdrawal of Life-Sustaining Treatment

BSD donation, the allocation process typically begins after brain death declaration. In DCD, allocation preparation must begin before WLST—during the donor workup phase [8]. Preliminary recipient matching, histocompatibility assessment, blood group confirmation, and transport planning must all be completed, or substantially advanced, before WLST is executed. This requires a fundamentally parallel rather than sequential workflow, and it demands that the NOTTO-ROTTO-SOTTO communication chain be activated simultaneously with—not after—the donor referral.

Principles of an Effective DCD Allocation System

An effective DCD allocation system must be governed by six core principles, reflecting both the clinical realities of DCD and the ethical obligations of the transplant community:

- *Equity*: Every suitable recipient on the waitlist must have fair access to available organs according to pre-defined, transparent allocation policies—without advantage to patients of better-resourced centers or states.

- *Utility*: Organs must be allocated to maximize graft survival, recipient survival, and overall transplant benefits, particularly important for DCD organs, where ischemic preconditioning already constrains the margin for suboptimal matching.
- *Timeliness*: Allocation must occur with sufficient speed to minimize warm and cold ischemia. In DCD, time is not a resource to be managed but it is the central constraint of the entire process.
- *Transparency*: All allocation decisions must be traceable, auditable, and should follow standardized protocols. Annual reports on DCD-specific outcomes may be published by the hospitals.
- *Organ Stewardship*: Every potentially transplantable organ must be evaluated appropriately, with DCD-specific acceptance criteria that neither over- nor under-utilize organs based on ischemia risk alone.
- *Collaboration*: DCD allocation cannot function as sequential communication but it requires continuous, real-time, parallel coordination between the donor hospital, NOTTO/ROTTO/SOTTO, histocompatibility laboratories, transport services, and recipient transplant centers.

Factors Affecting DCD Organ Utilization

DCD organ utilization is multifactorial, which is determined by donor factors, recipient factors, and logistical factors that differ in their relative weighting from BSD donation.

Donor Factors

Donor factors such as donor age, the nature and severity of the underlying illness or injury, hemodynamic stability in the ICU prior to WLST, oxygenation status, baseline organ function (particularly creatinine for kidney and AST/ALT for liver), the anticipated duration of the dying process after WLST, and the actual functional warm ischemia time determine the type of and number of transplantable organs from any given DCD donor.

Recipient Factors

Medical urgency particularly for liver recipients where Model for End-Stage Liver Disease (MELD) score predicts short-term mortality on the waitlist—blood group and size compatibility, immunological sensitization (panel reactive antibody status), the ability of the recipient to reach the transplant center rapidly, and the institutional expertise of the recipient center in managing DCD organs and their specific complications (delayed graft function for kidneys; ischemic cholangiopathy for livers) all govern the recipient selection.

Logistical Factors

Geographic distance, organ transport time and modality (road versus aviation), operation theater readiness at both donor and recipient hospitals, availability of retrieval teams trained in DCD procurement, determine whether a medically suitable organ can actually be transplanted within its acceptable ischemia window. Access to machine perfusion equipment is expected to improve the outcome of transplantation especially in marginal organs. Study (2025) demonstrated that NRP-procured DCD livers had a significantly lower 6-month ischemic cholangiopathy rate (1.2%) compared to static cold storage (9.5%), underscoring that logistical investment in machine perfusion translates directly into clinical outcomes [14].

Time-Critical Coordination and Communication

Communication Pathways

Communication is the operational backbone of DCD allocation. The underlying principle is that real-time communication reduces ischemia time and improves organ utilization. India's existing NOTTO infrastructure—the national waitlist and unique ID system—provides a foundation. It requires addition of DCD-specific real-time tracking modules, automated recipient matching triggered by donor referral, and a 24-h on-call escalation protocol at every ROTTO and SOTTO.

Backup Allocation Strategies

DCD allocation is inherently unpredictable. Delayed or absent circulatory arrest after WLST, which occurs in approximately 10–20% of cases even in experienced programs, organ quality deterioration, positive crossmatch, transport failures, and recipient unavailability are the possible causes of allocation failure [9]. Below are the strategies for these contingencies:

- *Backup Recipient Lists*: Alternative recipients must be identified and held on standby before WLST is initiated.
- *Backup Transport Pathways*: Alternative air or road transport arrangements must be confirmed and put on standby. Preplanned green corridor authorizations for road transport of DCD organs—a model already used in Indian BSD donation—must be extended to DCD retrievals.
- *Stand-Down Protocol*: If circulatory arrest does not occur within the clinically acceptable timeframe (typically 60–120 min post-WLST in kidney-only programs, shorter for liver/heart) [8], the patient is returned to the ICU and put on full supportive care. This stand-down possibility must be explained to the family before consent. The expectation that death may not occur within the operative window is a unique feature of cDCD that distinguishes it from BSD donation and requires explicit family counseling.

Organ Salvage Techniques: Feasibility and Cost in India

The degree to which DCD organs are exposed to warm ischemic injury and the degree to which that injury can be reversed or limited are determined by the organ salvage technique employed. Table 10.4 summarizes the three principal techniques, their feasibility in the Indian context, and their cost implications.

The evidence base for machine perfusion in DCD has strengthened considerably. Hosgood et al. demonstrated in a 2023 Nature Medicine randomized controlled trial that normothermic machine perfusion (NMP) significantly reduced delayed graft function compared to static cold storage in DCD kidney transplantation [15]. Oniscu et al. showed in a 2023 Transplantation analysis that in situ NRP improved organ utilization and transplant outcomes in cDCD across UK centers [11]. The 2024 systematic review confirms that both NMP and NRP are feasible strategies that may increase utilization of DCD kidneys while maintaining acceptable outcomes [15].

Table 10.4 Organ salvage techniques for DCD—feasibility and cost in the Indian context

Technique	Description	Feasibility in India	Cost implication
In situ cooling (rapid cold flush)	Cold preservation solution flushed via femoral cannulas immediately after stand-off period to cool abdominal organs in situ	High—feasible in most tertiary hospitals with standard OT/ICU infrastructure	Moderate—cannulas, HTK or UW solution, disposables
NRP	ECMO-based circuit restores warm oxygenated circulation to abdominal organs post-death; reverses ischemic injury; enables functional organ assessment before acceptance	Low to medium—Technically complex; requires ECMO, trained perfusionists, specialized teams	Very high—capital equipment + per-case consumables; currently limited to 3–4 centers
HMP	Oxygenated cold perfusion of procured organs ex vivo; standard for kidneys; increasingly used for livers. Reduces DGF rates by ~40% in randomized controlled trial data	Medium—Growing availability; requires portable perfusion devices	High—device cost; per-case consumables; trained personnel
NMP	Ex vivo warm oxygenated perfusion; allows real-time viability assessment (lactate, bile production, perfusion parameters) before transplantation	Low—highly specialized; very few Indian centers	Very high—most expensive strategy; best evidence for DCD liver viability assessment

DCD Donation after Circulatory Death, *DGF* Delayed Graft Function, *ECMO* Extracorporeal Membrane Oxygenation, *HMP* Hypothermic Machine Perfusion, *HTK* Histidine-Tryptophan-Ketoglutarate, *ICU* Intensive Care Unit, *NMP* Normothermic Machine Perfusion, *NRP* Normothermic Regional Perfusion, *OT* Operation Theater, *UW* University of Wisconsin preservation solution

For India's nascent DCD program, the practical starting point is in situ cooling—technically straightforward, feasible in any tertiary hospital with standard operation theater (OT) infrastructure equipped with cannulas, preservation solution, and basic surgical skills. As experience and funding allow, a phased introduction of Hypothermic Machine Perfusion (HMP) for kidneys (given the level-1 evidence for DGF reduction) and ultimately NRP for livers (given the ischemic cholangiopathy prevention data) should form the machine perfusion roadmap [13, 15].

Challenges, Controversies, and the Way Forward

Ethical and Legal Challenges

The most consistent ethical challenge in DCD is maintaining the absolute separation between the decision to withdraw life support and the consideration of organ donation. This is the foundation of public trust in the program. Any perception that a patient's care might be compromised, or a death hastened, for the benefit of a transplant recipient would be catastrophically damaging to deceased donation program.

The NRP controversy deserves specific mention. Critics argue that initiating NRP calls into question whether the "cessation of circulation" criterion used to declare death remains intact. The dominant international consensus says that NRP does not violate the DDR provided that: (a) cerebral and cardiac perfusion are occluded; (b) the no-touch period was fully observed before NRP initiation; and (c) the death declaration was made independently of and prior to NRP commencement [16]. Standardized NRP protocols, including the consensus statement from the Society of Thoracic Surgeons, provide the technical framework [17].

Operational and Infrastructural Challenges

India's operational challenges are substantial and should not be underestimated. Coordinating with ICU teams, transplant coordinators, retrieval surgeons, preservation equipment, operation theaters, and transport simultaneously and often under time pressure is not easy. Doing this in a system that has not previously run a DCD program is even more challenging. The timely consent process is particularly challenging given the very short window between WLST decision and potential donation during which families are dealing with profound grief while being asked to make complex decisions about multiple interventions posing an enormous emotional and practical burden. There are also some very practical hurdles. Limited experience with post-mortem ECMO, NRP, and normothermic perfusion is still limited. The costs are higher compared to BSD donation; and there are no clear mechanisms to manage financial risks when organs are not used or donors stand down. These issues require policy solutions including cost reimbursement frameworks and clear medico-legal guidance on donor management costs rather than clinical workarounds.

The Way Forward articulated in NOTTO's operational plan includes:

- Pilot DCD programs in major tertiary hospitals.
- National DCD guidelines and standard operating procedures aligned with THOTA.
- Streamlined medico-legal handling.
- Integrated awareness campaigns.
- Dedicated on-call retrieval teams with access to preservation fluids, operation theaters, and green corridor logistics [1].

DBD First, DCD Complementary

A crucial principle for India's program design is that DCD should be positioned as complementary to DBD donation but not as a replacement. Countries with established DCD programs achieved their donation rates in addition to DBD. The concern that an easier DCD pathway might reduce the aggressiveness of neurocritical care—thereby lowering BSD donation rates [18]—is a legitimate risk that India's program design must specifically address through training, incentives, and audits. Transplant coordinators and ICU staff must be equipped and motivated to pursue BSD pathways simultaneously and prioritize them when feasible.

The Role of Technology

Digital tools have the potential to transform DCD allocation in India. Real-time organ allocation software with automated recipient matching—triggered by donor referral rather than donation confirmation—would compress the allocation timeline substantially. Organ tracking systems, predictive analytics for expected fWIT based on donor hemodynamics, and AI-assisted logistics optimization for transport routing are all technologies that could be integrated into the NOTTO national registry platform at relatively low cost given existing IT infrastructure [1]. Machine perfusion systems with built-in organ viability assessment—lactate clearance, transaminase washout, bile production—provide real-time graft quality data that transform the organ acceptance decision from a clinical estimate into an evidence-based calculation.

Feasibility in India: Untapped Donor Pool

The epidemiological case for DCD in India is compelling. India has one of the world's highest burdens of road traffic accident trauma: over 1.73 lakh of *road accident fatalities* were reported by States/UTs as per the report "Road Accidents in India 2023" of Ministry of Road Transport and Highways.

A substantial proportion of these patients suffer catastrophic, non-survivable brain injuries that never progress to meet strict BSD criteria. They are precisely the population—young, previously healthy, hemodynamically supported in an ICU, with non-recoverable neurological injury—that constitutes the prototypical cDCD category III donor.

Even capturing 5–10% of this population for DCD—a conservative estimate by the experience of any functional program—would generate thousands of additional organ donors annually. The 2024 consensus paper estimated that if DCD were operationalized at India's existing transplant hospitals, the deceased donor rate could double within 5 years. India's transplant infrastructure—over 1000 registered hospitals, 26 SOTTOs, and a growing cadre of trained transplant coordinators—is not an obstacle to DCD; it is the platform on which DCD can be built.

NOTTO's Current DCD Initiatives

Working with legal and medical experts to establish a clearer national DCD framework within THOTA 1994.

Consulting with multidisciplinary experts to draft standardized National Operational Guidelines and SOPs for DCD.

Conducting training and sensitization workshops for ICU physicians and transplant coordinators on donor identification and WLST.

Integrating DCD messaging into national organ donation awareness campaigns.

Planning pilot DCD programmes in identified high-volume tertiary hospitals across India.

Required Amendments to India's Organ Allocation Policy for DCD

India's existing organ allocation framework under THOTA 1994 and the 2014 Rules was architected exclusively around DBD. Integrating DCD requires not a parallel system but a structured set of reforms across policy domains—each grounded in Indian consensus documents and validated by international society guidance and by the experience of established DCD allocation programs worldwide (Table 10.5). Table 10.5 summarizes the five leading DCD allocation programmes worldwide. Two features recur across all of them and directly inform the reforms proposed below: allocation and recipient matching are initiated *before* WLST, and geographic hierarchy is subordinated to ischemia-time limits.

- *Allocation Initiation*: The most consequential structural change is the shift in the allocation start point. Under DBD, allocation begins after brain death declaration. For DCD, recipient shortlisting, histocompatibility assessment, and transport logistics must all be initiated before WLST is executed—a parallel, pre-death

Table 10.5 Top five DCD organ allocation programs: comparative overview

Country/body	DCD start	DCD donors per million population	Kidney graft survival (5-year)	Allocation principle	Key guideline highlights	Allocation start point
Spain (ONT)	1989	19.6 (Ranked #1)	~88% to 90%	Medical urgency → waiting time → geography (hub-spoke)	Both cDCD and uDCD; only country transplanting all organ types from DCD; pioneer of NRP; 2024: 51% of donations were DCD	Before WLST Recipient matching activated during donor workup; parallel allocation workflow
Belgium (Eurotransplant)	1995	12.8	~86%	Urgency → HLA → waiting time (Eurotransplant protocol)	World's first DCD-V (euthanasia) donor in 2005; strong cDCD III program; national machine perfusion integration; DCD-V now ~8% of all DCD	Before WLST Eurotransplant match run pre-WLST; DCD-V allocation via Eurotransplant rules
Netherlands (NTS/ Eurotransplant)	Early 1980s	10.0	~85%	HLA matching → waiting time → geography (Eurotransplant)	First European DCD program (kidneys); since 2001 DCD/ DBD kidneys allocated indiscriminately; expanded to liver, lung & heart since 2020	Before WLST Eurotransplant pre-allocation matching run initiated after donor referral; recipient activated before circulatory death

(continued)

Table 10.5 (continued)

Country/body	DCD start	DCD donors per million population	Kidney graft survival (5-year)	Allocation principle	Key guideline highlights	Allocation start point
United Kingdom (NHSBT/BTS)	1990s	9.4	~85%	Geography-first; points for HLA, waitlist time, age & location	BTS guidelines (1st 2004, latest 2023); DCD now ~35% of all deceased donations; increasing NRP use; DCD hearts transplanted since 2015	Before WLST Recipient identified & on standby before withdrawal; national offering scheme with 3-h WLST window for logistics
United States (UNOS/OPTN)	1992 (Pittsburgh protocol)	~11 (Est.)	~82% to 85%	Acuity-based (sickest first) → geography (DSA/region circles) → waiting time	OPTN policy Ch. 18 governs DCD; 2020 acuity-circle reform for liver; DCD now 49% of all deceased donors (2025)	Before WLST OPTN acuity-circle policy mandates local DCD offers to reduce cold ischemia; recipient activated before WLST

BTS British Transplantation Society, *cDCD* Controlled DCD, *DCD* Donation after Circulatory Death, *DCD-V* DCD after euthanasia, *DSA* Donor service area, *HLA* Human leukocyte antigen, *NHSBT* NHS Blood and Transplant, *NRP* Normothermic Regional Perfusion, *NTS* Nederlandse Transplantatie Stichting, *ONT* Organización Nacional de Trasplantes, *OPTN* Organ Procurement and Transplantation Network, *uDCD* Uncontrolled DCD, *UNOS* United Network for Organ Sharing, *WLST* Withdrawal of life-sustaining treatment workflow fundamentally different from the current sequential model. This is endorsed by both the IJCCM 2022 consensus and the American Society of Transplant Surgeons (ASTS) 2023 best-practice recommendations [9, 16].

- *The Administrative Hierarchy of Hospital*: SOTTO → ROTTO → NOTTO must be subordinated to ischemia time limits for DCD organs: functional warm ischemia time (FWIT) ≤30 min for kidneys and ≤20 min for liver, beyond which organ viability is critically compromised [10]. Organ donation must shift from sequential to simultaneous multi-center notification, with revised acceptance windows of ≤20 min for kidneys and ≤10 min for liver, requiring a significant upgrade to the NOTTO digital platform.
- *Organ Preservation*: Static cold storage, used as standard in DBD, is insufficient for DCD organs. Hypothermic Machine Perfusion (HMP) for kidneys, which is supported by level-1 randomized controlled trial evidence demonstrating a 40% reduction in delayed graft function [14]—and Normothermic Regional Perfusion (NRP) for livers, reduces ischemic cholangiopathy from 9.5% to 1.2% [13], must be formally integrated into the allocation pathway with defined reimbursement mechanisms under the national organ transplant program.
- *Ethics and Consent*: Three separate, independently witnessed consent documents—for WLST, organ donation, and antemortem interventions (AMI)—must replace the single combined consent used in DBD donation. Although implied under THOTA, the separation between treating and transplant teams should be clearly defined in law, with specific and enforceable penalties for any breaches [8, 9, 19, 20].
- *Cost Framework*: AMI costs, machine perfusion costs, and stand-down donor ICU costs create tangible financial disincentives for institutional DCD participation. Mechanisms for covering these costs can be worked out in consultation with professional associations to make it a sustainable program.
- *Outcome Registry*: A mandatory DCD-specific registry capturing FWIT, DGF rates, ischemic cholangiopathy rates, and 12-month graft survival—published annually by NOTTO—is required to drive quality improvement and sustain public and regulatory approval in the program.

Conclusion

DCD in India is no longer distant possibility—it represents an immediate and actionable opportunity. The legal framework is already established, ethical boundaries are clearly defined, and essential clinical processes such as WLST, stand-off period, and organ preservation, are well-defined and adaptable within the Indian healthcare setting. The 2023 Supreme Court judgment has provided a procedural framework, while the 2022 joint position paper and 2024 consensus statements have strengthened the clinical and scientific foundation. At the same time, NOTTO is actively developing guidelines, building capacity, and planning pilot programmes. The next critical step is translating this groundwork into implementation. This includes initiating pilot programmes in high-volume centers; developing national

DCD guidelines through professional societies under the aegis of NOTTO; integrating a dedicated DCD component in the NOTTO digital platform; establishing financial models for interventions such as AMI, machine perfusion, and donor management; and sustaining a national awareness effort that frames WLST as a dignified choice and DCD as an act of generosity rather than a last recourse. In essence, the successful DCD allocation requires rapid and equitable allocation systems, early planning prior to WLST, continuous, parallel communication, stringent ethical oversight, real-time logistics management, and strong governance with transparency. All of these elements are achievable within India's existing institutional framework, with NOTTO well positioned to lead. The donor pool exists, as do the patients in need. The framework presented here serves as the crucial link between them.

Competing Interests The author(s) has no competing interests to declare that are relevant to the content of this manuscript.

Ethics Approval The author(s) declares that this manuscript does not include primary research with human participants.

The author(s) declares that this manuscript does not include primary studies involving animals.

References

1. National Organ and Tissue Transplant Organization (NOTTO). Annual report 2024. Ministry of Health and Family Welfare, Govt. of India. New Delhi: NOTTO; 2025. Available from: https://notto.mohfw.gov.in.
2. Zirpe K, Pandit R, Gurav S, Mani RK, Prabhakar H, Clerk A, Wanchoo J, Reddy KS, Ramachandran P, Karanth S, George N, Vaity C, Shetty RM, Samavedam S, Dixit S, Kulkarni AP. Management of potential organ donor: indian society of critical care medicine-position statement. Indian J Crit Care Med. 2024;28(Suppl 2):S249–78. https://doi.org/10.5005/jp-journals-10071-24698.
3. Martin F, Carmona M, Mahillo B, Alvarez M, Luengo A, Chatzixiros E, López-Fraga M, Domínguez-Gil B, Tullius SG. Organ donation and transplantation worldwide: the global observatory on donation and transplantation 2024 report. Transplantation. 2026;110(3):e655–69. https://doi.org/10.1097/TP.0000000000005657.
4. Transplantation of Human Organs and Tissues Act, 1994 (Act 42 of 1994), as amended by The Transplantation of Human Organs and Tissues (Amendment) Act, 2011. New Delhi: Ministry of Health and Family Welfare, Government of India; 2011.
5. Supreme Court of India. Common Cause (A Regd. Society) vs. Union of India and Others. Writ Petition (Civil) No. 215 of 2005. Judgment dated 24 January 2023.
6. Bernat JL. How the distinction between "irreversible" and "permanent" illuminates circulatory-respiratory death determination. J Med Philos. 2010;35(3):242–55. https://doi.org/10.1093/jmp/jhq018.
7. International Society for Organ Donation and Procurement (ISODP). TTS-ISODP position statement on DCD. 2024. Available from: https://www.tts.org/isodp-education.
8. Kootstra G, Daemen JH, Oomen AP. Categories of non-heart-beating donors. Transplant Proc. 1995;27(5):2893–4.
9. Seth AK, Mohanka R, Navin S, Gokhale AG, Sharma A, Balakrishnan K, Mirza D, Dhital K, Sahay M, Sundaram R, Gupta S, Kute VB, Shroff S. Organ donation after circulatory deter-

mination of death in India: a joint position paper. Indian J Crit Care Med. 2022;26(4):423–40. https://doi.org/10.5005/jp-journals-10071-24198.
10. Wind J, Faut M, van Smaalen TC, van Heurn EL. Variability in protocols on donation after circulatory death in Europe. Crit Care. 2013;17(5):R217. https://doi.org/10.1186/cc13034.
11. Alghannam K, Fine J, Howard B, Loza J, Goussous NM, Sageshima J, Mineyev NM, Wang AX, Perez RV, Than PA. Impact of warm ischemia time on donation after circulatory death kidney transplant outcomes. Clin Transpl. 2024;38(8):e15436. https://doi.org/10.1111/ctr.15436.
12. Oniscu GC, Mehew J, Butler AJ, Sutherland A, Gaurav R, Hogg R, Currie I, Jones M, Watson CJE. Improved organ utilization and better transplant outcomes with in situ normothermic regional perfusion in controlled donation after circulatory death. Transplantation. 2023;107(2):438–48. https://doi.org/10.1097/TP.0000000000004280.
13. Reddy MS, Varghese J, Mathur SK. Deceased donor program in India: listing and allocation practices and the legal process with respect to liver transplantation. J Clin Exp Hepatol. 2025;15(1):102408. https://doi.org/10.1016/j.jceh.2024.102408.
14. Bababekov YJ, Ha AH, Nydam TL, Goncalves C, Choudhury R, Shinsako J, Baimas-George M, Reynolds DM, Yoshida C, Racke CA, Grewal H, Pomposelli, Rodriguez IE, Hoffman JRH, Schold JD, Kaplan B, Pomfret EA, Pomposelli JJ. Thoracoabdominal normothermic regional perfusion: real-world experience and outcomes of DCD liver transplantation. Transplant Direct. 2025;11(3):e1767. https://doi.org/10.1097/TXD.0000000000001767.
15. Hosgood SA, Callaghan CJ, Wilson CH, Smith L, Mullings J, Mehew J, Oniscu GC, Phillips BL, Bates L, Nicholson ML. Normothermic machine perfusion versus static cold storage in donation after circulatory death kidney transplantation: a randomized controlled trial. Nat Med. 2023;29(6):1511–9. https://doi.org/10.1038/s41591-023-02376-7.
16. Hoffman JRH, Hartwig MG, Cain MT, Rove JY, Siddique A, Urban M, Mulligan MS, Bush EL, Balsara K, Demarest CT, Silvestry SC, Wilkey B, Trahanas JM, Pretorius VG, Shah AS, Moazami N, Pomfret EA, Catarino PA, American Society of Transplant Surgeons (ASTS), International Society of Heart and Lung Transplantation (ISHLT), Society of Thoracic Surgeons (STS), American Association for Thoracic Surgery (AATS). Consensus statement: technical standards for thoracoabdominal normothermic regional perfusion. Ann Thorac Surg. 2024;118(4):778–91. https://doi.org/10.1016/j.athoracsur.2024.07.002.
17. Tingle SJ, Thompson ER, Figueiredo RS, Moir JA, Goodfellow M, Talbot D, Wilson CH. Normothermic and hypothermic machine perfusion preservation versus static cold storage for deceased donor kidney transplantation. Cochrane Database Syst Rev. 2024;7(7):CD011671. https://doi.org/10.1002/14651858.CD011671.
18. Kute VB, Vanikar AV, Shah PR, Gumber MR, Patel HV, Modi PR, Rizvi SJ, Shah VR, Trivedi HL. Outcome of renal transplantation from deceased donors after cardiac death: a single-center experience from a developing country. Transplant Proc. 2013;45(6):2147–51. https://doi.org/10.1016/j.transproceed.2013.02.128.
19. Croome KP, Barbas AS, Whitson B, Zarrinpar A, Taner T, Lo D, MacConmara M, Kim J, Kennealey PT, Bromberg JS, Washburn K, Agopian VG, Stegall M, Quintini C, American Society of Transplant Surgeons Scientific Studies Committee. American Society of Transplant Surgeons recommendations on best practices in donation after circulatory death organ procurement. Am J Transplant. 2023;23(2):171–9. https://doi.org/10.1016/j.ajt.2022.10.009.
20. O'Neill S, Asgari E, Callaghan C, Gardiner D, Hartog H, Iype S, Manara A, Nasralla D, Oniscu GC, Watson C. The British transplantation society guidelines on organ donation from deceased donors after circulatory death. Transplant Rev (Orlando). 2023;37(4):100791. https://doi.org/10.1016/j.trre.2023.100791.

Part IV

Recipient Evaluation and Risk Stratification in DCD

Recipient Selection in DCD Transplantation: Criteria, Risk Stratification and Organ Specific Considerations

11

Sai Praneeth Reddy Perugu, Arun Panjathia, S. P. Shiva Kumar, Piyush Gupta, Amay Banker, and Ravi Mohanka

Abbreviations

AKI	Acute Kidney Injury
CIT	Cold Ischaemia Time
DBD	Donation after Brain Death
DCD	Donation after Circulatory Death
DGF	Delayed Graft Function
DSA	Donor Specific Antibodies
EPTS	Estimated Post-Transplant Survival
Fwit	functional Warm Ischaemia Time
HLA	Human Leukocyte Antigen
HMP	Hypothermic Machine Perfusion
KDPI	Kidney Donor Profile Index
KDRI	Kidney Donor Risk Index

S. P. R. Perugu · A. Panjathia · S. P. Shiva Kumar (✉)
Department of Renal Transplant Surgery, PGIMER, Chandigarh, India
e-mail: sp.shivakumar@pgimer.edu.in

P. Gupta
Medstar Georgetown Transplant Institute, Georgetown University Hospital, Washington, DC, USA

A. Banker
Department of Surgery, Miami Transplant Institute, University of Miami, Miami, FL, USA

R. Mohanka (✉)
Department of Liver Transplantation and HPB Sciences, Sir HN Reliance Foundation Hospital, Mumbai, India

Methodist Transplant Institute, University of Tennessee Health Science Centre, Memphis, TN, USA
e-mail: ravi.mohanka@rfhospital.org

S. P. Kolte et al. (eds.), *Organ Donation After Circulatory Death*,
https://doi.org/10.1007/978-981-92-6377-6_11

NMP	Normothermic Machine Perfusion
NRP	Normothermic Regional Perfusion
PAK	Pancreas after Kidney Transplant
PNF	Primary Non Function
PRA	Panel Reactive Antibody
PTA	Pancreas Transplant Alone Transplant
SPK	Simultaneous Pancreas and Kidney Transplant

Kidney and Pancreas

Sai Praneeth Reddy Perugu, Arun Panjathia, and S. P. Shiva Kumar

- Donation after circulatory death (DCD) has emerged as an important strategy to expand the donor pool and address the growing disparity between organ demand and availability.
- The physiological derangements associated with circulatory death, particularly hypotension and hypoxia, have been hypothesised to contribute significantly to the inferior graft function observed in DCD transplantation when compared with outcomes achieved using organs from DBD donors [1].
- The warm ischaemic injury, occurring from circulatory arrest to cold perfusion, directly impacts organ viability and function post-transplant.
- Despite comparable patient and graft survival, the high incidence of DGF remains a concern [2], as it increases postoperative morbidity, prolongs recovery and may adversely affect graft function and patient outcomes.
- This underscores the pivotal role of meticulous recipient selection in optimising outcomes and minimising post-transplant morbidity.
- Understanding and integrating the donor factors into allocation algorithms and recipient selection protocols are essential to maximise the benefit of DCD organs while ensuring patient safety.

- *Factors Affecting DCD–Recipient Selection*
  Key donor and recipient factors relevant to recipient selection are summarised in Table 11.1 and discussed in detail in the following sections.

Table 11.1 Recipient and donor characteristics affecting DCD-recipient selection [3–5]

Donor parameters	Recipient parameters
1. Donor age	Physiological reserve:
2. Donor BMI	Comorbidity burden:
3. fWIT	Immunological risk:
4. CIT injury	Urgency vs utility:
5. Donor comorbidities (AKI, pancreatitis)	

Donor Factors Affecting Recipient Selection

Donor Age

- Advanced donor age has consistently been associated with inferior graft outcomes, likely owing to reduced functional reserve and impaired microvascular resilience, which diminish the organ's capacity to tolerate ischaemia-related injury [6].
- The combination of advanced donor age with other adverse factors, high functional warm ischaemia time (fWIT), high cold ischaemia time (CIT) or a recipient with pre-existing comorbidities markedly worsens prognosis.
- In general, the use of older age donors may be considered acceptable, provided there is no cumulative burden of additional donor–related risk factors and prolonged warm or cold ischaemic times are avoided [7].
- For DCD kidney transplantation, older donors (aged >60 with a KDPI >85%) may still be acceptable, but preferably for recipients with a lower risk [8].
- In contrast, DCD pancreas grafts are less tolerant of donor age because the pancreas is highly sensitive to ischaemic injury, pancreatitis, thrombosis and technical failure and use stricter donor age limits (45–50 years) than for DBD donors [9, 10].

Implication for Recipient Selection

- Ideal preference should be given to *younger, lower-risk recipients* when using older DCD donors, avoiding marginal recipients (e.g. frail, high comorbidity burden).
- Older DCD kidney donors may be allocated to recipients in whom the survival benefit of transplantation outweighs the DGF risk.
- However, older DCD pancreas donors should be avoided in high-risk recipients.

Donor BMI

For Kidneys

- Donor BMI influences kidney graft quality through several mechanisms, like glomerulomegaly, focal segmental glomerulosclerosis, renal lipotoxicity and a proinflammatory milieu that exacerbates ischaemia-reperfusion injury.
- In DCD kidneys, donor obesity adds to the ischaemic injury and compounds the risk of DGF and long-term graft dysfunction.
- A BMI >30 kg/m^2 in the DCD donor has been associated with a higher burden of donor–derived nephron injury, and BMI >35 kg/m^2 is generally considered a relative contraindication [11].

For Pancreas

- BMI is particularly critical in DCD pancreas donation.
- Donor obesity is associated with pancreatic steatosis, reduced beta-cell mass, higher intraoperative technical difficulty, and elevated rates of post-transplant graft pancreatitis and thrombosis.

- In pancreas transplants, donor obesity (BMI >30) is associated with a significantly lower graft survival rate at 1-year post-transplant and increases surgical complications, for all recipient categories (SPK, PAK, PTA) [12].
- Most DCD pancreas programmes apply a maximum donor BMI threshold of <30 kg/m^2 [10, 13].

Functional Warm Ischaemia Time (fWIT)

- UNOS definition of fWIT, defined as systolic blood pressure <80 mmHg or oxygen saturation <80% sustained for a minimum of 5 min until core cooling, is initiated [14].
- fWIT is the most critical determinant of DCD graft quality associated with increased risk of DGF, PNF and Early graft loss and is the most common reason for higher discard rates.
- For kidneys, there are no defined cut-off values; however, earlier studies stated that prolonged that fWIT up to 60 min is not significantly associated with 1- and 5-year graft failure compared to lower fWIT & DBD with appropriate organ preservation method, donor and recipient selection and can be extended up to 90 min if it is from younger donors, with lower KDRI, absence of comorbidities and absence of acute kidney injury [14].
- Acceptable cardiorespiratory parameters for pancreas donation during this phase have not yet been clearly defined; however, the interval between withdrawal of life-sustaining treatment and organ perfusion has generally been limited to less than 30 min [15, 16].
- For pancreas transplantation, Maastricht Class III and IV DCD donors may be considered suitable when warm ischaemia time is restricted to a maximum of 30 min [4].
- *Implication for Recipient Selection*
  - Long fWIT grafts need to be allocated for stable recipients with low immunological risk.
  - Risk stratification using standard models (e.g. KDRI >1.14, indicating increased risk of death-censored graft failure) can improve the efficient use of DCD kidneys and lead to better recipient outcomes [17].
  - Donors with long fWIT should always be supplemented by short CIT to improve the overall outcomes.

Cold Ischaemia Time (CIT)

- Prolonged cold ischaemia appears to be particularly detrimental in organs retrieved from circulatory death donors, which have already been exposed to a period of warm ischaemia, with each additional hour of cold ischaemia time being associated with a significantly increased risk of graft failure and poorer patient survival [18].
- In DCD, this window is particularly hazardous for the pancreas as it already sustains warm ischaemia injury, so additional CIT amplifies reperfusion pancreatitis, endothelial activation and the risk of low-flow thrombosis.
- Donor risk stratification based on cold ischaemia time (CIT) is summarised below (Table 11.2).

Table 11.2 Donor risk stratification based on CIT

CIT—DCD kidneys		
<12 h	Acceptable range; DGF risk comparable to DBD; no significant risk of graft survival [19]	Ideal target
12–22 h	Increased DGF risk; eGFR starts declining significantly above 12 h in DCD (not seen in DBD) [20]	High risk
>24 h	Associated with increased DGF likelihood; however, recent UNOS mate-kidney analysis (2024) found no adverse allograft survival and transplantation is still preferred over discard, adopting strategies like careful recipient selection, organ preservation(machine perfusion), dual kidney transplants, etc. [21]	Very high risk
CIT—DCD pancreas		
< 8 h	DCD-specific target recommended with low risk of DGF, graft loss, and better patient survival [22]	Ideal target
12–20 h	CIT <12 h has been associated with the most favourable transplant outcomes, whereas CIT between 12 and 20 h is linked to intermediate results, and CIT >20 h is associated with the poorest outcomes. This adverse effect of prolonged CIT appears to be more pronounced in older donors (>25 years) and overweight donors (BMI >25 kg/m^2) [23]	High risk

Donor Comorbidities

- The chronic comorbidities, like hypertension and cardiovascular disease, contribute to chronic microvascular damage, compounding ischaemic injury.
- Kidneys procured from DCD donors with acute kidney injury (AKI) are associated with a significantly higher risk of DGF, although rates of PNF remain comparable to those of kidneys from DCD donors without AKI. Importantly, 1-year estimated eGFR and graft survival have been reported to be similar between the two groups [24].
- Hyperglycaemia and hyperamylasaemia were not considered absolute contraindications, whereas necrotising pancreatitis, chronic pancreatitis and diabetes mellitus should be ruled out for pancreas transplant [25].
- Implication for recipient selection:
  - Marginal donors should match with recipients having longer expected survival and lower competing risks.
  - Avoid high-risk recipients (elderly, severe cardiovascular disease).
  - AKI kidneys need to be allocated to recipients with low risk and fit enough to tolerate DGF (good physiological reserve, low immunological risk, stable dialysis access).

The aforementioned donor factors are summarised below within a DCD-specific donor risk stratification framework relevant to recipient selection (Table 11.3).

Table 11.3 DCD-Donor risk stratification influencing the recipient selection [6–19, 21–25]

	Kidney ideal donor	Kidney high-risk donor	Pancreas ideal donor	Pancreas high-risk donor
Age:	<60 years	>60 years	<45–50 years	>50 years
BMI:	<30	30–35	< 27–30	>30
Fwit:	<60 min	60 min	<30 min	30 min
CIT:	<12 h	12–22 h	<8 h	12–20 h
Donor comorbidities:	Nil	AKI+ Hypertension+ Haemodynamic instability+	Nil	Pancreatitis+ Haemodynamic instability+
	⇩	⇩	⇩	⇩
Recipient selection:	Low risk Extended risk recipients	Only low-risk recipients	Low risk Extended risk recipients	These grafts should be considered after careful assessment in only selected low-risk recipients If multiple risk factors + better to avoid DCD SPK/pancreas transplant

BMI Body mass index, *fWITt* functional warm ischaemia time, *CIT* cold ischaemia time

DCD Recipient Selection

- Successful transplantation of kidneys and pancreases obtained from DCD donors depends not only on donor organ quality, but critically on the careful selection of recipients who can derive the greatest benefit while tolerating the unique risks associated with DCD organs.
- Recipient selection for DCD transplantation is a multidimensional process that integrates clinical, immunological, functional and psychosocial parameters.
- DCD grafts should preferably be allocated to recipients in whom early graft dysfunction can be safely tolerated, and the guiding principle is to avoid combining a marginal DCD organ with a high-risk recipient and prolonged ischaemia time.
- Contemporary DCD allocation strategies increasingly stratify candidates according to four major domains (Table 11.4):
  1. Physiological reserve,
  2. Immunological risk,
  3. Comorbidity burden,
  4. Urgency versus utility balance.

Table 11.4 Recipient risk stratification for DCD kidney & pancreas transplant

Domain	Low risk	Intermediate risk	High risk
Physiological reserve:	Age <45–50, no frailty, good functional capacity	Age:50–65; mild frailty, reduced exercise tolerance	Age:>65 frailty, poor functional status, sarcopenia
Comorbidity burden:	Minimal comorbidities, BMI <28, no CAD, EF >55% Controlled diabetes with no complications	Controlled and stable CAD, EF:40–55%, mild PVD, controlled diabetes with minimal complications	Severe CAD, LV dysfunction, diffuse PVD, diabetes with end-organ damage
Immunological risk:	Low PRA (<20%), first transplant, no DSA	Moderate PRA (20–85%), prior transplant	Highly sensitised, cPRA>85%, DSA+, prior transplant
	⇩	⇩	⇩
DCD- kidney transplantation:	Ideal for standard or marginal DCD kidney donors	Ideal for standard DCD kidney donors	Only low-risk DCD kidney donors
DCD- SPK/pancreas transplantation:	Ideal for standard or marginal DCD pancreas	Only for an ideal DCD pancreas donor	Avoid DCD SPK/ pancreas

PRA panel reactive antibody, *DSA* donor specific antibody, *CAD* coronary artery disease, *EF* ejection fraction, *LV* left ventricle, *PVD* peripheral vascular disease

Physiological Reserve

Physiological reserve refers to the recipient's capacity to tolerate perioperative stress, ischaemia–reperfusion injury and early graft dysfunction. Given the higher incidence of DGF following DCD transplantation, recipients should possess adequate cardiovascular, metabolic and functional reserve to endure the postoperative recovery period and potential delays in graft function.

a. *Age*

Younger recipients generally tolerate DCD-related complications better and exhibit superior long-term graft survival. Elderly recipients with low reserve may not tolerate the ischaemia-reperfusion injury inherent in DCD grafts; and most centres preferentially allocate DCD pancreas grafts to young recipients, who are physiologically fit even if chronologically older. However, older recipients receiving older DCD kidneys have demonstrated acceptable outcomes in some registry analyses [26].

b. *Frailty*

Validated tools such as the Fried Frailty Phenotype, Clinical Frailty Scale (CFS), and Short Physical Performance Battery (SPPB) should be used. Recipients with CFS ≥5 (moderately frail) face 2–3× higher post-transplant mortality and prolonged DGF duration compared to non-frail recipients [27]. Advanced recipient age combined with frailty is associated with significantly worse outcomes, including prolonged hospitalisation, functional decline, and mortality.

Immunological Risk

DCD grafts are particularly vulnerable to immune-mediated injury because ischaemia–reperfusion injury enhances innate and adaptive immune activation. Highly sensitised recipients, including cPRA >80%, prior transplants, multiple transfusions, pregnancy sensitisation, HLA mismatch (A, B, DR) and higher DSA burden, are better avoided. Preformed DSAs, combined with DCD ischaemic injury, increase the risk of antibody-mediated rejection, microvascular inflammation and graft thrombosis.

Comorbidity Burden

- *Cardiovascular Risk*

Cardiovascular disease is the leading cause of death following kidney transplantation and a major determinant of tolerance to DGF. A structured cardiovascular workup is mandatory before listing any recipient for DCD kidney transplantation, and should be updated periodically (at least every 1–2 years) while on the waiting list. EF <40% is a significant risk factor for perioperative mortality. Recipients with poorly controlled cardiac disease (un-revascularised multi-vessel CAD, severe pulmonary hypertension with PASP >50 mmHg,

New York Heart Association Class IV heart failure) should not receive DCD kidneys until cardiological optimisation is achieved.

- *Obesity*

BMI >35 is associated with prolonged operative times, wound complications, and suboptimal immunosuppressive pharmacokinetics, compounding DGF risk in DCD transplantation. BMI <30 kg/m^2 is particularly recommended for DCD pancreas transplantation because ischaemia already predisposes to graft oedema and thrombosis.

- *Diabetes-Related Complications*

Important considerations include autonomic neuropathy, gastroparesis, severe vasculopathy, cerebrovascular disease, and recipients with advanced end-organ damage may have limited ability to recover from postoperative complications.

- *Dialysis Vintage and Metabolic Stability*

Long dialysis duration correlates with systemic sensitisation and rising PRA, progressive cardiovascular disease, left ventricular hypertrophy, malnutrition, sarcopenia and immune dysregulation and increases the risk of DGF-related complications. However, these patients also carry the greatest burden of dialysis-related harm and may derive the greatest absolute survival benefit from DCD transplantation. The net benefit calculation must therefore be individualised. Recipients with shorter dialysis vintage often demonstrate better DCD outcomes. For pancreas transplantation, brittle diabetes, severe hypoglycaemic unawareness and preserved rehabilitation potential favour transplantation despite moderate perioperative risk.

- Advanced liver disease or severe chronic lung disease markedly increases perioperative mortality and reduces suitability for DCD transplantation.
- As DCD recipients might require chronic ICU stay and invasive monitoring, any recipient with a history of chronic uncontrolled infections becomes a relative contraindication for DCD kidney and pancreas transplant.

Urgency Vs Utility

Modern allocation increasingly balances immediate recipient need (urgency) versus long-term graft utility and survival benefit.

Utility Principle

It prioritises maximising graft longevity, patient survival and quality-adjusted life years.

DCD organs, especially pancreas grafts, may therefore be preferentially allocated to recipients with:

- Good rehabilitation potential.
- Longer projected survival.
- Lower perioperative risk.

This approach aims to optimise the benefit derived from technically demanding grafts.

Urgency Principle
Some recipients may warrant transplantation despite elevated risk due to:

- Life-threatening dialysis complications.
- Lack of vascular access.
- Severe brittle diabetes.
- Recurrent hypoglycaemia.
- Rapidly deteriorating quality of life.

Studies have consistently demonstrated that recipients on dialysis for longer duration have inferior kidney graft survival compared to those transplanted earlier [28]. In such settings, accepting a DCD organ may still provide a substantial survival advantage.

Organ-Specific Criteria for Recipient Selection

DCD Kidney Transplantation

(a) *Ideal Recipient Criteria* [29, 30]
  - Age < 60 years.
  - Good cardiovascular reserve.
  - Non-sensitised (low PRA, no prior transplant).
  - Ability to tolerate DGF.
  - Not requiring immediate graft function.

(b) *Relative Contraindications*
  - age ≥ 65,
  - morbid obesity (BMI ≥ 35),
  - Bladder insufficiency requiring reconstruction/diversion/conduit,
  - frailty,
  - multiple medical comorbidities,
  - history of chronic and recurrent infections (eg; TB, UTI, Pneumonia, etc),
  - lack of financial and social support,
  - psychosocial issues.

DCD Pancreas Transplantation

(a) *Ideal Recipient Criteria* [10, 15, 31].
  - Young (preferably <50–55 years).
  - Low BMI (<30 kg/m^2 preferably <28 kg/m2).

- Low cardiovascular risk.
- Insulin-dependent diabetes with:
  - Low insulin requirement (<1 U/kg/day).
- No severe vascular disease.

(b) *Relative Contraindications*

- BMI >30.
- Poorly controlled Diabetes.
- Chronic active infections or open wounds.
- Multiple prior abdominal surgeries.
- Significant peripheral or cerebrovascular disease.
- Limited mobility or inability to participate in physical therapy.
- Limited financial & caregiver support.
- Poor 5-year life expectancy.

Strategies to Optimise Recipient Selection

- Recipient optimisation in DCD transplantation requires individualised risk stratification integrating physiological reserve, immunological risk, comorbidity burden and ischaemic exposure.
- Outcomes are optimised by balancing donor and recipient risk, minimising cold ischaemia time and aligning recipient complexity with institutional experience and organ quality.

Limiting Ischaemic Times

- Normothermic regional perfusion (NRP), utilising normothermic extracorporeal membrane oxygenation, has emerged as a promising strategy to restore perfusion and replenish cellular energy stores in donor organs prior to retrieval, thereby mitigating ischaemia–reperfusion injury at the time of transplantation [32].
- In situ cooling techniques have also been developed to minimise warm ischaemic injury to the donor pancreas, including the use of a double-balloon catheter-based regional organ cooling system to achieve rapid selective cooling before organ retrieval [33].
- Policies for local allocation of organs so as to avoid travelling logistic issues, increasing ischaemic times.

Safe Preservation

- Advancements in organ preservation techniques, particularly hypothermic machine perfusion (HMP) and normothermic machine perfusion (NMP), have demonstrated significant improvements in the utilisation of marginal organs and grafts retrieved from DCD donors by reducing rates of delayed graft function (DGF) and enabling assessment of organ viability prior to transplantation [34].
- These aim to restore cellular energetics and substrates, reducing the damaging ischaemic effect on the organs [13].
- High-risk donors may be used in expanded recipient pools if perfusion parameters are favourable.

Donor Kidney Biopsy

- Zero-hour kidney biopsy remains a complementary tool in DCD recipient selection, particularly when clinical parameters are borderline.
- Key histological features assessed include Glomerulosclerosis, IFTA, arterial hyalinosis reflecting chronic diminished functional reserve and ATN for DCD kidneys; severity correlates with fWIT and predicts DGF duration.
- Preimplantation biopsy is recommended for elderly DCD donors, with kidneys demonstrating a Remuzzi score ≤4 considered suitable for single-kidney transplantation, whereas those with scores of 5–7 may be allocated for dual-kidney transplantation in appropriately selected recipients [35, 36].

DCD Transplant—Risk Prediction Models

Recipient risk prediction in DCD kidney and pancreas transplantation requires an integrated assessment of recipient physiological reserve, cardiovascular risk, immunological profile, technical complexity and the capacity to tolerate ischaemia-related early graft dysfunction.

- *In DCD kidney transplantation*, risk models are primarily directed towards predicting delayed graft function, with validated tools incorporating donor age, DCD status, terminal creatinine, warm and cold ischaemia times, recipient dialysis duration, sensitisation and comorbidity.
- The Estimated Post-Transplant Survival (EPTS) score, developed by UNOS/OPTN, quantifies expected post-transplant longevity, and a lower EPTS score corresponds to a recipient expected to live longer post-transplant [37]. The Kidney Donor Profile Index (KDPI), derived from the Kidney Donor Risk Index (KDRI), is currently the most widely accepted scoring system in the United States for assessing the quality and risk profile of deceased donor kidneys and serves as a reliable predictor of donor–recipient transplant outcomes. Despite comparable KDPI scores, kidneys procured from DCD donors have consistently been associated with higher rates of delayed graft function (DGF) than those from DBD donors [38, 39]. The principle underlying EPTS-based allocation is that high-quality kidneys (low KDPI) should preferentially be offered to recipients who will benefit for the longest time (low EPTS), while marginal donor kidneys (high KDPI, including high-risk DCD kidneys) may be preferentially allocated to recipients with higher EPTS (shorter expected survival), for whom any functioning graft represents meaningful benefit.
  - Low KDPI DCD kidneys (KDPI <35%): May be allocated as per standard criteria, preferring low-EPTS recipients.
  - High KDPI DCD kidneys (KDPI >85%): Allocated preferentially to high-EPTS recipients (typically older, diabetic, on dialysis longest), where the survival benefit of transplantation over dialysis remains positive, but shorter graft life is acceptable.
- *In DCD pancreas* and SPK transplantation, there are no robust recipient-specific prediction models; and available tools such as PDRI and P-PASS

primarily estimate donor or graft suitability rather than recipient tolerance [40, 41]. Therefore, DCD pancreas grafts should be preferentially allocated to physiologically robust, low-BMI, low-cardiovascular-risk, low-immunological-risk recipients with favourable iliac vessels and anticipated short operative time. While marginal DCD kidneys may be acceptable in recipients capable of tolerating delayed graft function, DCD pancreas grafts require a narrower safety margin, and the accumulation of donor and recipient risk factors should be avoided.

- *Recent AI Algorithms*
  Expanding the application of artificial intelligence in the stratification and selection of DCD donors may optimise donor evaluation, expand the donor pool and improve transplant outcomes. Emerging tools such as predictive modelling and organ quality assessment (OrQA) have the potential to address critical challenges in donor selection, facilitate personalised decision-making strategies and enhance the feasibility and success of pancreas transplantation using DCD donors [34].

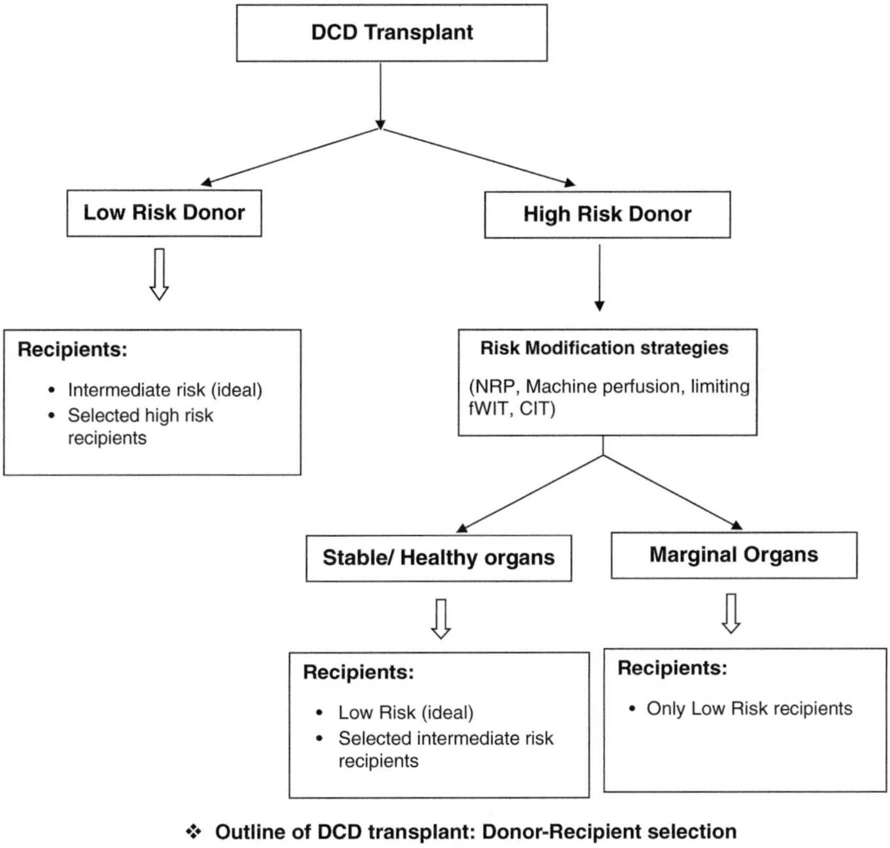

Outline of DCD transplant: Donor-Recipient selection

Recipient Consent for DCD Transplant

- Valid consent requires that the prospective transplant recipient is adequately informed about the risks and benefits of the proposed intervention, including transplantation using a DCD-donor organ.
- Following an organ offer, the final risk–benefit discussion with the recipient should clearly outline the comparative risks of remaining on the transplant waiting list versus proceeding with transplantation using a DCD organ.
  - *DCD Specific Recipient Counselling*
    - The biological distinction between DBD and DCD donors, including the mechanism of warm ischaemia and why it matters for graft function.
    - Organ-specific DCD risks (DGF rates of DCD vs DBD; surgical complications, prolonged hospital stay, etc.) have to be disclosed in detail.
    - The potential for machine perfusion (normothermic or hypothermic) and how this modifies but does not eliminate risk.
    - The patient's right to express preferences—e.g. willingness to accept only certain DCD Maastricht categories (cDCD vs uDCD), or only machine-perfused grafts.
    - Long-term graft survival data stratified by organ and donor category.
    - Any donor comorbidities or intraoperative findings that elevate risk (e.g. donor obesity, steatosis in liver, donor history of cardiac arrest with resuscitation).
    - The explicit right to decline this specific organ offer without losing waitlist position or prejudicing future offers—this is both ethically mandatory and legally required in most jurisdictions. The BTS guidance (2019) and the UNOS policy both clearly stipulate this.
    - The NHSBT and BTS recommend a two-stage consent process for DCD transplantation suggesting the first stage at the time of registration on the national deceased donor transplant waiting list during which patients receive both verbal and written information from the multidisciplinary team regarding the risks and benefits of transplantation and the second stage to take place at the time of organ offer, when consent for DCD transplantation is reconfirmed by the transplant surgeon upon the patient's admission [31].

  The Time-Pressure Problem
    - Organ offers must be accepted or declined within hours. This compresses the consent process in ways that may compromise voluntariness.

  Best practice includes:
    - Pre-emptive 'decision planning' at annual review, where patients state their DCD preferences in advance so they are not making a genuinely novel decision at midnight under duress.
    - Involving next of kin or healthcare proxy in line with the patient's expressed wishes.
    - Using transplant coordinators trained specifically in DCD risk communication, not just surgical team members.
    - Avoiding what has been termed 'therapeutic privilege'—the temptation to withhold unfavourable organ data to prevent the patient from declining an organ the surgeon believes is adequate.

Liver

Piyush Gupta, Amay Banker, and Ravi Mohanka

Introduction

Donation after circulatory death (DCD) liver transplantation occupies a unique position in the spectrum of deceased donation. The graft arrives bearing an obligate, quantifiable warm-ischaemic insult and the choice of recipient determines whether that insult is tolerated or amplified. In donation after brain death (DBD), recipient selection is dominated by waiting-list mortality and post-transplant survival considerations; in DCD, selection must additionally absorb the donor's biological burden—most prominently the risks of primary non-function (PNF, 2–8% in DCD versus 1–2% in DBD), early allograft dysfunction (EAD, 25–40%) and ischaemic cholangiopathy (IC, historically 10–30% in static-cold-stored DCD livers) [42, 46, 48]. Selecting the wrong recipient for a DCD graft creates the now well-recognised 'double jeopardy'—a marginal organ implanted into a marginal patient, in whom small physiological perturbations cascade into graft loss and death [46].

For emerging health systems such as India, where the deceased-donation rate remains below 1 per million population (NOTTO 2023–24: ~1000 deceased donor transplants nationally; ≈0.8 pmp), the prospect of DCD adds a much-needed organ stream but also imports a steeper learning curve. Indian recipients differ systematically from European or North-American cohorts: median MELD at transplant tends to be higher (often 22–28 in deceased donor recipients), tropical and chronic infections (HBV, HCV, tuberculosis, dengue, leptospirosis) are prevalent, alcohol-associated liver disease (ALD) and metabolic dysfunction-associated steatohepatitis (MASH) increasingly dominate the aetiological mix, and out-of-pocket financing of transplantation is the rule rather than the exception [64, 66].

This chapter addresses recipient selection exclusively. Donor and machine-perfusion considerations are covered elsewhere in this volume; outcomes data are cited only insofar as they are necessary to justify thresholds for selection.

Conceptual Framework: The Graft–Recipient Interaction in DCD

The DCD liver carries irreversible mitochondrial injury accumulated during functional warm ischaemia (donor systolic blood pressure <50 mmHg or SpO_2 <70% to cessation of cold flush) and during the obligate 'no-touch' period. Reperfusion in the recipient triggers oxidative burst, sterile inflammation and microvascular cholangiocyte injury [73]. The recipient's capacity to tolerate this insult depends on cardiopulmonary reserve, renal function, coagulation balance, immune set-point and surgical complexity (re-do field, portal vein thrombosis, prior TIPS). Conceptually, DCD-LT selection should be regarded as an additive risk equation: total risk = donor warm-ischaemic burden + cold-ischaemic time + recipient physiological reserve deficit + surgical complexity. Each axis contributes independently and, beyond a threshold, multiplicatively [42, 46]. Recipient selection is the only one of these axes fully under the transplant team's deliberate control once an organ is offered.

Recipient Factors Influencing DCD Candidacy

MELD Score

The recipient laboratory MELD is consistently the single most important recipient predictor in DCD. In the derivation of the UK DCD Risk Score (Schlegel et al., 1153 UK DCDs 2000–2015), recipient lab MELD >25 was independently associated with 1-year graft loss and assigned 2 points in the additive score [42]. In the UNOS validation cohort ($n = 1617$), recipients with MELD >25 had approximately a doubling of graft-loss hazard when combined with prolonged donor warm ischaemia [42, 44]. Historically, MELD ≥30 was considered a relative contraindication to DCD-LT, with US registry data showing 1-year graft survival falling below 75% [46].

This dogma has, however, been challenged. Meier et al. (UCSF/UNOS, *Front Immunol* 2023) analysed 41 UCSF and 375 UNOS DCD-LT recipients with lab-MELD ≥35 and reported a 5-year patient survival of 85% in the UCSF cohort, statistically equivalent to matched DBD recipients (86%, $p = 0.84$), provided strict donor selection (donor age <50, fWIT <20 min) and modern preservation were applied [47]. Multivariate analysis showed younger donor age and contemporary era (2011–2021 vs 1999–2010) were the dominant survival modifiers, with the adjusted hazard ratio for DCD vs DBD becoming non-significant in propensity-matched cohorts [47]. The implication is that high-MELD per se is no longer an absolute exclusion, but it raises the bar for donor quality and machine-perfusion support.

For programmes early in their DCD trajectory—including most Indian centres—a pragmatic threshold of MELD ≤25 (with serum sodium ≥130, and not on renal-replacement therapy) is recommended for DCD candidacy in the absence of normothermic regional perfusion (NRP) or hypothermic oxygenated perfusion (HOPE).

Recipient Age

Age >60 years contributes 3 points in the UK DCD Risk Score and is a robust predictor of graft loss (HR ≈ 1.6, 95% CI 1.2–2.1 in pooled analyses) [42, 43]. However, biological rather than chronological age matters: in subgroup analyses, recipients >60 with a cumulative score ≤10 retained acceptable 5-year graft survival (>75%) [43]. For Indian recipients, where average life expectancy at LT remains lower than in Western cohorts, an age cap of 65 years for DCD candidacy is reasonable, with case-by-case consideration up to 70 years for biologically robust patients (Karnofsky ≥80, no significant cardiopulmonary comorbidity).

BMI and Obesity

Obesity (BMI >30) increases surgical complexity, cold-ischaemic time, and post-reperfusion haemodynamic instability. While BMI in the UK DCD Risk Score is a donor variable, recipient BMI >35 is independently associated with EAD (OR 1.4, 95% CI 1.1–1.8 in UNOS analyses) and prolonged ICU stay [42, 44]. In Indian populations, BMI thresholds should be interpreted alongside body composition — sarcopenic obesity is increasingly recognised, particularly in MASH cirrhosis, where mortality is substantially elevated (pooled HR 1.76, 95% CI 1.33–2.33; multivariate HR 2.33, 95% CI 1.34–4.04) [71].

Cardiovascular Reserve

DCD reperfusion is haemodynamically more turbulent than DBD. All candidates require formal cardiac assessment: transthoracic echocardiography, dobutamine stress echocardiography or coronary angiography for those >50 years or with cardiovascular risk factors and right heart catheterisation when porto-pulmonary hypertension is suspected (mean pulmonary artery pressure >35 mmHg is a relative contraindication; >45 mmHg an absolute contraindication for any LT, more so DCD). Cardiopulmonary exercise testing (CPET) with anaerobic threshold <9 mL/kg/min and peak VO_2 <14 mL/kg/min identifies a high-risk group whose 90-day mortality after LT exceeds 20% in published series, and such patients should generally not receive a DCD graft outside an NRP/HOPE setting.

Renal Function

Pre-transplant renal dysfunction interacts adversely with DCD reperfusion injury. In UNOS analyses, recipients on renal-replacement therapy at the time of DCD-LT had a 1-year graft survival 8–12 percentage points lower than non-dialysed recipients [44, 46]. Estimated GFR <40 mL/min/1.73 m^2 and dialysis dependence should prompt strong consideration of simultaneous liver-kidney transplantation, or deferral to a DBD allocation, unless NRP/HOPE is available.

Frailty and Sarcopenia

The Liver Frailty Index (LFI; grip strength, chair stands, balance) categorises patients as robust (<3.2), pre-frail (3.2–4.5), or frail (>4.5). Frail status independently predicts waitlist mortality (HR 2.2, 95% CI 1.6–3.0) and 1-year post-LT mortality [69, 70]. Radiographic sarcopenia, quantified as L3 psoas muscle index <50 cm^2/m^2 (males) or <39 cm^2/m^2 (females), correlates with LFI but predicts post-LT outcomes somewhat less well than functional frailty [72]. In the DCD context, frailty should be regarded as a particularly strong relative contraindication: the additive insult of DCD reperfusion in a deconditioned recipient frequently exceeds physiological reserve. Pre-habilitation programmes—feasible even in resource-limited Indian settings—should be embedded into DCD candidacy.

Re-transplantation

Re-transplantation contributes 9 points (the largest single weight) in the UK DCD Risk Score and effectively places almost any recipient into the 'futile' category (>10 points) when combined with even moderate donor risk [42]. The original UCLA cohort reported an HR of 11.6 for re-transplantation in DCD-LT graft loss [80]. Re-LT with a DCD organ should be regarded as a near-absolute contraindication outside dedicated machine-perfusion programmes.

Prior Abdominal Surgery and Portal Vein Thrombosis

Yerdel grade III–IV portal vein thrombosis (PVT) and extensive prior upper-abdominal surgery prolong cold-ischaemic time (CIT) and increase intraoperative blood loss. In DCD, where every additional hour of CIT progressively magnifies cholangiopathy risk (HR for IC $\approx$ 1.34 per hour beyond 6 h) [73], Yerdel III–IV PVT is a relative contraindication. Recipients with high surgical-complexity scores should be matched only with low-risk DCD donors and, ideally, with NRP-recovered grafts.

Aetiology of Liver Disease

- *Hepatocellular Carcinoma (HCC)*: A meta-analysis of five comparative studies (487 DCD vs 973 DBD HCC recipients) demonstrated equivalent 1-year (RR 0.99, 95% CI 0.95–1.03) and 3-year (RR 0.99, 95% CI 0.89–1.09) recurrence-free survival, equivalent 1-year and 3-year patient survival, and equivalent graft survival [75]. HCC recipients within Milan or expanded criteria are appropriate DCD candidates and may benefit disproportionately given waitlist drop-out risk.
- *Alcohol-Associated Liver Disease (ALD)*: Acceptable if abstinence and psychosocial criteria are satisfied. Sarcopenia is common and must be assessed.
- *MASH*: Often coexists with cardiovascular and renal comorbidity; assess accordingly.
- *Viral hepatitis (HBV, HCV)*: With contemporary direct-acting antivirals and HBIG/nucleoside-analogue prophylaxis, HBV/HCV recipients are appropriate DCD candidates [67].
- *Acute liver failure (ALF)*: Generally avoid DCD; coagulopathy, cerebral oedema and haemodynamic instability create a milieu in which DCD reperfusion injury is poorly tolerated [46].
- *Autoimmune hepatitis, PBC, PSC*: Acceptable. PSC carries an inherent biliary-tree vulnerability and DCD adds risk—preferably with HOPE/NRP.

Psychosocial Readiness

DCD candidacy demands explicit, documented understanding of the elevated and qualitatively different risk profile. Cognitive impairment, active substance use, unstable housing and absent caregiver support are stronger relative contraindications in DCD than DBD because of the longer and more complex post-LT trajectory.

Risk Prediction Models

Risk Scores transform implicit clinical judgement into explicit, auditable thresholds. None is perfect; transportability across health systems is limited. We summarise the four most widely used.

UK DCD Risk Score (Schlegel 2018)

Seven variables are summed additively (Table 11.5). Performance: derivation c-statistic 0.79; UNOS validation 0.71; Birmingham 0.64 [42]. Subsequent US re-validation by Wu et al. on a contemporary UNOS cohort reported a degraded c-statistic of 0.611—though graft-loss hazards retained directional consistency: HR 0.79 (95% CI 0.68–0.93, $p = 0.004$) for 0–5 vs 6–10 and HR 1.26 (95% CI 1.01–1.56, $p = 0.04$) for 11–20 vs 6–10 [44]. The drop in discrimination reflects improved overall outcomes (compression of variance) and broader use of marginal grafts, not failure of the score's underlying logic.

A statistical critique by Schwab and colleagues noted unusually large effect sizes (notably for re-transplantation and fWIT) and questioned model overfitting [45]; for clinical use, the score remains the best-validated DCD-specific instrument worldwide and is endorsed by the ILTS 2021 consensus [46].

US-DCD Risk Index (DCD-RSI)

Eight variables, weighted; predicts 3-month survival; c-statistic 0.6971 in derivation. Strongest recipient predictors: serum sodium >150 mEq/L at transplant, albumin <2.0 g/dL, history of PVT. It outperformed BAR, RRI and SOFT in selecting optimal DCD candidates pre-transplant [61].

UC-DCD Score (UCSF)

Ten variables including donor warm ischaemia time, donor heparinisation, recipient mechanical ventilation, TIPS, aetiology, MELD, BMI, donor/recipient age and CIT. UNOS validation AUC 0.635, outperforming all prior scores in that contemporary US cohort [60].

BAR Score (Dutkowski 2011)

Six variables (recipient MELD, recipient age, donor age, CIT, life support, re-LT), range 0–27. Originally derived in DBD (UNOS, $n = 37{,}255$), excluding DCDs. Cut-off 18 separates acceptable from unacceptable risk [56, 57]. In external Spanish

Table 11.5 UK DCD Risk Score—variables, weights and risk bands

Variable	Cut-off	Points
Donor age	>60 years	2
Donor BMI	>25 kg/m^2	3
Functional warm ischaemia	20–30 min	3
Functional warm ischaemia	>30 min	6
Cold ischaemia	>6 h	2
Recipient lab MELD	>25	2
Recipient age	>60 years	3
Re-transplantation	Yes	9

Risk bands: Low risk 0–5 (1-year graft survival >95%); high risk 6–10 (>85%); futile >10 (~50% at 1 year; <20% at 5 year)

Abbreviations: *BMI* body mass index, DCD donation after circulatory death, MELD model for end-stage liver disease

DCD-inclusive cohorts, AUROC was 0.62 for 5-year survival; in living-donor cohorts 0.6–0.7. BAR is best regarded as a generic donor–recipient match score, not DCD-specific.

Donor Risk Index and Eurotransplant DRI

DRI was derived in DBD; DCD status itself is an input variable (HR 1.51) [58]. Pure DRI has a c-statistic of only ~0.50 to 0.55 for short-term outcomes in DCD cohorts and is not recommended as a stand-alone DCD selection tool.

SOFT and D-MELD

SOFT (18 variables) and D-MELD (donor age × recipient MELD) provide adjunctive information [59]. D-MELD >1600 is associated with markedly inferior outcomes in DBD; in DCD the threshold is intuitively lower (~1200) but not formally validated.

Comparative Performance

The comparative performance of the various validated DCD/LT Risk Scores is presented in Table 11.6.

Donor Selection Criteria for DCD Liver Transplantation

Donor selection is the upstream complement to recipient selection: cumulative donor–recipient risk, not either side alone, drives PNF and IC after DCD-LT. ILTS-endorsed routine thresholds are donor age ≤60 year, BMI ≤30 kg/m^2, macrovesicular steatosis ≤30%, fDWIT ≤30 min (≤20 min preferable) and CIT ≤8 h [46, 73]. Donors above these limits may still be acceptable if quantified by the UK or US-DCD Risk Score and used with machine perfusion; conversely, no preservation strategy reliably rescues a graft with open-ended fDWIT or severe steatosis.

Table 11.6 Comparative performance of validated DCD/LT risk scores

Score	Population	Derivation c-stat	External c-stat	Key finding
UK DCD (2018)	UK DCD	0.79	0.71 (UNOS); 0.611 (US 2022)	Futile band (>10 pts) → 5-year graft survival <20%
DCD-RSI (2023)	UNOS DCD	0.697	–	Recipient Na >150 strongest single recipient predictor
UC-DCD (2022)	UCSF / UNOS	0.64	0.635 (UNOS)	Outperformed prior scores in contemporary US cohort
BAR (2011)	UNOS DBD	0.70	0.62 (Spain DCD-incl.)	Cut-off 18; generic match score, not DCD-specific
DRI (2006)	UNOS	0.58	~0.50–0.55 (DCD)	Limited stand-alone utility in DCD; DCD itself is an input

Abbreviations: *BAR* balance of risk, *c-stat* concordance statistic, *DBD* donation after brain death, *DCD* donation after circulatory death, *DCD-RSI* donation after circulatory death risk selection index, *DCD-incl.* donation after circulatory death-inclusive, *DRI* donor risk index, *UNOS* united network for organ sharing, *UC-DCD* University of California Donation after circulatory death score, *UCSF* University of California, San Francisco

The same donor liver may be unacceptable under static cold storage (SCS), borderline under hypothermic oxygenated perfusion (HOPE) and confidently transplantable under in situ NRP or ex situ NMP once functional viability is demonstrated. Beyond perfusate lactate and transaminases, viability adjudication uses hepatocyte glucose utilisation (insulin-responsive fall in perfusate glucose) for PNF risk and biliary bicarbonate, pH and glucose for IC risk [82, 83]. Table 11.7 summarises the principal numerical thresholds. The operational rule is simple: an SCS-only programme should hold tighter donor limits than a perfusion-capable one, and machine perfusion converts donor acceptance from a binary decision into a graded one [46, 52, 53, 82].

Calibration, Reclassification and Machine Learning

Hosmer–Lemeshow calibration of the UK DCD score in the original derivation was acceptable ($p > 0.05$); however, no formal Net Reclassification Improvement (NRI) or Integrated Discrimination Improvement (IDI) metrics have been published comparing it head-to-head with newer scores [42, 60]. Recent machine-learning approaches using NMP perfusate biomarkers (lactate clearance, transaminase trajectory, perfusate pH) have produced AUROCs of 0.80–0.88 for prediction of EAD in single-centre studies, though external validation and class imbalance remain concerns [49, 51]. Heterogeneity across published validations is high ($I^2 > 60\%$ in pooled analyses of c-statistic shifts), reflecting era effects, allocation differences and variable preservation strategies.

Donor–Recipient Matching to Avoid Double Jeopardy

The cardinal principle: *a marginal DCD graft must not be allocated to a marginal recipient*. Operationally, this is best expressed as a 3 × 3 matrix (Table 11.8) that combines donor and recipient risk strata and indicates the perfusion intervention required for marginal combinations to be acceptable. This formalises the ILTS 2021 recommendation that DCD-LT outcomes depend on cumulative donor–recipient risk and that the UK DCD Risk Score should be used to define thresholds for declining certain combinations [46].

Special Populations

HCC Equivalent oncologic outcomes (Section "Aetiology of Liver Disease"). Active candidates with rising AFP or progression on bridging therapy are particularly appropriate for DCD given waitlist drop-out risk [46, 75].

Acute Liver Failure Generally avoid. The combination of cerebral oedema, vasoplegia and coagulopathy makes DCD reperfusion injury poorly tolerated. Reserve only for situations in which no DBD organ is available within the projected survival window.

Table 11.7 Comparative numerical viability thresholds for SCS, NMP, and NRP—markers most relevant to PNF and IC prevention

Parameter	SCS	Ex situ NMP	In situ NRP
Functional viability window	–	4–6 h ex vivo	1–4 h in situ post-arrest
Perfusate lactate	–	≤2.5 mmol/L by 2–4 h [82, 83]	Downward trend; DO_2-normalised clearance [52]
Transaminases (peak perfusate)	Donor ALT/AST screen only	ALT <6000 IU/L (Cambridge); rising trajectory predicts EAD [51, 82, 83]	AST/ALT <1000 IU/L by 2 h NRP; >1000 IU/L at 2 h is the leading discard reason [52]
Perfusate pH	–	>7.30 [82]	Maintained physiologic range
Glucose utilisation (hepatocyte)	–	Fall in perfusate glucose, augmented by insulin; failure to metabolise glucose is rare and concerning [82, 83]	Perfusate glucose trend; insulin-responsiveness less standardised
Bile pH (cholangiocyte/ IC)	–	>7.48 [83]	Not directly measurable; IC reduced via peribiliary-plexus reperfusion [52, 53, 76]
Bile bicarbonate	–	>18 mmol/L [83]	Not measurable in situ
Bile glucose / bile-perfusate ratio	–	Bile glucose <16 mmol/L; bile/ perfusate glucose ratio < 0.67 [83]	Not measurable in situ
Flavin mononucleotide (FMN)[a]	–	–	<10.6 ng/mL low-risk; >23.5 ng/mL high-risk (HOPE/D-HOPE) [84]
Routine donor cut-offs	Tight: Age ≤ 60, BMI ≤30, steatosis ≤30%, fDWIT ≤30 min, CIT ≤8 h [46, 73]	Selectively extendable when ex vivo criteria met [51, 82]	Selectively extendable when in situ criteria met [46, 52, 53]

[a]FMN is validated for hypothermic oxygenated perfusion (HOPE/D-HOPE); included for completeness given increasing use of sequential HOPE→NMP and HOPE-after-NRP protocols. ITBL, ischaemic-type biliary lesion

Abbreviations: *ALT* alanine aminotransferase, *AST* aspartate aminotransferase, *BMI* body mass index, *CIT* cold ischaemia time, *D-HOPE* dual hypothermic oxygenated perfusion, *DO_2* oxygen delivery, *EAD* early allograft dysfunction, *FMN* flavin mononucleotide, *fDWIT* functional donor warm ischaemia time, *HOPE* hypothermic oxygenated perfusion, *IC* ischaemic cholangiopathy, *IU/L* international units per litre, *NMP* normothermic machine perfusion, *NRP* normothermic regional perfusion, *SCS* static cold storage

Table 11.8 Donor–recipient matching matrix to avoid double jeopardy

Donor risk × Recipient risk	Low-risk recipient (MELD ≤20, age <55, no PVT, robust)	Intermediate recipient (MELD 21–28, age 55–65, mild co-morbidity)	High-risk recipient (MELD >28, age >65, frail, Yerdel III–IV, re-LT)
Low-risk DCD donor (age <50, fWIT <20 min, BMI <25)	Acceptable	Acceptable	Acceptable only with NRP/HOPE
Intermediate DCD donor (age 50–60, fWIT 20–30 min, BMI 25–30)	Acceptable	Acceptable with HOPE/NRP	Avoid
High-risk DCD donor (age >60, fWIT >30 min, steatosis >30%)	Acceptable only with HOPE/NRP	Avoid	Futile — do not transplant

Abbreviations: *BMI* body mass index, *DCD* donation after circulatory death, *fWIT* functional warm ischaemia time, *HOPE* hypothermic oxygenated perfusion, *MELD* model for end-stage liver disease, *NRP* normothermic regional perfusion, *PVT* portal vein thrombosis, *re-LT* re-transplantation

Re-transplantation Relative-to-absolute contraindication outside dedicated programmes with NRP/HOPE; UK score weighting (9 points) effectively excludes these patients from "low-risk" categorisation [42, 46].

Paediatric DCD paediatric LT remains uncommon. Where used (largely with split or reduced grafts), donor age ≤40, fWIT <20 min and recipient stability are mandatory. Indian centres should not embark on paediatric DCD-LT until adult DCD programmes mature [65].

HIV/HBV/HCV HIV-positive recipients with controlled disease (CD4 > 200, undetectable viral load) are candidates. HBV and HCV are not contraindications. For HBV-positive recipients, low-dose HBIG plus a high-genetic-barrier nucleoside-analogue strategy is appropriate [67].

Ethical Considerations

The four-principle framework—autonomy, beneficence, non-maleficence, justice—is recalibrated in DCD-LT.

Equipoise and Equity Are similarly placed waitlist patients offered DCD on similar terms? Programmatic offer–acceptance audits should be routine.

Utility Versus Urgency A high-MELD recipient may have the greatest urgency, but allocating a marginal DCD graft to that recipient maximises double-jeopardy risk. Most allocation systems (UNOS, Eurotransplant, UK NHSBT) explicitly permit 'centre discretion' to refuse a DCD offer for a high-MELD recipient—this discretion should be exercised transparently and documented [46].

Marginal-Graft Acceptance and the Duty of Disclosure Once a DCD organ is provisionally accepted, the recipient (or surrogate) must be told that the graft carries a higher risk profile. Failing to disclose breaches autonomy and exposes the programme to medico-legal risk. In Indian practice, where family-centred decision-making is the norm, disclosure should be made to the recipient and to the financially responsible family member jointly.

Indian-Specific Issues Out-of-pocket financing creates the risk of financial coercion—patients may feel obligated to accept a marginal organ rather than continue paying ICU costs while waiting. Programmes must counter this by explicitly stating that refusal of a particular DCD offer does not affect future DBD allocation. The ISOT–ISCCM 2022 joint position paper explicitly mandates that the decision to withdraw life-sustaining treatment in a potential DCD donor must be entirely independent of and prior to any organ-donation discussion [62]; the same firewall principle should apply on the recipient side regarding organ acceptance.

Informed Consent for DCD Recipients

Disclosure must be DCD-specific, written, signed at a non-emergency timepoint (i.e. during candidacy evaluation, not at the moment of organ offer), and reaffirmed at the time of acceptance (Table 11.9). Quantitative

Table 11.9 Mandatory disclosure elements for DCD-specific informed consent

Mandatory disclosure element	Quantitative anchor (where available)
Definition of DCD and difference from DBD	Lay-language explanation
Risk of primary non-function (PNF)	2–8% (DCD) vs 1–2% (DBD)
Risk of early allograft dysfunction (EAD)	25–40% (DCD) vs 15–25% (DBD)
Risk of ischaemic cholangiopathy	10–30% (static cold storage); ~3% with NRP/HOPE
Risk of biliary stricture requiring ERCP	20–30% over 5 years
Risk of re-transplantation	8–15% within 5 years
1-year graft survival expectation	85–95% (low–/high-risk bands of UK score)
5-year graft survival expectation	70–80% (selected populations)
Alternative options	Continued waitlist for DBD; LDLT; declining transplant
Right to refuse this specific offer	Explicit statement; future allocation unaffected

Abbreviations: *DBD* donation after brain death, *DCD* donation after circulatory death, *EAD* early allograft dysfunction, *ERCP* endoscopic retrograde cholangiopancreatography, *HOPE* hypothermic oxygenated perfusion, *LDLT* living donor liver transplantation, *NRP* normothermic regional perfusion, *PNF* primary non-function communication ('approximately 1 in 5 risk of biliary complication requiring further procedures') consistently outperforms verbal qualifiers ('uncommon', 'occasional') in patient-comprehension studies. Indian centres should provide consent documents in the recipient's primary language and engage trained transplant coordinators rather than surgical residents for the consent conversation.

Worked Clinical Examples

Example 1: A 'Borderline Acceptable' Indian Recipient

Patient Mr. A, 52-year-old male, ALD-cirrhosis, abstinent 14 months, MELD 22, BMI 28, eGFR 78 mL/min/1.73 m^2, LFI 3.6 (pre-frail), echocardiogram normal, CPET peak VO_2 18 mL/kg/min, no PVT, first transplant.

Donor Offer 58-year-old controlled DCD donor, BMI 27, fWIT 24 min, anticipated CIT 5.5 h, no significant steatosis on biopsy. NRP not available; HOPE available.

UK DCD Risk Score Calculation

- Donor age > 60: 0 (donor is 58).
- Donor BMI >25: 3.
- fWIT 20–30 min: 3.
- CIT >6 h: 0 (anticipated 5.5 h).
- Recipient MELD >25: 0 (MELD 22).
- Recipient age > 60: 0 (age 52).
- Re-LT: 0.
- *Total: 6 points → high-risk band (1-yr graft survival ~ 85%)* [42].

BAR Score MELD 22 (4 pts), recipient age 52 (1 pt), donor age 58 (1 pt), CIT 5.5 h (0), no life support (0), no re-LT (0) = 6 points (well below the 18-point cutoff) [56, 57].

Decision Accept with HOPE preservation. The high-risk UK score band predicts adequate but not excellent survival; HOPE is expected to reduce ischaemic cholangiopathy from ~18% (DHOPE-DCD trial control arm) to ~6% (intervention arm; van Rijn et al., NEJM 2021) [49, 50]. Pre-frailty is addressed with intensified prehabilitation. Consent documentation must explicitly include the high-risk band classification.

Example 2: A 'Futile' Combination to Refuse

Patient Mr. B, 64-year-old male, MASH cirrhosis, MELD 28, BMI 33, eGFR 42 mL/min/1.73 m^2, Yerdel grade III PVT, prior cholecystectomy and TIPS, LFI 4.7 (frail), peak VO_2 11 mL/kg/min.

Donor Offer 62-year-old DCD donor, BMI 28, fWIT 32 min, anticipated CIT 7 h.

UK DCD Risk Score Donor age > 60 (2) + Donor BMI >25 (3) + fWIT >30 min (6) + CIT >6 h (2) + Recipient MELD >25 (2) + Recipient age > 60 (3) + Re-LT (0) = *18 points* → *futile band* [42].

Decision Decline. Predicted 1-year graft survival <50%; the combination of high-risk donor and high-risk recipient creates archetypal double jeopardy. The recipient should be considered for living-donor LT (Indian context), prioritised for DBD or—if a low-risk DCD donor with NRP support becomes available—re-evaluated. Even with NRP, the recipient's frailty and surgical complexity make this a marginal candidate; multidisciplinary review is mandatory before any future DCD offer is accepted for this patient.

Indian Context: Regulatory Framework, Recipient Pool and Practical Recommendations

The Transplantation of Human Organs Act (THOTA) 1994 and its 2011 amendment provide the legal framework for both DBD and DCD in India. The ISOT–ISCCM 2022 joint position paper (Seth, Mohanka, Navin et al.) explicitly endorses controlled DCD (Maastricht III), uncontrolled DCD (categories I, II, V), and category IV (cardiac arrest during brain-death determination), and specifies ethical, legal and procedural safeguards including the firewall between withdrawal-of-life-sustaining-treatment (WLST) decisions and donation discussions, the no-touch period and antemortem-intervention consent (Table 11.10) [62]. Allocation occurs through SOTTOs and ROTTOs under the NOTTO umbrella; DCD organs follow the same allocation logic as DBD organs in most states.

Indian Recipient-Pool Reality

- Median MELD at deceased donor LT is high (often 22–28); DCD candidacy must be calibrated accordingly [64, 66].
- HBV remains prevalent (5–10% of cirrhosis); HCV is declining post-DAA but remains relevant; tuberculosis screening (IGRA, chest CT) is mandatory pre-LT, and active TB precludes DCD-LT until treated [67].
- ALD and MASH together now constitute over half of LT indications in most major Indian centres [66, 68].
- The first reported DCD liver transplant in India was performed at BLK Super Speciality Hospital; subsequent isolated cases and small series have been reported from Apollo, Global, Reliance, Medanta and Rela Institute. The total Indian DCD-LT experience remains in low double digits as of 2025 [64, 65].
- Out-of-pocket financing (typical adult LT cost ₹20–35 lakh) creates pressure for rapid decision-making; programmes must build in a structured 'cooling-off' interval for DCD consent. Additional cost of NRP should be considered which can range from Rs.50,000 to Rs.120,000 depending on the type of equipment used [85].

Table 11.10 Indian-context summary: regulatory, epidemiological, and practical considerations for DCD recipient selection

Domain	Indian context	Implication for DCD recipient selection
Legal framework	THOTA 1994 (amended 2011, 2014); ISOT-ISCCM 2022 DCD position paper recognises Maastricht I, II, III, IV, V	Begin programmes with controlled (Maastricht III); operationalise the WLST/donation firewall
Allocation	NOTTO/SOTTO criteria; no DCD-specific allocation algorithm yet	Centre-level recipient selection is the principal safeguard
Consent	Form-8 family consent; WLST framework consolidating after 2018/2023 supreme court guidance	DCD-specific written consent in primary language; structured cooling-off
MELD distribution	Median MELD at deceased donor LT 22–28	Pool of low-risk recipients limited; HOPE/NRP highly desirable
Infection burden	HBV 5–10%; HCV declining post-DAA; TB endemic; tropical infections common	Stringent screening; avoid DCD in active viraemia or untreated TB
Aetiology mix	ALD and MASH together >50% of LT indications	Rigorous cardiac/renal workup; address sarcopenic obesity
Cost	Predominantly out-of-pocket; HOPE/NMP largely unreimbursed. Cost of NRP ranging from Rs. 50,000 to 120,000 depending on location of withdrawal of care and use of ECMO circuit vs a modified cardiopulmonary bypass circuit.	Address financial coercion in consent; phased machine-perfusion adoption
Geography	Long inter-city distances; variable green-corridor reliability	Prioritise local allocation; minimise CIT
Centre experience	Total DCD-LT national experience in low double digits as of 2025	Restrict early DCD-LT to high-volume LDLT/DDLT centres

Abbreviations: *ALD* alcohol-associated liver disease, *CIT* cold ischaemia time, *DAA* direct-acting antiviral, *DCD* donation after circulatory death, *DDLT* deceased donor liver transplantation, *ECMO* extracorporeal membrane oxygenation, *HBV* hepatitis B virus, *HCV* hepatitis C virus, *HOPE* hypothermic oxygenated perfusion, *ISCCM* Indian Society of Critical Care Medicine, *ISOT* Indian Society of Organ Transplantation, *LDLT* living donor liver transplantation, *LT* liver transplantation, *MASH* metabolic dysfunction-associated steatohepatitis, *MELD* model for end-stage liver disease, *NMP* normothermic machine perfusion, *NOTTO* National Organ and tissue transplant organisation, *NRP* normothermic regional perfusion, *SOTTO* state organ and tissue transplant organisation, *TB* tuberculosis, *THOTA* transplantation of human organs and tissues act, *WLST* withdrawal of life-sustaining treatment

Practical Recommendations for Indian Centres

1. Begin with low-risk DCD donors (age < 50, fWIT <20 min, BMI <25, anticipated CIT <6 h) only.
2. Match initial DCD organs to low-risk recipients (MELD 15–20, age < 60, no PVT, robust LFI <3.2, normal cardiopulmonary reserve).

3. Apply the UK DCD Risk Score formally to every offer; refuse all combinations >10 points until at least 25 DCD-LTs have been performed and outcomes audited [42].
4. Invest in HOPE before NRP (lower complexity, lower cost, demonstrable Class I evidence from the DHOPE-DCD trial) [49, 50].
5. Maintain a centre-level DCD registry feeding into the proposed ISOT national DCD registry; report outcomes against UK and US benchmarks [54].
6. Implement structured DCD-specific consent in the local language with a quantitative risk-communication template.
7. Address financial coercion proactively through transparent counselling and, where possible, philanthropic or insurance support.

Future Directions

Three trajectories will reshape DCD recipient selection over the next decade. *First, dynamic risk reassessment with machine perfusion*—the perfusate lactate, transaminase, pH and bile composition during NMP/HOPE allow real-time graft viability assessment, in effect replacing static recipient-side risk thresholds with intraoperative go/no-go decisions; recipient selection becomes a probabilistic, conditional process rather than a binary pre-acceptance one [49, 51, 55]. *Second, AI-based donor–recipient matching—neural-network* and gradient-boosted models trained on registry and perfusion data are achieving AUROCs of 0.80+ for EAD prediction; their fairness, calibration and transportability to Indian populations require deliberate validation. *Third, biomarker-augmented selection*—recipient mitochondrial function (peripheral blood ATP synthesis), inflammatory signatures (IL-6, sTNFR1) and gut-microbiome composition may emerge as adjunctive selection variables, particularly for high-MELD candidates. Indian centres should actively contribute to international validation cohorts to ensure these tools are calibrated for South-Asian physiology.

Conclusion

DCD liver transplantation can be a force multiplier for India's organ supply, but only if recipient selection is executed with discipline. The UK DCD Risk Score, supplemented by the BAR and emerging US-DCD scores, provides an explicit, validated framework. Avoiding the futile band (>10 points), recognising the disproportionate weight of re-transplantation and prolonged warm ischaemia and refusing to compound marginal grafts onto marginal recipients are the cardinal rules [42, 46]. In emerging programmes, conservatism is not timidity—it is the foundation on which a credible DCD record is built. As Indian centres extend their DCD experience, the integration of HOPE, NRP and dynamic perfusion-based risk reassessment will progressively widen the acceptable donor–recipient envelope. Throughout, the ethical core remains constant: the recipient must understand the additional risk, must consent to it freely and must be selected because the graft can plausibly serve them—not because the system needs them to serve the graft.

Conflict of Interest The authors have no conflicts of interest to disclose.

Competing Interests The author(s) has no competing interests to declare that are relevant to the content of this manuscript.

Ethics Approval The author(s) declares that this manuscript does not include primary research with human participants.

The author(s) declares that this manuscript does not include primary studies involving animals.

References

1. Scalea JR, Redfield RR, Arpali E, Leverson GE, Bennett RJ, Anderson ME, Kaufman DB, Fernandez LA, D'Alessandro AM, Foley DP, et al. Does DCD donor time-to-death affect recipient outcomes? Implications of time-to-death at a high-volume Center in the United States. Am J Transplant. 2017;17(1):191–200.
2. Bellingham JM, Santhanakrishnan C, Neidlinger N, Wai P, Kim J, Niederhaus S, Leverson GE, Fernandez LA, Foley DP, Mezrich JD, et al. Donation after cardiac death: a 29-year experience. Surgery. 2011;150(4):692–702.
3. Gruessner AC, Saggi SJ, Gruessner RWG. Pancreas transplantation from donors after cardiac death – the US experience. Transplant Rep. 2022;7(2):100099.
4. Leemkuil M, Leuvenink HGD, Pol RA. Pancreas transplantation from donors after circulatory death: an irrational reluctance? Curr Diab Rep. 2019;19(11):129.
5. Yao Z, Kuang M, Li Z. Risk factors for delayed graft function in patients with kidney transplantation: a systematic review and meta-analysis. BMJ Open. 2025;15(3):e087128.
6. Summers DM, Johnson RJ, Hudson A, Collett D, Watson CJ, Bradley JA. Effect of donor age and cold storage time on outcome in recipients of kidneys donated after circulatory death in the UK: a cohort study. Lancet. 2013;381(9868):727–34.
7. Boggi U, Vistoli F, Andres A, Arbogast HP, Badet L, Baronti W, Bartlett ST, Benedetti E, Branchereau J, Burke GW 3rd, et al. First World Consensus Conference on pancreas transplantation: Part II – recommendations. Am J Transplant. 2021;21:17–59.
8. Prunster J, Wong G, Larkins N, Wyburn K, Francis R, Mulley WR, Ooi E, Pilmore H, Davies CE, Lim WH. Kidney donor profile index and allograft outcomes: interactive effects of estimated post-transplant survival score and ischaemic time. Clin Kidney J. 2023;16(3):473–83.
9. Gruessner AC, Sutherland DE. Pancreas transplant outcomes for United States (US) and non-US cases as reported to the United Network for Organ Sharing (UNOS) and the International Pancreas Transplant Registry (IPTR) as of June 2004. Clin Transpl. 2005;19(4):433–55.
10. Muthusamy ASR, Mumford L, Hudson A, Fuggle SV, Friend PJ. Pancreas transplantation from donors after circulatory death from the United Kingdom. Am J Transplant. 2012;12(8):2150–6.
11. Nicoletto B, Fonseca N, Manfro R, Gonçalves L, Leitão C, Souza G. Effects of obesity on kidney transplantation outcomes: a systematic review and meta-analysis. Transplantation. 2014;98:167–76.
12. Humar A, Ramcharan T, Kandaswamy R, Gruessner RWG, Gruessner AG, Sutherland DER. The impact of donor obesity on outcomes after cadaver pancreas transplants. Am J Transplant. 2004;4(4):605–10.

13. Mittal S, Gilbert J, Friend PJ. Donors after circulatory death pancreas transplantation. Curr Opin Organ Transplant. 2017;22(4):372–6.
14. Alghannam K, Fine J, Howard B, Loza J, Goussous NM, Sageshima J, Mineyev NM, Wang AX, Perez RV, Than PA. Impact of warm ischemia time on donation after circulatory death kidney transplant outcomes. Clin Transpl. 2024;38(8):e15436.
15. Qureshi MS, Callaghan CJ, Bradley JA, Watson CJE, Pettigrew GJ. Outcomes of simultaneous pancreas–kidney transplantation from brain-dead and controlled circulatory death donors. Br J Surg. 2012;99(6):831–8.
16. El Sabagh A, Mohamed IB, Aloor FZ, Abdelwahab A, Hassan MM, Jalal PK. Current status of biomarkers and molecular diagnostic tools for rejection in liver transplantation: light at the end of the tunnel? J Clin Exp Hepatol. 2023;13(1):139–48.
17. Chumdermpadetsuk RR, Alvino DML, Kaul S, Fleishman A, Eckhoff DE, Pavlakis M, Lee DD. Impact of donor warm ischemia time on graft survival for donation after circulatory death kidney transplantation. Transplantation. 2025;109(3):504–10.
18. Debout A, Foucher Y, Trébern-Launay K, Legendre C, Kreis H, Mourad G, Garrigue V, Morelon E, Buron F, Rostaing L, et al. Each additional hour of cold ischemia time significantly increases the risk of graft failure and mortality following renal transplantation. Kidney Int. 2015;87(2):343–9.
19. Luo Y, Dong Z, Hu X, Tang Z, Zhang J, Deng W, Wei X, Miao B, Qin F, Na N. Donor death category is an effect modifier between cold ischemia time and post-transplant graft function in deceased-donor kidney transplant recipients. Front Med (Lausanne). 2021;8:743085.
20. Peters-Sengers H, Houtzager JHE, Idu MM, Heemskerk MBA, van Heurn ELW, Homan van der Heide JJ, Kers J, Berger SP, van Gulik TM, Bemelman FJ. impact of cold ischemia time on outcomes of deceased donor kidney transplantation: an analysis of a national registry. Transplant Direct. 2019;5(5):e448.
21. Cojuc-Konigsberg G, Rivera B, Cañizares S, Pavlakis M, Eckhoff D, Chopra B. Impact of cold ischemia time and donor age on donation after circulatory death kidney transplant outcomes: a UNOS mate-kidney analysis. Clin Transpl. 2024;38(12):e70051.
22. Muñoz-Bellvís L, López-Sánchez J. Donor risk factors in pancreas transplantation. World J Transplant. 2020;10(12):372–80.
23. Rudolph EN, Dunn TB, Sutherland DER, Kandaswamy R, Finger EB. Optimizing outcomes in pancreas transplantation: impact of organ preservation time. Clin Transpl. 2017;31(9)
24. Trachsel C, Kalt F, Jonas JP, Rössler F, Lopez-Lopez V, Hübel K, Schneider M, Kron P, Gerdes S, Stratta R, et al. Outcomes of kidney transplants from donors after circulatory death with acute kidney injury: a systematic review. Curr Transplant Rep. 2025;12(1):40.
25. Fernandez LA, Di Carlo A, Odorico JS, Leverson GE, Shames BD, Becker YT, Chin LT, Pirsch JD, Knechtle SJ, Foley DP, et al. Simultaneous pancreas-kidney transplantation from donation after cardiac death: successful long-term outcomes. Ann Surg. 2005;242(5):716–23.
26. Walls DO, Lee-Riddle GS, Bover Manderski M, Sawinski DL, Abt PL. Kidney transplant outcomes from donation after circulatory death donors of advanced age. Clin Transpl. 2020;34(7):e13881.
27. McAdams-DeMarco MA, Olorundare IO, Ying H, Warsame F, Haugen CE, Hall R, Garonzik-Wang JM, Desai NM, Walston JD, Norman SP, et al. Frailty and postkidney transplant health-related quality of life. Transplantation. 2018;102(2):291–9.
28. Meier-Kriesche HU, Kaplan B. Waiting time on dialysis as the strongest modifiable risk factor for renal transplant outcomes: a paired donor kidney analysis. Transplantation. 2002;74(10):1377–81.
29. Summers DM, Johnson RJ, Allen J, Fuggle SV, Collett D, Watson CJ, Bradley JA. Analysis of factors that affect outcome after transplantation of kidneys donated after cardiac death in the UK: a cohort study. Lancet. 2010;376(9749):1303–11.
30. Cooper JT, Chin LT, Krieger NR, Fernandez LA, Foley DP, Becker YT, Odorico JS, Knechtle SJ, Kalayoglu M, Sollinger HW, et al. Donation after cardiac death: the University of Wisconsin experience with renal transplantation. Am J Transplant. 2004;4(9):1490–4.

31. Society BT: Guidelines relating to solid organ transplants from non-heart beating donors: British Transplantation Society; 2005.
32. Berney T, Boffa C, Augustine T, Badet L, de Koning E, Pratschke J, Socci C, Friend P. Utilization of organs from donors after circulatory death for vascularized pancreas and islet of Langerhans transplantation: recommendations from an expert group. Transpl Int. 2016;29(7):798–806.
33. Nagata H, Matsumoto S, Okitsu T, Iwanaga Y, Noguchi H, Yonekawa Y, Tanaka K. In situ cooling of pancreata from non–heart-beating donors prior to procurement for islet transplantation. Transplant Proc. 2005;37(8):3393–5.
34. Chassot M, Scheen M, Wassmer C-H, Compagnon P, Peloso A, Haidar F. Donor after circulatory death in pancreas transplantation: a scoping review of the literature. Front Transplant. 2025;4:2025.
35. Kosmoliaptsis V, Salji M, Bardsley V, Chen Y, Thiru S, Griffiths MH, Copley HC, Saeb-Parsy K, Bradley JA, Torpey N, et al. Baseline donor chronic renal injury confers the same transplant survival disadvantage for DCD and DBD kidneys. Am J Transplant. 2015;15(3):754–63.
36. Summers DM, Watson CJE, Pettigrew GJ, Johnson RJ, Collett D, Neuberger JM, Bradley JA. Kidney donation after circulatory death (DCD): state of the art. Kidney Int. 2015;88(2):241–9.
37. Vanin AA, Valderrama Cometa LA, Acuña Roldan CF, Alhajj NA, Devia Santacruz CJ. Graft and patient survival in kidney transplant with deceased donor using KDRI (kidney donor risk index), KDPI (kidney donor profile index), and EPTS (estimated post-transplant survival) in Colombia. Ann Transplant. 2023;28:e940522.
38. Zens TJ, Danobeitia JS, Leverson G, Chlebeck PJ, Zitur LJ, Redfield RR, D'Alessandro AM, Odorico S, Kaufman DB, Fernandez LA. The impact of kidney donor profile index on delayed graft function and transplant outcomes: a single-center analysis. Clin Transpl. 2018;32(3):e13190.
39. Dahmen M, Becker F, Pavenstädt H, Suwelack B, Schütte-Nütgen K, Reuter S. Validation of the kidney donor profile index (KDPI) to assess a deceased donor's kidneys' outcome in a European cohort. Sci Rep. 2019;9(1):11234.
40. Axelrod DA, Sung RS, Meyer KH, Wolfe RA, Kaufman DB. Systematic evaluation of pancreas allograft quality, outcomes and geographic variation in utilization. Am J Transplant. 2010;10(4):837–45.
41. Campsen J, Zimmerman MA. Pancreas transplantation following donation after circulatory death. Transplant Rep. 2022;7(4):100120.
42. Schlegel A, Kalisvaart M, Scalera I, Laing RW, Mergental H, Mirza DF, et al. The UK DCD risk score: a new proposal to define futility in donation-after-circulatory-death liver transplantation. J Hepatol. 2018;68(3):456–64.
43. Kalisvaart M, Muiesan P, Schlegel A. The UK-DCD-risk-score—practical and new guidance for allocation of a specific organ to a recipient? Expert Rev Gastroenterol Hepatol. 2019;13(8):771–83.
44. Wu DD, Vargas C, Lozano P, McAlister V, Skaro AI, Bhat M, et al. Applicability of the UK DCD risk score in the modern era of liver transplantation: a U.S. update. Clin Transpl. 2022;36(3):e14579.
45. Schwab S, Banz V, Held U, Hoessly L, Magini G. Does the UK DCD risk score have statistical flaws? J Hepatol. 2025;83(2):e84–5. https://doi.org/10.1016/j.jhep.2025.04.030. PMID: 40328364.
46. Schlegel A, Foley DP, Savier E, Flores Carvalho M, De Carlis L, Heaton N, Taner CB. Recommendations for donor and recipient selection and risk prediction: working group report from the ILTS consensus conference in DCD liver transplantation. Transplantation. 2021;105(9):1892–903.
47. Meier RPH, Nunez M, Syed SM, Feng S, Tavakol M, Freise CE, et al. DCD liver transplant in patients with a MELD over 35. Front Immunol. 2023;14:1246867.
48. Croome KP, Mathur AK, Aqel B, et al. Classification of distinct patterns of ischemic cholangiopathy following DCD liver transplantation. Transplantation. 2022;106(6):1206–14.

49. van Rijn R, Schurink IJ, de Vries Y, DHOPE-DCD Trial Investigators, et al. Hypothermic machine perfusion in liver transplantation—a randomized trial. N Engl J Med. 2021;384(15):1391–401.
50. van Rijn R, Endo C, Küçükerbil EH, et al. Long-term follow-up after hypothermic oxygenated machine perfusion in DCD liver transplantation: results of a randomized controlled Multicenter trial (DHOPE-DCD). Ann Surg. 2025;282(5):717–24. https://doi.org/10.1097/SLA.0000000000006483.
51. Markmann JF, Abouljoud MS, Ghobrial RM, Bhati CS, Pelletier SJ, et al. Impact of portable normothermic blood-based machine perfusion on outcomes of liver transplant: the OCS liver PROTECT randomized clinical trial. JAMA Surg. 2022;157(3):189–98.
52. Hessheimer AJ, de la Rosa G, Gastaca M, Ruíz P, Otero A, et al. Abdominal normothermic regional perfusion in controlled donation after circulatory determination of death liver transplantation: outcomes and risk factors for graft loss. Am J Transplant. 2022;22(4):1169–81.
53. Brubaker AL, Sellers MT, Abt PL, Croome KP, Merani S, Wall A, et al. US liver transplant outcomes after normothermic regional perfusion vs standard super rapid recovery. JAMA Surg. 2024;159(6):677–85.
54. Schlegel A, van Reeven M, Croome K, Parente A, Dolcet A, Widmer J, et al. A multicentre outcome analysis to define global benchmarks for donation after circulatory death liver transplantation. J Hepatol. 2022;76(2):371–82.
55. Eden J, Brüggenwirth IMA, Berlakovich G, et al. Long-term outcomes after hypothermic oxygenated machine perfusion and transplantation of 1,202 donor livers in a real-world setting (HOPE-REAL study). J Hepatol. 2025;82(1):97–106.
56. Dutkowski P, Oberkofler CE, Slankamenac K, Puhan MA, Schadde E, Müllhaupt B, et al. Are there better guidelines for allocation in liver transplantation? A novel score targeting justice and utility in the model for end-stage liver disease era. Ann Surg. 2011;254(5):745–53.
57. Dutkowski P, Schlegel A, Slankamenac K, Oberkofler CE, Adam R, Burroughs AK, et al. The use of fatty liver grafts in modern allocation systems: risk assessment by the balance of risk (BAR) score. Ann Surg. 2012;256(5):861–9.
58. Feng S, Goodrich NP, Bragg-Gresham JL, et al. Characteristics associated with liver graft failure: the concept of a donor risk index. Am J Transplant. 2006;6(4):783–90.
59. Rana A, Hardy MA, Halazun KJ, et al. Survival outcomes following liver transplantation (SOFT) score: a novel method to predict patient survival following liver transplantation. Am J Transplant. 2008;8(12):2537–46.
60. Meier RPH, Braun HJ, Roll GR, Ascher NL. Advantages and limitations of clinical scores for donation after circulatory death liver transplantation. Front Surg. 2021;8:808733. (UC-DCD score).
61. Wu DD, Mathur AK, et al. Selecting DCD recipients using predictive indices. Transplant Direct. 2023;9(4):e1455.
62. Seth AK, Mohanka R, Navin S, Gokhale AGK, Sharma A, Kumar A, et al. Organ donation after circulatory determination of death in India: a joint position paper. Indian J Crit Care Med. 2022;26(4):423–40.
63. Zirpe K, Pandit R, Gurav S, et al. Management of Potential Organ Donor: Indian Society of Critical Care Medicine—position statement. Indian J Crit Care Med. 2024;28(S2):S249–78.
64. Pamecha V, Kumar S, Bharathy KGS, Sinha PK, Sasturkar SV, et al. Deceased donor liver transplantation in India: first report of 5-y outcomes. Transplantation. 2024;108(10):2109–16.
65. Cherukuru R, Reddy MS, Shanmugam NP, et al. Feasibility and safety of split-liver transplantation in a nascent framework of deceased donation. Liver Transpl. 2019;25(3):450–8.
66. Yadav SK, Saraf N, Choudhary NS, et al. High MELD score does not adversely affect outcome of living donor liver transplantation: experience in 1000 recipients. Clin Transpl. 2017;31(7):e12969.
67. Choudhary NS, Saraf N, Saigal S, Mohanka R, et al. Low-dose short-term hepatitis B immunoglobulin with high genetic-barrier antivirals: the ideal post-transplant hepatitis B prophylaxis? Transpl Infect Dis. 2015;17(3):329–33.

68. Rela M, Reddy MS. Living donor liver transplant (LDLT) is the way forward in Asia. Hepatol Int. 2017;11:148–51.
69. Lai JC, Feng S, Terrault NA, et al. Frailty predicts waitlist mortality in liver transplant candidates. Am J Transplant. 2014;14(8):1870–9.
70. Lai JC, Covinsky KE, Dodge JL, et al. Development of a novel frailty index to predict mortality in patients with end-stage liver disease (liver frailty index). Hepatology. 2017;66(2):564–74.
71. Huang HB, Zhu YB, Yu DX. Sarcopenic obesity is significantly associated with poorer overall survival after liver transplantation: a systematic review and meta-analysis. Front Nutr. 2024;11:1387602.
72. Bhanji RA, Takahashi N, Moynagh MR, Narayanan P, Angirekula M, Mara KC, et al. The evolution and impact of sarcopenia pre- and post-liver transplantation. Aliment Pharmacol Ther. 2019;49(6):807–13.
73. Kalisvaart M, Croome KP, Hernandez-Alejandro R, Pirenne J, Cortés-Cerisuelo M, Miñambres E, Abt PL. Donor warm ischemia time in DCD liver transplantation – working group report from the ILTS DCD, liver preservation, and machine perfusion consensus conference. Transplantation. 2021;105(6):1156–64.
74. Mehta N, Bhangui P, Yao FY, et al. Liver transplantation for hepatocellular carcinoma—working group report from the ILTS transplant oncology consensus conference. Transplantation. 2020;104(6):1136–42.
75. Anwar A, et al. Outcomes of liver transplantation for HCC in DCD vs DBD: systematic review and meta-analysis. Ann Hepatol. 2024;29:101484.
76. Wall AE, Adams BL, Brubaker A, et al. The American Society of Transplant Surgeons consensus statement on normothermic regional perfusion. Transplantation. 2024;108(2):312–8.
77. Hessheimer AJ, Coll E, Torres F, et al. Normothermic regional perfusion vs super-rapid recovery in controlled donation after circulatory death liver transplantation. J Hepatol. 2019;70(4):658–65.
78. European Association for the Study of the Liver. EASL clinical practice guidelines on liver transplantation. J Hepatol. 2024;81(6):1040–86. https://doi.org/10.1016/j.jhep.2024.07.032. PMID: 39487043.
79. Croome KP, Lee DD, Burns JM, Musto K, Paz D, Nguyen JH, et al. Improving outcomes of DCD liver transplantation: a 20-year single-center experience. Curr Transplant Rep. 2020;7:194–204.
80. Hong JC, Yersiz H, Kositamongkol P, et al. Liver transplantation using organ donation after cardiac death: a clinical predictive index for graft failure-free survival (UCLA score). Arch Surg. 2011;146(9):1017–23.
81. Khorsandi SE, Giorgakis E, Vilca-Melendez H, et al. Developing a donation after cardiac death risk index for adult and paediatric liver transplantation (KCH score). World J Transplant. 2017;7(3):203–12.
82. Mergental H, Laing RW, Kirkham AJ, Perera MTPR, Boteon YL, Attard J, et al. Transplantation of discarded livers following viability testing with normothermic machine perfusion. Nat Commun. 2020;11(1):2939.
83. Watson CJE, Kosmoliaptsis V, Pley C, Randle L, Fear C, Crick K, et al. Observations on the ex situ perfusion of livers for transplantation. Am J Transplant. 2018;18(8):2005–20.
84. Muller X, Schlegel A, Kron P, Eshmuminov D, Wurdinger M, Meierhofer D, et al. Novel real-time prediction of liver graft function during HOPE using flavin mononucleotide. J Hepatol. 2019;71(2):269–78.
85. Sheth A, Mohanka R, Haji J, et al. Consensus statement of the National Consortium on normothermic regional perfusion for organ donation after circulatory determination of death in India. Indian J Transplant. 2026;20(1):23–35. https://doi.org/10.4103/ijot.ijot_81_25.

Part V

Organ-Specific Transplant Outcomes in DCD

Kidney Transplantation from Donors After Circulatory Death (DCD) Donors

12

Richard J. Baker

Background

Although the increasing proportion of DCD organs in deceased donation is a relatively recent phenomenon, it is worth remembering that the earliest cadaveric transplants were indeed DCDs due to the lack of perfusion technology. This includes the first attempts at deceased donor kidney transplantation in the UK [1]. As transplantation became more commonplace, bioethical debate focused on deciding the exact moment of death which in turn led to the development of brainstem death criteria and the adoption of donation after brainstem death (DBD) as normal practice [2]. Inevitably, the demand for transplanted organs far outstripped the supply of DBD organs, and there was renewed interest in DCD donors at the end of the last century. There was also substantial advocacy by donor families who felt that their loved one's right to donate was being denied. This led to considerable ethical and legal debate and eventually the generation of a policy document published by the University of Pittsburgh proposing the judicious use of DCD organs [3].

In Europe, the use on DCD kidneys was pioneered by the group in Maastricht, and they soon developed the categories of donor that are still in use today as shown in Table 12.1 [4].

The shortage of donor organs also renewed interest in DCD donation in the UK and while DCD accounted for only 3% of deceased kidney donation in 2000, it had risen to 32% by 2009 [5]. This percentage has continued to rise, and DCD kidneys now represent the majority of deceased donor organs (see Fig. 12.1). However globally DCD donation only takes place 23 of the 91 countries reporting to the WHO and rates vary enormously, revealing a potentially vast unexploited resource [6] (see Fig. 12.2).

R. J. Baker (✉)
Department of Renal Medicine, St. James's University Hospital, Leeds, UK
e-mail: richard-j.baker@nhs.net

S. P. Kolte et al. (eds.), *Organ Donation After Circulatory Death*,
https://doi.org/10.1007/978-981-92-6377-6_12

Table 12.1 Maastricht categories of DCD organs

Maastricht category	Clinical correlate
1	Dead on arrival at A and E
2	Death with failed resuscitation
3	Awaiting cardiac death
4	Cardiac arrest when brain dead
5	Unexpected cardiac arrest in a hospitalised patient
N/A	Donation after medically assisted dying

Modified from Detry et al. [8]

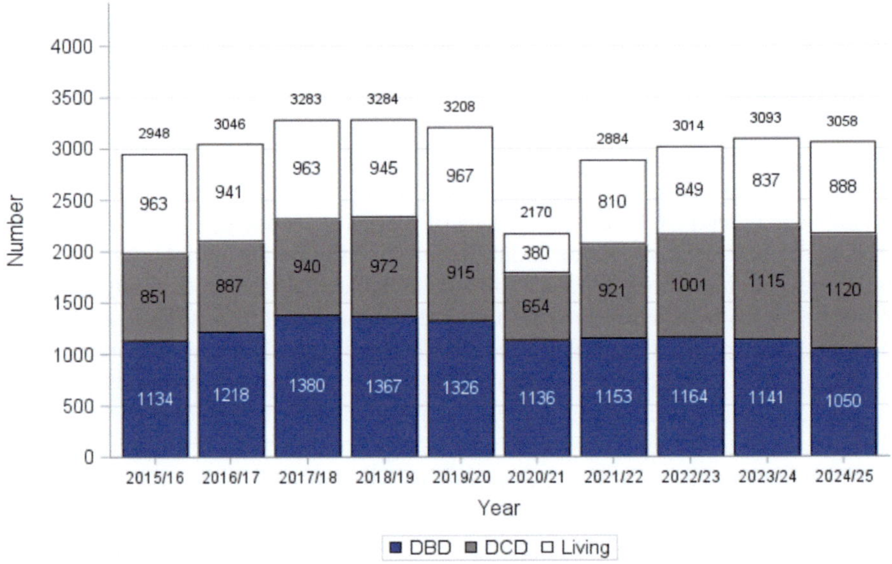

Fig. 12.1 Adult kidney only transplants in the UK 2015–2025—over a decade the proportion of DCD/Total Cadaveric kidneys rose from 42.8% to 51.6%. (Figure courtesy of NHSBT, extracted from Annual Report on Kidney Transplantation 2024/25, NHS Blood and Transplant—https://nhsbtdbe.blob.core.windows.net/umbraco-assets-corp/38526/nhsbt-kidney-transplantation-report-2425-v2.pdf)

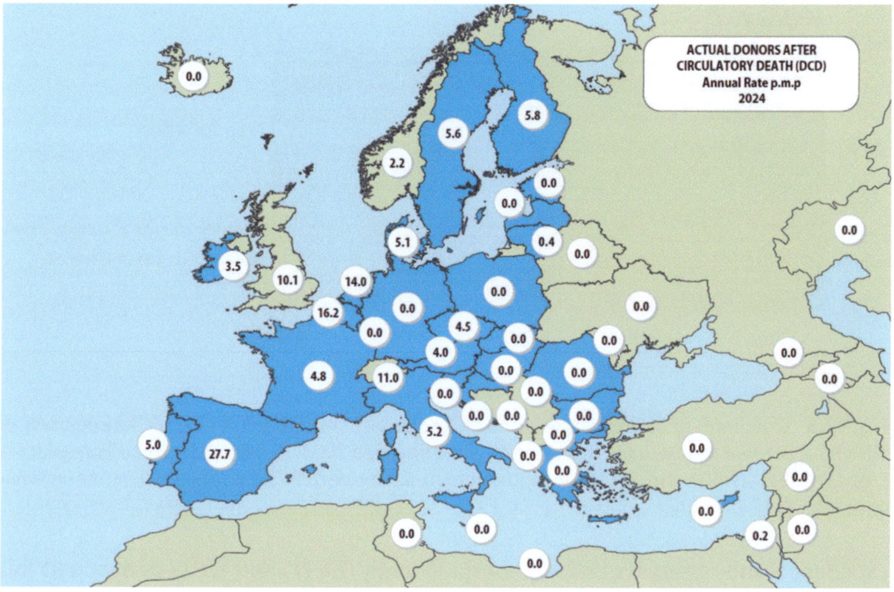

Fig. 12.2 DCD kidney transplantation rates (patients per million population) for countries in Europe 2024. (Reproduced with permission from the Newsletter Transplant, October 2025 published by the European Directorate for the Quality of Medicines and Healthcare—https://freepub.edqm.eu/publications/PUBSD-87/detail)

DCD Development in the UK

Historically, the numbers of deceased donors in the UK had been relatively low at around 750 per annum (population c. 60 million—13 pmp). In 2006, an Organ Donation Taskforce was established and published a momentous report 2 years later, 'Organs for Transplants' with the goal of increasing organ donors by 50% within 5 years [7]. The report recommended 14 key action points including the establishment of organ donation as a normal part of end-of-life care. Retrieval surgery was provided around the clock in the UK by seven abdominal retrieval teams commissioned centrally by the National Organ Retrieval Service (NORS) and there were Specialist Nurses in Organ Donation (SNOD) embedded in all critical care units. In addition, a legal and ethical framework was established to enable routine DCD donation [8]. These guidelines have recently been updated and form the basis for contemporary practice in the UK [9]. Within 5 years, these changes did indeed generate a 50% increase in deceased donor numbers but not the expected increase in numbers of transplants. This was because the increase in donors consisted of predominantly elderly DBD and DCDs. Unfortunately, decline rates increased and there was considerable clinical caution. Over the last decade, more emphasis has been placed on increasing organ utilisation as studies reveal substantial regional variation across the UK [10]. Clinical caution has been countered by publicising the

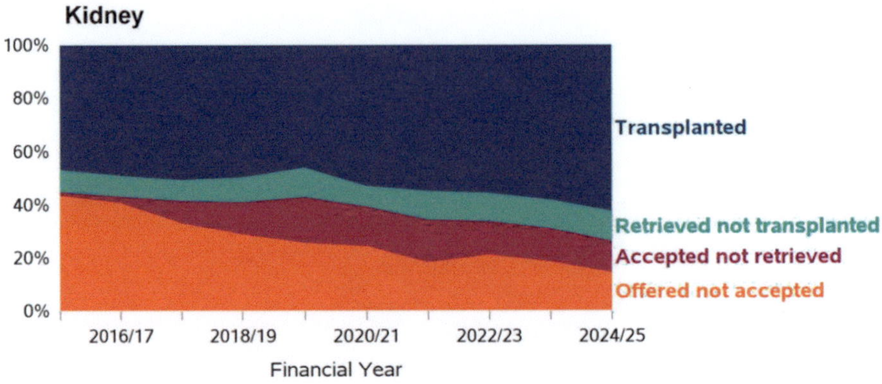

Fig. 12.3 Outcomes of offered organs from DCD donors in the UK 2015–2025. (Data courtesy of NHSBT, extracted from Annual Report on Organ Utilisation 2024/25, NHS Blood and Transplant—https://nhsbtdbe.blob.core.windows.net/umbraco-assets-corp/37330/organ-utilisation-annual-report-2024-25-final.pdf)

excellent results from Extended Criteria Donors (ECD) and DCD donors and this illustrates the importance of education and peer support in promoting the utilisation of DCD organs [11]. Figure 12.3 shows that utilisation rates for DCD kidneys have slowly improved over the last decade in the UK. It should be borne in mind that for most patients on the renal transplant waiting the riskiest option is not being transplanted and remaining on the waiting list. This has been demonstrated in the USA where it has been shown that accepting a DCD kidney from a donor over 50 yields a substantial survival benefit [12].

Outcomes of Transplanted DCD Kidneys

Initially, there were concerns over the quality of DCD kidneys, largely because of the extended period of warm ischaemia that occurs after the circulation ceases until the time that the organ is perfused with cold preservation fluid. A paper from Zurich published in 2002 compared outcomes in 122 DCD transplants with historic risk matched DBD recipients [13]. They showed that Delayed Graft Function (DGF) rates were significantly higher in DCD transplants vs. DBD (48.4% vs. 23.8%) but importantly that graft survival at 10 years was equivalent (78.7% vs. 76.7%, respectively). In the same year, a large retrospective analysis from the USA demonstrated similar results with approximately double the rate of DGF in DCD transplants but similar six-year graft and patient survival [14]. They also identified significant risk factors for allograft loss in DCD transplants as:

- Increasing donor age.
- Female recipient sex.
- Second or subsequent transplants.

- Donor cause of death (head injury worst).
- Delayed Graft Function.

Although delayed graft function was associated with worse outcomes for both groups, the markedly increased DGF rates in DCD were not sufficiently influential to cause worse long-term outcomes. This was an interesting finding and contradicted the strong correlation in between DGF and poor outcomes in DBD transplantation [15, 16]. There was a suggestion that DCD kidneys were less susceptible to damage by DGF than their DBD counterparts. Over the next decade, a number of other groups confirmed these findings, and it is widely acknowledged that DGF rates are roughly double those of DBD donors but that overall long-term outcomes are similar [17–21].

In 2010, Summers et al. published a landmark paper which detailed the outcomes of kidney transplantation in the UK from DCD donors. Using national registry data they compared outcomes across all 22 adult kidney transplant centres from 6759 DBD donors versus 739 DCD donors in adult recipients of first renal transplants transplanted between 2000 and 2007 [5]. Primary non-function (PNF) rates were similar for first transplants at 3% but DGF was significantly higher in the DCD kidneys (49% vs. 24%—$P < 0.0001$). There was no difference in graft survival up to 5 years, and the eGFR values were similar at all time points after 1 year. Factors associated with worse outcomes were increasing donor and recipient age, repeat transplantation and a cold ischaemia time longer than 12 h.

The same group published a further paper looking at an overlapping cohort which demonstrated once again similar graft survival but poorer graft outcomes in older donors (>60) a finding that was consistent across both DBD and DCD groups [22]. They also showed that DCD kidneys were more vulnerable to prolonged cold ischaemia with worse outcomes after more than 12 h, a trend that was not observed in DBD kidneys. Initially, DCD kidneys were offered regionally within allocation system in the UK to minimise cold ischaemia times. However, as DCD donation has increased, relative to DBD, it has been gradually integrated into the national allocation system since 2014, albeit with some priority for local use.

The most recent UK data is shown in Table 12.2 [8]. Risk factors for poor outcomes in the UK cohort include:

Table 12.2 Outcomes of first adult deceased donor kidney transplants in the UK—patients transplanted between 2001 and 2012

	DCD	DBD	P value
n	3626	9684	
PNF	3.2%	2.6%	0.06
DGF	48.5%	24.9%	<0.0001
eGFR 1 year	47.4	48.7	0.005
eGFR 5 years	49.6	48.1	0.06
Death-censored graft survival 5 years	85.9%	84.5%	0.22
Death-censored graft survival 10 years	74.9%	74.3%	0.20

Adapted from Summers et al. [8]

- Donor age (risk is similar for DBD and DCD).
- History of donor hypertension.
- Antemortem serum creatinine level.
- Recipient age.
- Primary cause of renal failure.
- Increased HLA mismatch.
- Longer CIT.

Under these circumstance, it is remarkable that overall UK graft survival data after deceased donation has remained constant with no appreciable drop in graft survival rates despite increasing donor age and increasing proportions of DCD grafts [23]. The available evidence in the UK would suggest that decisions over utilisation of organs should not include whether DBD or DCD in origin.

A comprehensive systematic review of the available international trial data in 2020 also revealed similar survival data in DCD and DBD kidneys [24]. When compared to DBD kidneys, DCD kidneys had:

- Higher rates of PNF (3.3% vs. 2.5%).
- Higher rates of DGF (44% vs. 31%).
- Lower rates of rejection (9.5% vs. 17%).
- Increase prevalence of ECD risk factors.

Rijkse et al. have conducted a systemic review of international studies and concluded that outcomes with DCD kidneys are equivalent to DBD kidneys in terms of graft and patient survival [25]. They considered 51 studies including 73,454 DCD kidney transplants versus 518,229 DBD transplants. DCD transplants had a 43% increased chance of PNF and twice the risk of DGF. They also described a 13% reduction in graft survival in the first year but similar long-term graft survival and equivalent renal function.

There has been a great deal of interest in the use of preimplantation biopsies in the UK generated by studies that have suggested benefit [26]. To test this hypothesis, a stepped-wedge randomised controlled trial was carried out to look at the use of preimplantation biopsies in deceased donors over 60 years of age [27]. However, biopsy provision did not improve utilisation rates or graft function at 1 year. There is a great deal of interest in markers that might help predict which DCD kidneys organs will function well after transplantation and this area remains an area of active research.

Types of DCD

It is noteworthy that nearly all of the DCD donors in the UK were Maastricht Category 3, that is controlled donation after circulatory death. These are almost exclusively patients who have suffered catastrophic brain injuries who are admitted to critical care units but who do not fulfil the criteria for brainstem death. Supportive care is withdrawn, usually inotropic and ventilatory support, and death is certified after cessation of circulatory function. In the UK, no antemortem interventions are permitted (e.g. femoral cannulation or intravenous heparinisation) and a period of 5 min of observation is observed after circulatory arrest, when brainstem death has occurred. In a small minority of cases (<10%) DCD retrieval occurs after brainstem death (usually when the donor family do not wish donation to take place with a beating heart). In these cases, interventions may take place as the donor is legally brainstem dead and no observation period is required [8].

In the France and Spain, there is more experience of uncontrolled DCD donation (Maastricht Categories 1 and 2). The main cause of concern in these programmes is the elevated rate of primary non-function (PNF) at around 8% despite judicious selection of donors and the use on normothermic regional perfusion [28]. However, ten-year graft survival rates have been good (>70%), and it is estimated that this form of donation could provide a substantial increase in donors. Results from the Netherlands suggest that uncontrolled DCD donation can provide outcomes indistinguishable from controlled donation [29]. Spanish results have also been encouraging with better outcomes than with extended criteria standard DBD donors but with a higher PNF rate [30]. Factors predicting primary non-function were prolonged CPR times both in and out of hospital and pulmonary embolism as a cause of death. Results from uncontrolled DCD studies have recently been reviewed and suggest considerable untapped potential [31].

Withdrawal of Life Sustaining Treatment (WLST)

After WLST, the clinical course in the donor is highly unpredictable although 60% of potential donors die within 3 h [32]. Understandably, there was originally a great deal of caution regarding the effects of warm ischaemia prior to cold perfusion. Reassurance was provided by the team in Cambridge who studied 173 potential donors following WLST [33]. 117 became kidney donors and yielded a total of 190 kidneys. In the transplants from the 23% of donors who died more than 1 h after WLST there was no correlation between either degree or duration of haemodynamic instability and outcomes in terms of graft function at either 3 or 12 months.

A detailed analysis of UK registry data considered 7183 recipients of DCD kidneys [34]. Of these, the Time to Death (TTD) was greater than 1 h in 885 donors and greater than 2 h in 303. The TTD did not correlate with DGF rates, graft function at 1 year or overall graft survival. However, the authors acknowledged that this study only included kidneys that were eventually transplanted and so there may be some selection bias. The results do support the UK practice of waiting a minimum of 3 h post WLST. The same group has also recently extended their findings to the US registry data with similar findings [35].

Another widely used concept is functional warm ischaemia time, defined as the interval between systolic blood pressure falling below an ischaemic threshold and the initiation of in situ perfusion. Most centres agree that this time commences when the donor systolic blood pressure drops below 50 mmHg and this value has been adopted in the UK national guidelines [9, 36]. However, recent analysis of a large US database did not demonstrate any association between longer warm ischaemia times (>60 min) and poor outcomes including PNF as long as asystole time was short [37].

Alternatives to Static Cold Perfusion

The high incidence of DGF in DCD kidneys, and also the low levels of utilisation for other abdominal organs, has generated a great deal of interest in using machine perfusion techniques for DCD donors. These can broadly be divided in two groups;

- In situ techniques—Normothermic Regional Perfusion (NRP).
- Ex situ techniques—Hypothermic (HMP) or normothermic machine perfusion (NMP) +/– Oxygenation.

Normothermic Regional Perfusion (NRP)

In the UK until recently the vast majority of kidneys were retrieved with cold perfusion and then transported by static cold storage (SCS), as opposed to perfusion devices. Retrieval surgery is provided 24 h a day by the seven abdominal teams of the National Organ Retrieval Service (NORS). However, over the last 15 years, teams from Cambridge and Edinburgh have championed Normothermic Regional Perfusion (NRP) and this has become widely established as the standard of care.

NRP is usually abdominal but can also be thoracoabdominal if the heart and lungs are included in the perfusion circuit (TANRP). NRP is carried out "in situ" in the donor after death with the use of machinery that provides extracorporeal respiratory and circulatory support via a femoral catheter. This allows the abdominal organs to be supplied with oxygen, nutrients and possibly therapeutic agents prior to retrieval. The first attempts at using this technology demonstrated a reduced incidence of DGF in DCD donor kidneys [25]. Techniques for this process have been in regular use in the UK for the last 15 years, with promising results in DCD donors [38]. This has led to the widespread introduction of regional NRP services with supporting teams of Organ Perfusion Specialists [39]. The latest results from these teams show significantly improved results in DCD liver donation. In DCD kidneys, NRP increased utilisation rates by 50%. In addition, NRP kidneys had 35% lower chance of developing DGF and they had a significantly better eGFR at 12 months (+ 6.3 ml/min/1.73m^2, $p < 0.0001$). It should be acknowledged that this was retrospective registry analysis including all DCD donors both with or without NRP and there may have been some selection bias. An analysis of the UNOS database looked at the use of NRP in 21,010 recipients of DCD kidneys in the USA, compared with standard retrieval [40]. NRP was associated with reduced DGF rates (30.3% vs. 49.7%), shorter hospital stay (median 4 vs. 5 days) and significantly improved patient and graft survival particularly in higher risk donors. US data also suggests reduced rates of DGF and better early renal function after TANRP [41].

Clearly, this is a very promising technique, and it allows for dynamic functional testing of the organ during perfusion. It may also offer the opportunity to use therapeutics to rejuvenate donor organs prior to implantation, and this remains an area of keen interest [42].

Ex Situ Perfusion—Hypothermic and Normothermic Machine Perfusion

A landmark European study in 2009 demonstrated that the provision of pulsatile cold perfusion fluid (HMP) after retrieval could significantly reduce both DGF and increase transplant survival when compared to SCS [43]. However, a multicentre randomised study in the UK showed no benefit to HMP over SCS and to this day SCS predominates in the UK, in contrast to continental Europe [44]. A further study which randomised donor kidneys to undergo HMP with or without oxygenation suggested that the addition of oxygen might further improve graft function [45]. This had led some countries, for example Belgium, to adopt widespread machine perfusion with demonstrable economic benefits and increased utilisation [46].

A recent Cochrane analysis suggested that there may be some benefit from HMP with a 22% reduction in DGF and probably greater benefit if the perfusion was provided from the point of retrieval [47]. It was estimated that nearly eight kidneys need to be perfused to prevent one episode of DGF in DCD donors.

There is also interest in normothermic machine perfusion which can be delivered from the point of retrieval or when the organ reaches the implanting hospital. This has been carried in several units and in the future may facilitate therapeutic interventions during NMP. A recent UK study demonstrated that NMP after SCS and prior to implantation was safe but there was no advantage in terms of DGF rates [48]. However, in future, this process may pave the way for therapeutic interventions and viability assessment prior to implantation [49].

Organisation and Infrastructure

The excellent results in DCD kidneys which are being reported in the USA and some European countries are the result of more than 30 years of evolution and refinement. Success requires coherent efforts by several teams who are highly trained and working together with a common purpose. They rely on the security provided by a clear ethical and legal framework in which to work. Novel perfusion techniques have added to the complexity and cost of DCD retrieval, but the potential benefits are tantalising as we enter the era of possible assessment and therapeutics during perfusion. Other simpler logistical hurdles remain, for example, the rates of DCD kidneys implanted within 12 h differ greatly across the UK. There are 22 adult transplant centres, and there is variation between 5% and 85% in DCD transplants performed with CIT under 12 h [23]. Previous UK data suggests that 5-year graft survival was 88.6% in recipients with CIT <12 h but drops to 82.6% for kidneys >24 h [8]. Given the UK data about worse performance with prolonged CIT time it emphasises the importance of mobilising resources to ensure optimal DCD performance.

Conclusions

DCD transplantation remains a largely untapped resource in many parts of the world. Experience derived from Western Europe and the USA has clearly demonstrated that DCD kidney transplants can make a major contribution to deceased donor numbers with excellent medium- and long-term outcomes. There is also emerging evidence that new technologies may offer the opportunity to improve DCD utilisation rates and hopefully long-term outcomes.

The establishment of a successful national DCD programme requires a solid foundation in clinical practice including:

- Establishment of a clear and consensual ethical and legal framework regarding donor death.
- Consideration of donation as part of the end-of-life pathway within intensive care units.
- A sympathetic and unhurried approach to donor families by properly trained professionals.
- Education both within the medical profession and to the general public.
- Fair and equitable allocation of donor organs.
- Well-organised and uniform retrieval practice with effective clinical governance.
- Timely access to operating theatres at recipient hospitals to minimise recipient cold ischaemic times.
- Peer support and mentorship for clinical teams starting DCD programmes.
- Judicious and evidence-based use of new perfusion technologies.
- Further research into parameters that affect outcomes in particular PNF and DGF.
- National registries to monitor and disseminate outcomes.

Globally, DCD donors remain a largely untapped resource, despite robust evidence that these organs can provide substantial benefits to patients when compared to remaining on the waiting list. Hopefully, over the next decade steps can be taken to improve utilisation of these organs for the benefit of patients across the world with end-stage renal failure.

Competing Interests The author(s) has no competing interests to declare that are relevant to the content of this manuscript.

Ethics Approval The author(s) declares that this manuscript does not include primary research with human participants.

The author(s) declares that this manuscript does not include primary studies involving animals.

References

1. Joekes AM, Porter KA, Dempster WJ. Immediate post-operative anuria in a human renal homotransplant. Br J Surg. 1957;44(188):607–15.
2. Wijdicks EFM. The history of donation after circulatory death (DCD): backlash and boomerang. Neurocrit Care. 2024.
3. DeVita MA, Snyder JV. Development of the University of Pittsburgh Medical Center policy for the care of terminally ill patients who may become organ donors after death following the removal of life support. Kennedy Inst Ethics J. 1993;3(2):131–43.
4. Detry O, Le Dinh H, Noterdaeme T, De Roover A, Honoré P, Squifflet JP, et al. Categories of donation after cardiocirculatory death. Transplant Proc. 2012;44(5):1189–95.
5. Summers DM, Johnson RJ, Allen J, Fuggle SV, Collett D, Watson CJ, et al. Analysis of factors that affect outcome after transplantation of kidneys donated after cardiac death in the UK: a cohort study. Lancet. 2010;376(9749):1303–11.
6. Vidgren M, Delorme C, Oniscu GC. Challenges and opportunities in organ donation after circulatory death. J Intern Med. 2025;297(2):124–40.
7. ODT. Organs for transplants; a report from the Organ Donation Taskforce. London: Department of Health; 2008.
8. Summers DM, Watson CJ, Pettigrew GJ, Johnson RJ, Collett D, Neuberger JM, et al. Kidney donation after circulatory death (DCD): state of the art. Kidney Int. 2015;88(2):241–9.
9. Phillips B, Asgari E, Berry M, Callaghan C, Cerisuelo MC, Johnson P, et al. British Transplantation Society guidelines on abdominal organ transplantation from deceased donors after circulatory death. Transplant Rev (Orlando). 2024;38(1):100801.
10. Summers DM, Johnson RJ, Hudson AJ, Collett D, Murphy P, Watson CJ, et al. Standardized deceased donor kidney donation rates in the UK reveal marked regional variation and highlight the potential for increasing kidney donation: a prospective cohort study†. Br J Anaesth. 2014;113(1):83–90.
11. Ibrahim M, Greenhall GHB, Summers DM, Mumford L, Johnson R, Baker RJ, et al. Utilization and outcomes of single and dual kidney transplants from older deceased donors in the United Kingdom. Clin J Am Soc Nephrol. 2020;15(9):1320–9.
12. Yu S, Long JJ, Yu Y, Bowring MG, Motter JD, Ishaque T, et al. Survival benefit of accepting kidneys from older donation after cardiac death donors. Am J Transplant. 2021;21(3):1138–46.
13. Weber M, Dindo D, Demartines N, Ambühl PM, Clavien PA. Kidney transplantation from donors without a heartbeat. N Engl J Med. 2002;347(4):248–55.
14. Rudich SM, Kaplan B, Magee JC, Arenas JD, Punch JD, Kayler LK, et al. Renal transplantations performed using non-heart-beating organ donors: going back to the future? Transplantation. 2002;74(12):1715–20.
15. Shoskes DA, Cecka JM. Deleterious effects of delayed graft function in cadaveric renal transplant recipients independent of acute rejection. Transplantation. 1998;66(12):1697–701.
16. Quiroga I, McShane P, Koo DD, Gray D, Friend PJ, Fuggle S, et al. Major effects of delayed graft function and cold ischaemia time on renal allograft survival. Nephrol Dial Transplant. 2006;21(6):1689–96.
17. Doshi MD, Hunsicker LG. Short- and long-term outcomes with the use of kidneys and livers donated after cardiac death. Am J Transplant. 2007;7(1):122–9.
18. Locke JE, Segev DL, Warren DS, Dominici F, Simpkins CE, Montgomery RA. Outcomes of kidneys from donors after cardiac death: implications for allocation and preservation. Am J Transplant. 2007;7(7):1797–807.
19. Tojimbara T, Fuchinoue S, Iwadoh K, Koyama I, Sannomiya A, Kato Y, et al. Improved outcomes of renal transplantation from cardiac death donors: a 30-year single center experience. Am J Transplant. 2007;7(3):609–17.
20. Barlow AD, Metcalfe MS, Johari Y, Elwell R, Veitch PS, Nicholson ML. Case-matched comparison of long-term results of non-heart beating and heart-beating donor renal transplants. Br J Surg. 2009;96(6):685–91.

21. Kokkinos C, Antcliffe D, Nanidis T, Darzi AW, Tekkis P, Papalois V. Outcome of kidney transplantation from nonheart-beating versus heart-beating cadaveric donors. Transplantation. 2007;83(9):1193–9.
22. Summers DM, Johnson RJ, Hudson A, Collett D, Watson CJ, Bradley JA. Effect of donor age and cold storage time on outcome in recipients of kidneys donated after circulatory death in the UK: a cohort study. Lancet. 2013;381(9868):727–34.
23. NHSBT. Annual report on kidney transplantation 2026.
24. Gavriilidis P, Inston NG. Recipient and allograft survival following donation after circulatory death versus donation after brain death for renal transplantation: a systematic review and meta-analysis. Transplant Rev (Orlando). 2020;34(4):100563.
25. Rijkse E, Ceuppens S, Qi H, IJzermans JNM, Hesselink DA, Minnee RC. Implementation of donation after circulatory death kidney transplantation can safely enlarge the donor pool: a systematic review and meta-analysis. Int J Surg. 2021;92:106021.
26. Gandolfini I, Buzio C, Zanelli P, Palmisano A, Cremaschi E, Vaglio A, et al. The Kidney Donor Profile Index (KDPI) of marginal donors allocated by standardized pretransplant donor biopsy assessment: distribution and association with graft outcomes. Am J Transplant. 2014;14(11):2515–25.
27. Summers DM, Ayorinde JOO, Neil DA, Hemming K, Smith L, Mehew J, et al. Evaluation of a national digital pre-implantation biopsy service for deceased-donor kidney transplantation in the UK (Pithia trial); a stepped-wedge cluster randomised registry trial. Lancet Reg Health Eur. 2025;56:101390.
28. Summers DM, Pettigrew GJ. Kidney transplantation following uncontrolled donation after circulatory death. Curr Opin Organ Transplant. 2020;25(2):144–50.
29. Peters-Sengers H, Homan van der Heide JJ, Heemskerk MBA, Ten Berge IJM, Ultee FCW, Idu MM, et al. Similar 5-year estimated glomerular filtration rate between kidney transplants from uncontrolled and controlled donors after circulatory death – a Dutch cohort study. Transplantation. 2017;101(6):1144–51.
30. Sánchez-Fructuoso AI, Pérez-Flores I, Del Río F, Blázquez J, Calvo N, Moreno de la Higuera M, et al. Uncontrolled donation after circulatory death: a cohort study of data from a long-standing deceased-donor kidney transplantation program. Am J Transplant. 2019;19(6):1693–707.
31. Pionnier Y, Darius T, Penaloza A, Steenebruggen F, Dupriez F, Neyrinck A, et al. Solid organ transplantation originating from uncontrolled donation after circulatory death in Europe: a narrative review. Scand J Trauma Resusc Emerg Med. 2024;32(1):130.
32. Bradley JA, Pettigrew GJ, Watson CJ. Time to death after withdrawal of treatment in donation after circulatory death (DCD) donors. Curr Opin Organ Transplant. 2013;18(2):133–9.
33. Reid AWN, Harper S, Jackson CH, Wells AC, Summers DM, Gjorgjimajkoska O, et al. Expansion of the kidney donor pool by using cardiac death donors with prolonged time to cardiorespiratory arrest. Am J Transplant. 2011;11(5):995–1005.
34. Tingle SJ, Chung NDH, Malik AK, Kourounis G, Thompson E, Glover EK, et al. Donor time to death and kidney transplant outcomes in the setting of a 3-h minimum wait policy. JAMA Netw Open. 2024;7(11):e2443353.
35. Amarnath DR, Kalpana TSR, Kourounis G, Malik AK, Philip J, Thompson ER, et al. Time to death and donation after circulatory death kidney transplant outcomes: opportunities for improved utilization in the United States. Clin Transpl. 2026;40(4):e70548.
36. Eden J, Sousa Da Silva R, Cortes-Cerisuelo M, Croome K, De Carlis R, Hessheimer AJ, et al. Utilization of livers donated after circulatory death for transplantation – an international comparison. J Hepatol. 2023;78(5):1007–16.
37. Ong OY, Munoz N, Schaubel DE, Jackson KR, Parsons RF, Abt PL, et al. Do prolonged donor warm ischemic times correlate with kidney transplant outcomes? The largest study of donation after circulatory death donors in the United States. Transplantation. 2026;110(8):e1711–e9.
38. Oniscu GC, Randle LV, Muiesan P, Butler AJ, Currie IS, Perera MT, et al. In situ normothermic regional perfusion for controlled donation after circulatory death—the United Kingdom experience. Am J Transplant. 2014;14(12):2846–54.

39. Hunt F, Johnston CJC, Coutts L, Sherif AE, Farwell L, Stutchfield BM, et al. From haphazard to a sustainable normothermic regional perfusion service: a blueprint for the introduction of novel perfusion technologies. Transpl Int. 2022;35:10493.
40. Kusakabe J, Fernandes E, Refaai K, Hussein A, Kumar K, Abdalla A, et al. Impact of normothermic regional perfusion on clinical outcomes in kidney transplantation from donors after circulatory death: a US nationwide analysis of 38,048 cases. Ann Surg. 2026;283:915.
41. Merani S, Urban M, Westphal SG, Dong J, Miles CD, Maskin A, et al. Improved early post-transplant outcomes and organ use in kidney transplant using normothermic regional perfusion for donation after circulatory death: national experience in the US. J Am Coll Surg. 2024;238(1):107–18.
42. Kayumov M, Song Z, Martin F, Tsou S, Xiao Y, Zhou H, et al. The promise of organ rejuvenation to overcome the shortage in organ transplantation. Nat Commun. 2025;16(1):11259.
43. Moers C, Smits JM, Maathuis MH, Treckmann J, van Gelder F, Napieralski BP, et al. Machine perfusion or cold storage in deceased-donor kidney transplantation. N Engl J Med. 2009;360(1):7–19.
44. Watson CJ, Wells AC, Roberts RJ, Akoh JA, Friend PJ, Akyol M, et al. Cold machine perfusion versus static cold storage of kidneys donated after cardiac death: a UK multicenter randomized controlled trial. Am J Transplant. 2010;10(9):1991–9.
45. Jochmans I, Brat A, Davies L, Hofker HS, van de Leemkolk FEM, Leuvenink HGD, et al. Oxygenated versus standard cold perfusion preservation in kidney transplantation (COMPARE): a randomised, double-blind, paired, phase 3 trial. Lancet. 2020;396(10263):1653–62.
46. Darius T, Jochmans I, Foguenne M, Hoste E, Randon C, Bracke B, et al. Nationwide hypothermic machine perfusion for ECD and DCD kidney transplantation in Belgium: one-year outcomes and impact on transplant rates and budget impact analysis. Transpl Int. 2025;38:15282.
47. Tingle SJ, Thompson ER, Figueiredo RS, Moir JA, Goodfellow M, Talbot D, et al. Normothermic and hypothermic machine perfusion preservation versus static cold storage for deceased donor kidney transplantation. Cochrane Database Syst Rev. 2024;7(7):Cd011671.
48. Hosgood SA, Callaghan CJ, Wilson CH, Smith L, Mullings J, Mehew J, et al. Normothermic machine perfusion versus static cold storage in donation after circulatory death kidney transplantation: a randomized controlled trial. Nat Med. 2023;29(6):1511–9.
49. Hosgood SA, Callaghan CJ, Wilson CH, Phillips BL, Thompson ER, Bates L, et al. Utilization and transplantation of unused kidneys after assessment using normothermic machine perfusion technology. Transplantation. 2026;110(2):e505–e6.

Liver Transplantation Outcomes from DCDD Donors

13

Amay Banker, Piyush Gupta, and Ravi Mohanka

Introduction

Liver transplant is now the standard of care of for patients with end-stage liver disease, acute liver failure, and patients with malignant liver cancer [1]. Despite steady growth in both living-donor liver transplantation and donation after neurological determination of death (DNDD), the number of patients requiring a liver transplant still exceeds the available donor pool. Donation after circulatory determination of death (DCDD) is an important and ethically acceptable strategy to expand access to liver transplantation. In 2021, an estimated 38,156 deceased donations were performed worldwide, of which 8545 (22.39%) were from DCDD donors [2].

Although the basic premise of DCDD is straightforward—organ recovery after irreversible cessation of circulation—its clinical application is complex. A major challenge in DCDD procurement is the unavoidable period of warm ischemia time (WIT) that occurs between withdrawal of life-sustaining treatment (WLST) and initiation of organ perfusion. During this WIT, interruption of blood supply and oxygen delivery can initiate a cascade of ischemic injury

A. Banker
Abdominal Transplant Surgery Fellow, Department of Surgery, Miami Transplant Institute, University of Miami, Miami, FL, USA

P. Gupta
Medstar Georgetown Transplant Institute, Georgetown University Hospital, Washington, DC, USA

R. Mohanka (✉)
Department of Liver Transplantation and HPB Sciences, Sir HN Reliance Foundation Hospital, Mumbai, India

Methodist Transplant Institute, University of Tennessee Health Science Centre, Memphis, TN, USA
e-mail: ravi.mohanka@rfhospital.org

S. P. Kolte et al. (eds.), *Organ Donation After Circulatory Death*,
https://doi.org/10.1007/978-981-92-6377-6_13

characterized by cellular edema, endothelial activation, and microvascular damage that can cause injury to the biliary epithelium [3–6]. Overcoming this procurement-related ischemic injury has been the principal barrier to broader adoption of DCDD liver grafts.

With refinement in donor and recipient selection, advances in surgical technique, and advancement of preservation technologies, clinical outcomes of liver transplantation performed using DCDD allografts have improved over time. Preservation technologies such as normothermic regional perfusion (NRP), and ex situ machine perfusion [normothermic machine perfusion (NMP), and/or hypothermic machine perfusion (HMP)] have played an important role in increasing DCDD utilization. As a result, DCDD now contributes a significant proportion of deceased donation in several countries, including nearly 40% of deceased donor liver transplantation (DDLT) in the USA [7]. In this chapter, we review the outcomes of liver transplantation using DCDD donors, with particular focus on complications pertinent to DCDD transplantation and the impact of different preservation strategies.

Complications Pertinent to DCDD Liver Transplantation

Ischemic cholangiopathy (IC) represents one of the most significant complications after DCDD liver transplantation. IC refers to a spectrum of non-anastomotic biliary strictures that develop within the first 12 months of transplantation, in the absence of hepatic artery thrombosis. Rather than being a single entity, IC represents a spectrum of biliary injury, ranging from mild radiologic irregularities to diffuse destruction of the biliary tree.

The pathophysiology of IC is associated with procurement related ischemic injury. Unlike hepatocytes, the biliary epithelium relies primarily on the hepatic arterial blood supply alone making it more prone to ischemic injury. Preservation injury to the biliary epithelium involves two key components: the combined effects of ischemia during procurement, and the harmful effects of rewarming due to reperfusion. During the donor WIT, there is reduced Na-K-ATPase activity and adenosine triphosphate (ATP) depletion. This leads to cellular edema, build-up of toxic metabolites, and increased free reactive oxygen species (ROS) generation. During reperfusion, because of rewarming and restoration of blood flow there is excessive release of ROS, and this causes injury to the cholangiocytes. Damage to the peribiliary vascular plexus during procurement further compromises blood flow to the bile ducts. All of this leads to biliary ischemia, epithelial necrosis, and impaired cholangiocyte function. This alters bile composition, promotes biliary stasis and sludge formation, and ultimately predisposes to stricture formation [8–10].

Croome and colleagues categorized IC into four main radiologic phenotypes based on severity and pattern of involvement:

- minor,
- confluence dominant,

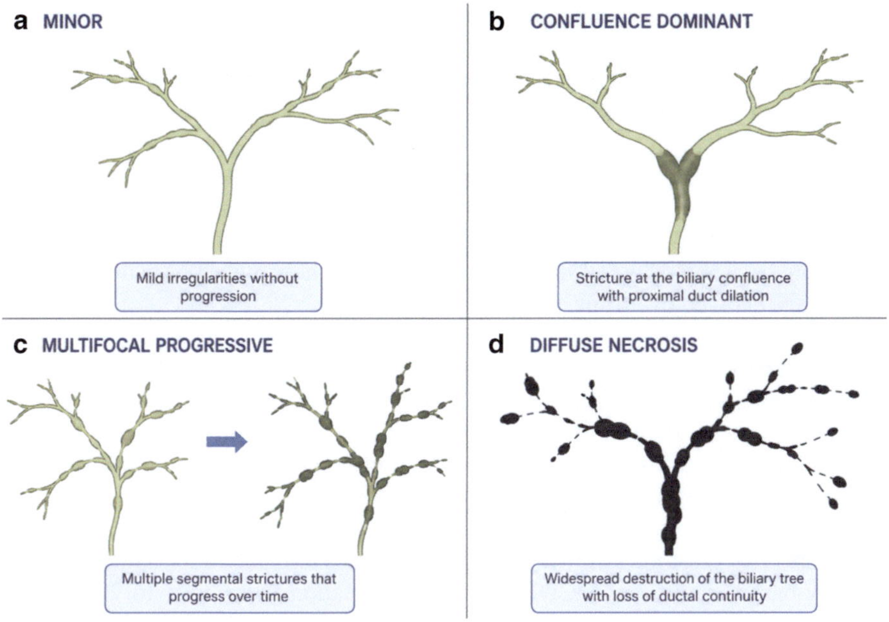

Fig. 13.1 Types of ischemic cholangiopathy

- multifocal progressive,
- diffuse necrosis (Fig. 13.1).

The minor form is characterized by mild biliary irregularities without progression and is generally associated with good outcomes. Confluence-dominant disease involves strictures at the biliary confluence with a significant percentage of patients requiring biliary intervention but has low re-transplantation rates. Multifocal progressive disease is more severe, with multiple strictures that worsen over time, leading to high rates of stent dependence and a significant risk of graft failure. The most severe phenotype is diffuse necrosis, which involves widespread destruction of the biliary tree and is associated with the poorest outcomes—nearly all patients require long-term stenting, and the majority ultimately need re-transplantation [11].

Historically, IC was a major limitation of DCDD liver transplantation, with early studies reporting incidence rates as high as 30% [9]. However, outcomes have improved significantly over time. Advances in donor selection, including stricter limits on WIT and improved donor-recipient matching, have helped reduce risk. In addition, the adoption of machine perfusion strategies to mitigate ischemic injury has improved rates of IC. As a result, more recent studies at experienced centers utilizing machine perfusion report IC rates in the range of 2–5%, approaching those seen in DNDD liver transplantation [6, 12–14].

Clinical Outcomes of DCDD Liver Transplantation

Clinical Outcomes After Utilization of DCDD Liver Allografts Using Super-Rapid Recovery

Super-rapid recovery (SRR), also referred to as static cold storage (SCS), represents the traditional approach to DCDD organ procurement, in which the liver is flushed and cooled in situ as rapidly as possible after circulatory arrest, then preserved on ice during transport. The following sections describe how outcomes using this technique have evolved over time.

Early Experience

Early experience with DCDD liver grafts in the 1990s was generally marked by inferior outcomes, such as lower patient and graft survival, higher rates of primary nonfunction (PNF), and greater need for re-transplantation [15–17]. In one of the earliest national registry studies using UNOS data from 1993 to 2001, 144 DCDD liver transplants were analyzed, and graft survival was 70.2% at 1 year and 63.3% at 3 years [18]. Over the following decade, outcomes remained suboptimal. Another registry-based analysis of DCDD liver transplantation from 2001 to 2009 found that, at 3 years after transplant, the graft survival rate was 64.9%, with a re-transplantation rate of 13.6% and a patient mortality rate of 21.6% which were significantly poorer compared to a similar DNDD cohort [19]. In a single-center series of 141 DCDD liver transplants, graft survival was found to be 69%, 56%, and 44% at 1, 5, and 10 years, respectively. PNF and biliary complications were major causes of graft loss. Worse outcomes were associated with donor WIT >20 min, cold ischemia time >8 h, and donor age >60 years [20]. They also demonstrated a lack of survival benefit in DCDD livers utilized for patients with model for end-stage liver disease score (MELD) ≤30. Other reports noted a 31.6% higher incidence of biliary complications and a 35.8% higher incidence of ischemic cholangiopathy in recipients of DCDD allografts and a threefold increase in hepatic artery stenosis compared with DNDD allografts (16.6% vs. 5.4%) [16, 21].

Therefore, toward the end of 2000s, there was a consensus of DCDD graft inferiority and the implementation of DCDD in liver transplant programs slowed down.

Recent Experience

Following the early DCDD experience, considerable efforts were directed toward improving outcomes through better donor selection, more refined donor–recipient matching, research focused on minimizing procurement, and preservation-related ischemic injury. There was also improvement in procurement and surgical techniques, and more effective management of DCDD-related complications [11, 22–24]. Together, these advances led to meaningfully improved clinical outcomes over the last decade.

In a study of 137 DCDD liver transplants, Frasco and colleagues found similar length of hospital stay, similar rates of re-transplantation, graft survival, and 1-year mortality as compared to DNDD graft recipients [25]. In 2021, another registry analysis was published which evaluated results of DCDD transplants before and they noticed that in after 2009 the patient survival at 10 years between DCDD and DNDD recipients was similar. By 2019, rates of re-transplantation of DCDD recipients differed from DNDD recipients by only 1.2%. Ischemic cholangiopathy-related graft failure declined sharply from 9.1% in 2002 to 0.92% in 2019 [26]. Scalea and others proved that outcomes with carefully selected DCDD livers were even superior to those achieved with using older DNDD livers [27]. Some centers also incorporated thrombolytics during DCDD procurement, with encouraging results. In one study of 100 consecutive DCDD liver transplants, graft survival was comparable to DNDD at both 1- and 3-years follow-up: 92% vs. 93.3% and 91.4% vs. 88.2%, respectively [28].

International Liver Transplant Society Recommendations to Improve Clinical Outcomes in DCDD Liver Transplantation

With promising recent experiences, the interest in DCDD transplantation has increased. In 2020, the International Liver Transplant Society organized a consensus conference and provided recommendations about various aspects of DCDD liver transplantation to optimize clinical outcomes [29–31].

Clinical Outcomes After Utilization of DCDD Liver Allografts in Era of Machine Perfusion

In recent years, increasing attention has been directed toward improving preservation techniques to improve clinical outcomes and utilization of DCDD allografts. One important approach is in situ or ex vivo machine perfusion technologies, which aim to actively control perfusion, temperature, and oxygen delivery to the allograft to reduce organ injury and to better assess graft function.

Machine perfusion techniques are categorized based on perfusate temperature (Table 13.1) [32–38]:

Table 13.1 Summary of recommendations from the International Liver Transplant Society for use of donation after circulatory determination of death allografts

Definitions	
DWIT definition	Report *total DWIT* from withdrawal of treatment to cold flush/NRP; report *functional DWIT* from SpO_2 <80% or MAP <60 mmHg to cold flush/NRP
Donor hepatectomy time	Define DHT as time from cold flush to liver out of body
Monitoring during DWIT	Monitor BP, SpO_2, and heart rate minute-by-minute; use arterial line BP and reliable pulse oximetry when possible
Procurement setting	Withdrawal of life-sustaining treatment should occur in the operating room when permitted to minimize fDWIT; experienced DCDD procurement surgeons are required
Domain	**ILTS recommendation**

(continued)

Table 13.1 (continued)

Donor age	Routine use of controlled DCDD livers from donors ≤*60 years*; selective use if >*60 years* considering other risks
Donor BMI	Routine use if donor BMI ≤*30* kg/m^2; selective use if >*30* $kg/m^2$with risk assessment
Steatosis	Avoid DCDD grafts with *macrovesicular steatosis* >*30%* unless machine perfusion/viability assessment is available
Cold ischemia time	Ideally implant DCDD livers within *8 h*; avoid expected CIT >*12 h*
Recipient selection	Allocate DCDD livers considering total medical risk, disease etiology, waitlist mortality, and ability to survive re-transplantation
Recipient age/BMI	No fixed recipient age or BMI cutoff is recommended
MELD score	Routine DCDD use is recommended for candidates with laboratory *MELD* ≤*25*; MELD >25 requires careful donor-risk limitation
Disease indication	DCDD grafts are *not contraindicated* for PSC, PBC, or HCC; MASH recipients should be selected carefully, especially for cardiovascular risk
Re-transplantation/ complex surgery	Use DCCD grafts selectively in re-transplantation or prior complex upper abdominal surgery
Portal vein thrombosis	Routine DCCD use is *not recommended* in recipients with complex portal vein thrombosis
Acute liver failure	DCCD grafts may be used selectively for ALF or super-urgent candidates
Combined liver-kidney transplant	Selective use of DCDD donors is recommended
DWIT threshold	If *functional DWIT* >*30 min*, increased graft-loss risk should be considered with donor, graft, recipient, and preservation factors

Abbreviations: *ALF* Acute Liver Failure, *BMI* Body Mass Index, *BP* Blood Pressure, *CIT* Cold Ischemia Time, *DCDD* Donation after Circulatory Determination of Death, *DHT* Donor Hepatectomy Time, *DWIT* Donor Warm Ischemia Time, *fDWIT* Functional Donor Warm Ischemia Time, *HCC* Hepatocellular Carcinoma, *MAP* Mean Arterial Pressure, *MELD* Model for End-Stage Liver Disease, *MASH* Metabolic syndrome associated Steatohepatitis, *NRP* Normothermic Regional Perfusion, *PBC* Primary Biliary Cholangitis, *PSC* Primary Sclerosing Cholangitis, SpO_2 Peripheral Oxygen Saturation

- hypothermic machine perfusion (HMP) (2–10 °C),
- sub-normothermic machine perfusion (SNMP) (20–25 °C),
- normothermic machine perfusion (NMP) (35–37.5 °C).

Clinical Outcomes After Utilization of DCDD Liver Allografts After Ex Situ Hypothermic Perfusion

Hypothermic machine perfusion (HMP), including hypothermic oxygenated perfusion (HOPE), is one of the earliest machine perfusion strategies implemented in clinical practice. It works by maintaining continuous circulation of the liver allograft using non-blood-based solutions ex situ which preserves endothelial function and prevents dysregulation of nitric oxide homeostasis. It also facilitates the clearance of metabolic waste. Delivery of oxygen, nutrients, and other substrates during perfusion helps in repaying the "oxygen debt" incurred during the period of donor warm ischemia and therefore minimize or even reverse procurement-related ischemic injury to the liver.

Most of the evidence for HMP comes from clinical trials performed in Europe. In a landmark randomized trial, van Rijn et al. demonstrated that HOPE significantly reduced non-anastomotic biliary strictures (6% vs. 18%) compared with SCS, with lower peak transaminases and better early graft function [39]. Other studies showed that HOPE was associated with reduced ischemia-reperfusion injury, lower rates of early allograft dysfunction [40]. Another long-term study from Europe evaluated 50 HOPE-treated DCDD liver transplants performed between 2012 and 2017 and compared them with 50 matched DNDD liver transplants and 50 SCS DDCD liver transplants. Despite longer donor WIT, HOPE-treated DCDD grafts achieved graft survival similar to DNDD grafts and superior to SCS preserved DCDD grafts (94% vs. 78%) [4].

Meta-analyses have reinforced benefits of HOPE particularly in reducing rates of non-anastomotic biliary strictures and early allograft dysfunction when compared with SCS alone in DCDD allografts. Some studies have also suggested improved graft survival and a reduced risk of PNF, particularly in higher-risk DCDD grafts, although these benefits have not been observed consistently [41, 42].

A major advantage of HMP strategies is their relative simplicity. There is no need for back-table preparation of the liver in most HMP devices. HMP also allows safer graft transport, as device malfunction does not expose the liver to a warm ischemic insult that could result in graft loss. In addition, these systems are generally less expensive and may be more practical in resource-limited settings.

Clinical Outcomes After Utilization of DCDD Liver Allografts After Ex Situ Normothermic Perfusion

Normothermic machine perfusion (NMP) is a preservation strategy in which the liver is maintained with continuous circulation of blood at near-physiologic temperature which allows for functional assessment prior to implantation.

In a randomized trial by Nasralla et al., NMP was associated with lower rates of early allograft dysfunction, and lower discard rates compared with SCS liver allografts. They also reported lower rates of non-anastomotic biliary strictures in the DCDD subgroup (11.1% vs. 26.3%) [43]. The PROTECT trial, a randomized trial in the USA reported similar findings, with lower rates of early allograft dysfunction (18% vs. 31%), decreased ischemic biliary complications (2.6% vs. 9.9%), and increased DCDD liver utilization (51% vs. 26%) after using NMP [44]. However, literature regarding NMP in DCDD liver transplantation is still limited and warrants further investigation.

There have been very few studies that have evaluated NMP against other preservation strategies. Gaurav et al. compared NMP with NRP and found that while both approaches improved outcomes in DCDD transplantation, NRP was associated with lower rates of ischemic cholangiopathy, and NMP offered the advantage of viability assessment and graft salvage [45]. Another recent study compared outcomes of NMP preserved DCDD livers to DNDD transplants and reported similar rates of early allograft dysfunction, biliary complications, and graft survival [46].

Current evidence suggests that NMP is useful in reducing early allograft injury, improving utilization of marginal DCDD grafts, and it allows for objective viability assessment prior to implantation. However, there is variability in outcomes across studies, particularly with regard to biliary complications, and further data is needed to evaluate NMP relative to other perfusion strategies such as NRP [47].

Clinical Outcomes After Utilization of DCDD Liver Allografts After In-Situ Normothermic Regional Perfusion

Normothermic regional perfusion (NRP) is a technique that restores oxygenated blood flow to organs after withdrawal of life-sustaining treatment and confirmed circulatory death. It is performed by rapidly cannulating the donor and initiating in situ perfusion, while ensuring that circulation is limited only to the organs intended for recovery. Multiple studies have demonstrated improved outcomes in DCDD transplantation after use of NRP. In a Spanish cohort of 545 NRP and 258 super rapid recovery (SRR) cases, Hessheimer et al. demonstrated significantly lower rates of early allograft dysfunction, hepatic artery thrombosis, biliary complications (12% vs. 29%), re-transplantation, and graft loss with NRP (Table 13.2) [48]. Similarly, a UK retrospective study comparing 43 NRP livers with 187 non-NRP-DCDD livers found significantly lower rates of early allograft dysfunction (12% vs. 32%), ischemic cholangiopathy (0% vs. 27%), and anastomotic strictures (7% vs. 27%) with NRP, along with a trend toward reduced 30-day graft loss (2% vs. 12%) [49]. Experience in the USA echoed similar findings of shorter hospital stays, fewer biliary complications, and lower rates of primary nonfunction [13, 50].

Outcomes with NRP were also found to be comparable to those after DNDD transplantation. Savier et al. matched 50 NRP cases with 100 DNDD transplants and reported similar complication rates and similar two-year graft and patient survival (88% vs. 85%; 90% vs. 88%, respectively) [51]. Ruiz et al. likewise found similar rates of early allograft dysfunction, acute kidney injury, and biliary complications in a matched cohort of 100 NRP and 200 DNDD transplants. In fact, they concluded that DCDD donors recovered using NRP should no longer be considered as "marginal donors." [14] NRP has also shown similar outcomes when compared with other machine perfusion strategies. In a multicenter analysis of NRP against HOPE, NRP was associated with lower rates of early allograft dysfunction (20% vs. 68%) [52, 53]. As mentioned in the previous section, NRP has also been shown to compare favorably when compared to ex situ NMP preservation, particularly with regards to reducing biliary complications [45, 46].

Another crucial benefit of NRP is its ability to improve utilization of liver allografts from DCDD donors, including grafts with prolonged donor WIT. In the USA, Bekki et al. found that thoracoabdominal NRP was associated with significantly higher liver utilization from DCD donors compared with non-NRP recovery, 70.6% versus 39.0% [54].

Benchmark Outcomes in DCDD Liver Transplantation

The study by Schlegel et al. attempted to establish "benchmark outcomes" for DCDD liver transplantation by analyzing over 2200 transplants across 17 international centers. Around 1012 low-risk donor–recipient pairs were used to define the *best achievable outcomes* in clinical practice (Table 13.3) [55]. It is important to

Table 13.2 Key studies comparing outcomes in DCDD liver transplantation

Author	Comparison	Biliary complications	Graft survival	Other key outcomes
De Vera et al. [20]	Single-center DCDD vs. DNDD	PNF and biliary complications accounted for 67% of early graft failures	DCDD: 1-, 5-, 10-year graft survival 69%, 56%, 44%; DBD: 82%, 73%, 63%	Worse outcomes associated with donor WIT >20 min, CIT >8 h, and donor age >60.
van Rijn et al. [39]	D-HOPE vs. SCS in DCDD	NAS: 6% vs. 18%	–	HOPE reduced non-anastomotic biliary strictures and improved early graft function.
Schlegel et al. [4]	HOPE-DCDD vs. untreated DCDD and DNDD	IC: 0% vs. 10%	Death-censored 5-year graft survival: HOPE-DCDD 94% vs. untreated DCDD 78%	HAT: 4% vs. 12%
Nasralla et al. [43]	NMP vs. SCS *(cohort included DNDD and DCDD transplants)*	DCDD subgroup NAS: 11.1% vs. 26.3%; clinically relevant ischemic cholangiopathy occurred in 1 patient in each arm	No significant difference in graft or patient survival	Overall, EAD: 10.1% vs. 29.9%; discard rate 11.7% vs. 24.1%; post-reperfusion syndrome 12.4% vs. 33.0%.
Markmann et al. [44]	NMP vs. ischemic cold storage *(cohort included DNDD and DCDD transplants)*	Ischemic biliary complications: 1.3% vs. 8.5% at 6 months; 2.6% vs. 9.9% at 12 months	30-day graft survival: 99.3% vs. 99.3%	Increased DCD liver utilization 51% vs. 26%.
Hessheimer et al. [48]	A-NRP vs. SRR in DCDD	Overall biliary complications: 12% vs. 29%; ITBL: 1% vs. 9%	1-year graft survival 90% vs. 79%; 3-year graft survival 87% vs. 68%	Patient survival 92% vs. 86% at 1 year and 89% vs. 76% at 3 years; adjusted HR for graft loss 0.435.
Watson et al. [49]	NRP vs. non-NRP-DCDD	IC 0% vs. 27%; anastomotic strictures 7% vs. 27%	30-day graft loss 2% vs. 12%	NRP independently associated with freedom from ischemic cholangiopathy.
Brubaker et al. [50]	NRP vs. SRR, US multicenter cohort	IC 0% vs. 9.0%; biliary anastomotic strictures 6.7% vs. 22.4%	Patient and graft survival comparable	LOS 7 vs. 10 days; PNF 0 vs. 1.5%; EAD 36.4% vs. 56.1%.
Savier et al. [51]	NRP-DCDD vs. DNDD	Similar biliary complications	2-year graft survival 88% vs. 85%	2-year patient survival 90% vs. 88%.

(continued)

Table 13.2 (continued)

Author	Comparison	Biliary complications	Graft survival	Other key outcomes
Ruiz et al. [14]	NRP-DCDD vs. DNDD	No ischemic-type biliary lesions in NRP-DCDD group	1-year 99% vs. 92%; 3-year 93% vs. 87%	Similar EAD, AKI, and biliary complications
Muller et al. [52]	NRP vs. HOPE in DCDD	No significant difference in NAS, PNF, or HAT; IC 4.5% vs. 8.6%	Recipient and graft survival >85% in both groups	EAD lower with NRP: 20% vs. 68%.

Abbreviations: *AKI* Acute Kidney Injury, *A-NRP* Abdominal Normothermic Regional Perfusion, *CIT* Cold Ischemia Time, *DBD* Donation after Brain Death, *DCDD* Donation after Circulatory Determination of Death, *D-HOPE* Dual Hypothermic Oxygenated Perfusion, *DNDD* Donation after Neurological Determination of Death, *EAD* Early Allograft Dysfunction, *HAT* Hepatic Artery Thrombosis, *HOPE* Hypothermic Oxygenated Perfusion, *HR* Hazard Ratio, *IC* Ischemic Cholangiopathy, *ITBL* Ischemic-Type Biliary Lesions, *LOS* Length of Stay, *NAS* Non-Anastomotic Strictures, *NMP* Normothermic Machine Perfusion, *NRP* Normothermic Regional Perfusion, *PNF* Primary Nonfunction, *SCS* Static Cold Storage, *SRR* Super-Rapid Recovery, *WIT* Warm Ischemia Time

Table 13.3 Benchmark outcomes in DCDD liver transplantation

Outcome measure	Benchmark value
In hospital complications	
Intensive care unit stay	≤3 days
Hospital stay	≤16 days
Bleeding	<10.3%
Primary nonfunction	≤2.5%
Renal replacement therapy	≤9.6%
Biliary complications	
Ischemic cholangiopathy	≤16.8%
Anastomotic biliary strictures	≤28.4%
Bile leak	≤8.3%
One-year outcomes	
Any complication	<95%
Comprehensive complication index at 1 year	≤38.9
1-year graft loss	≤14.4%
Re-transplant	≤6.9%
1-year mortality	≤9.6%

note that these benchmarks were derived before the widespread adoption of machine perfusion, and as machine perfusion becomes the standard of care, updated benchmark analyses will be needed.

Conclusion

Outcomes after DCDD liver transplantation have improved significantly over the past two decades, to the point where DCDD grafts—when carefully selected and managed—can achieve results comparable to those from DNDD donors. The introduction of machine perfusion techniques, including HMP/HOPE, NMP, and NRP, has played a crucial role in mitigating ischemic injury, improving graft utilization, and expanding the donor pool. Among these, NRP has emerged as particularly promising in reducing ischemic cholangiopathy and improving utilization, while NMP offers the advantage of ex situ viability assessment of the liver, and HMP/HOPE provides a simpler and more cost-effective alternative with decent evidence for reducing biliary complications.

Conflict of Interest The authors have no conflicts of interest to disclose.

Competing Interests The author(s) has no competing interests to declare that are relevant to the content of this manuscript.

Ethics Approval The author(s) declares that this manuscript does not include primary research with human participants.

The author(s) declares that this manuscript does not include primary studies involving animals.

References

1. Meirelles Júnior RF e, Salvalaggio P, de Rezende MB r, et al. Liver transplantation: history, outcomes and perspectives. Einstein. 2015;13(1):149. https://doi.org/10.1590/S1679-45082015RW3164.
2. 2021 Global report – GODT. https://www.transplant-observatory.org/2021-global-report-5/. Accessed 20 Apr 2026.
3. Schlegel A, De Rougemont O, Graf R, Clavien PA, Dutkowski P. Protective mechanisms of end-ischemic cold machine perfusion in DCD liver grafts. J Hepatol. 2013;58(2):278–86. https://doi.org/10.1016/J.JHEP.2012.10.004.
4. Schlegel A, Muller X, Kalisvaart M, et al. Outcomes of DCD liver transplantation using organs treated by hypothermic oxygenated perfusion before implantation. J Hepatol. 2019;70(1):50–7. https://doi.org/10.1016/J.JHEP.2018.10.005.
5. Banker A, Bhatt N, Rao PS, et al. A review of machine perfusion strategies in liver transplantation. J Clin Exp Hepatol. 2023;13(2):335–49. https://doi.org/10.1016/J.JCEH.2022.08.001.
6. Currie IS, Hunt FM. Donation after circulatory death; cholangiopathy in the machine age. Curr Opin Organ Transplant. 2025;30(4):337. https://doi.org/10.1097/MOT.0000000000001222.
7. Bekki Y, Loszko A, Endo Y, et al. Embracing liver transplantation from donation after circulatory death in the United States in the era of perfusion technology. Transplantation. 2026;110(2):e416–24. https://doi.org/10.1097/TP.0000000000005537.
8. Chan EY, Olson LC, Kisthard JA, et al. Ischemic cholangiopathy following liver transplantation from donation after cardiac death donors. Liver Transpl. 2008;14(5):604–10. https://doi.org/10.1002/LT.21361.
9. Sanchez-Urdazpal L, Gores GJ, Ward EM, et al. Ischemic-type biliary complications after orthotopic liver transplantation. Hepatology. 1992;16(1):49–53. https://doi.org/10.1002/HEP.1840160110.
10. de Vries Y, von Meijenfeldt FA, Porte RJ. Post-transplant cholangiopathy: Classification, pathogenesis, and preventive strategies. Biochim Biophy Acta Mol Basis Dis. 2018;1864(4):1507–15. https://doi.org/10.1016/J.BBADIS.2017.06.013.
11. Croome KP, Mathur AK, Aqel B, et al. Classification of distinct patterns of ischemic cholangiopathy following DCD liver transplantation: distinct clinical courses and long-term outcomes from a multicenter cohort. Transplantation. 2022;106(6):1206–14. https://doi.org/10.1097/TP.0000000000003928.
12. Eden J, Brüggenwirth IMA, Berlakovich G, et al. Long-term outcomes after hypothermic oxygenated machine perfusion and transplantation of 1,202 donor livers in a real-world

setting (HOPE-REAL study). J Hepatol. 2025;82(1):97–106. https://doi.org/10.1016/J.JHEP.2024.06.035.
13. Sellers MT, Nassar A, Alebrahim M, et al. Early United States experience with liver donation after circulatory determination of death using thoraco-abdominal normothermic regional perfusion: a multi-institutional observational study. Clin Transpl. 2022;36(6):e14659. https://doi.org/10.1111/CTR.14659.
14. Ruiz P, Valdivieso A, Palomares I, et al. Similar results in liver transplantation from controlled donation after circulatory death donors with normothermic regional perfusion and donation after brain death donors: a case-matched single-center study. Liver Transpl. 2021;27(12):1747–57. https://doi.org/10.1002/lt.26281.
15. Jay CL, Lyuksemburg V, Ladner DP, et al. Ischemic cholangiopathy after controlled donation after cardiac death liver transplantation: a meta-analysis. Ann Surg. 2011;253(2):259–64. https://doi.org/10.1097/SLA.0B013E318204E658.
16. Foley DP, Fernandez LA, Leverson G, et al. Donation after cardiac death: the University of Wisconsin experience with liver transplantation. Ann Surg. 2005;242(5):724–31. https://doi.org/10.1097/01.SLA.0000186178.07110.92.
17. Abt P, Crawford M, Desai N, Markmann J, Olthoff K, Shaked A. Liver transplantation from controlled non-heartbeating donors: an increased incidence of biliary complications. Transplantation. 2003;75(10):1659–63. https://doi.org/10.1097/01.TP.0000062574.18648.7C.
18. Abt PL, Desai NM, Crawford MD, et al. Survival following liver transplantation from non-heart-beating donors. Ann Surg. 2004;239(1):87–92. https://doi.org/10.1097/01.SLA.0000103063.82181.2C.
19. Mathur AK, Heimbach J, Steffick DE, Sonnenday CJ, Goodrich NP, Merion RM. Donation after cardiac death liver transplantation: predictors of outcome. Am J Transplant. 2010;10(11):2512–9. https://doi.org/10.1111/J.1600-6143.2010.03293.X.
20. De Vera ME, Lopez-Solis R, Dvorchik I, et al. Liver transplantation using donation after cardiac death donors: long-term follow-up from a single center. Am J Transplant. 2009;9(4):773–81. https://doi.org/10.1111/J.1600-6143.2009.02560.X.
21. Skaro AI, Jay CL, Baker TB, et al. The impact of ischemic cholangiopathy in liver transplantation using donors after cardiac death: the untold story. Surgery. 2009;146(4):543–53. https://doi.org/10.1016/J.SURG.2009.06.052.
22. Eden J, Sousa Da Silva R, Cortes-Cerisuelo M, et al. Utilization of livers donated after circulatory death for transplantation—an international comparison. J Hepatol. 2023;78(5):1007–16. https://doi.org/10.1016/j.jhep.2023.01.025.
23. Croome KP, Lee DD, Keaveny AP, Burcin Taner C. Improving national results in liver transplantation using grafts from donation after cardiac death donors. Transplantation. 2016;100(12):2640–7. https://doi.org/10.1097/tp.0000000000001483.
24. De Carlis R, Muiesan P, Taner B. Donation after circulatory death: novel strategies to improve the liver transplant outcome. J Hepatol. 2023;78(6):1169–80. https://doi.org/10.1016/J.JHEP.2023.04.008/ATTACHMENT/9F87F636-F0FD-41E5-ACCE-3894838E2E64/MMC1.PDF.
25. Frasco PE, Mathur AK, Chang YH, et al. Days alive and out of hospital after liver transplant: comparing a patient-centered outcome between recipients of grafts from donation after circulatory and brain deaths. Am J Transplant. 2023;23(1):55–63. https://doi.org/10.1016/J.AJT.2022.10.007.
26. Haque OJ, Roth EM, Fleishman A, Eckhoff DE, Khwaja K. Long-term outcomes of early experience in donation after circulatory death liver transplantation: outcomes at 10 years. Ann Transplant. 2021;26:e930243. https://doi.org/10.12659/AOT.930243.
27. Scalea JR, Redfield RR, Foley DP. Liver transplant outcomes using ideal donation after circulatory death livers are superior to using older donation after brain death donor livers. Liver Transpl. 2016;22(9):1197–204. https://doi.org/10.1002/LT.24494.
28. Bohorquez H, Seal JB, Cohen AJ, et al. Safety and outcomes in 100 consecutive donation after circulatory death liver transplants using a protocol that includes thrombolytic therapy. Am J Transplant. 2017;17(8):2155–64. https://doi.org/10.1111/AJT.14261.

29. Kalisvaart M, Croome KP, Hernandez-Alejandro R, et al. Donor warm ischemia time in DCD liver transplantation – working group report from the ILTS DCD, liver preservation, and machine perfusion consensus conference. Transplantation. 2021;105(6):1156–64. https://doi.org/10.1097/TP.0000000000003819.
30. Hessheimer AJ, Kalisvaart M. Creation of the ILTS consensus statements on DCD and liver perfusion: defining the future of liver transplantation by returning to the past. Transplantation. 2021;105(4):695–6. https://doi.org/10.1097/TP.0000000000003631.
31. Schlegel A, Foley DP, Savier E, et al. Recommendations for donor and recipient selection and risk prediction: working group report from the ILTS consensus conference in DCD liver transplantation. Transplantation. 2021;105(9):1892–903. https://doi.org/10.1097/TP.0000000000003825.
32. Boteon YL, Martins PN, Muiesan P, Schlegel A. Machine perfusion of the liver: putting the puzzle pieces together. World J Gastroenterol. 2021;27(34):5727–36. https://doi.org/10.3748/wjg.v27.i34.5727.
33. Ceresa CDL, Nasralla D, Pollok JM, Friend PJ. Machine perfusion of the liver: applications in transplantation and beyond. Nat Rev Gastroenterol Hepatol. 2022;19(3):199–209. https://doi.org/10.1038/s41575-021-00557-8.
34. Weeder PD, Van Rijn R, Porte RJ. Machine perfusion in liver transplantation as a tool to prevent non-anastomotic biliary strictures: rationale, current evidence and future directions. J Hepatol. 2015;63(1):265–75. https://doi.org/10.1016/J.JHEP.2015.03.008.
35. Detelich D, Markmann JF. The dawn of liver perfusion machines. Curr Opin Organ Transplant. 2018;23(2):151–61. https://doi.org/10.1097/MOT.0000000000000500.
36. Karimian N, Raigani S, Huang V, et al. Subnormothermic machine perfusion of steatotic livers results in increased energy charge at the cost of anti-oxidant capacity compared to normothermic perfusion. Meta. 2019;9(11):246. https://doi.org/10.3390/metabo9110246.
37. Czigany Z, Tacke F, Lurje G. Evolving trends in machine liver perfusion: comments on clinical end points and selection criteria. Gastroenterology. 2019;157(4):1166–7. https://doi.org/10.1053/J.GASTRO.2019.02.051.
38. Sousa Da Silva RX, Weber A, Dutkowski P, Clavien PA. Machine perfusion in liver transplantation. Hepatology. 2022;76(5):1531–49. https://doi.org/10.1002/HEP.32546.
39. van Rijn R, Schurink IJ, de Vries Y, et al. Hypothermic machine perfusion in liver transplantation – a randomized trial. N Engl J Med. 2021;384(15):1391–401. https://doi.org/10.1056/NEJMOA2031532.
40. Dutkowski P, Polak WG, Muiesan P, et al. First comparison of hypothermic oxygenated PErfusion versus static cold storage of human donation after cardiac death liver transplants: an international-matched case analysis. Ann Surg. 2015;262(5):764–71. https://doi.org/10.1097/SLA.0000000000001473.
41. Risbey CWG, Thomas C, Niu A, Liu K, Crawford M, Pulitano C. Hypothermic oxygenated machine PErfusion for high-risk liver grafts for transplantation: a systematic review and meta-analysis. Artif Organs. 2024;48(10):1085–99. https://doi.org/10.1111/AOR.14814.
42. Patrono D, Del Prete L, Eden J, et al. Machine perfusion of liver grafts: hypothermic versus normothermic versus normothermic regional perfusion. Int J Surg. 2025;111(9):5768. https://doi.org/10.1097/JS9.0000000000002648.
43. Nasralla D, Coussios CC, Mergental H, et al. A randomized trial of normothermic preservation in liver transplantation. Nature. 2018;557(7703):50–6. https://doi.org/10.1038/S41586-018-0047-9.
44. Markmann JF, Abouljoud MS, Ghobrial RM, et al. Impact of portable normothermic blood-based machine perfusion on outcomes of liver transplant: the OCS liver PROTECT randomized clinical trial. JAMA Surg. 2022;157(3):189. https://doi.org/10.1001/JAMASURG.2021.6781.
45. Gaurav R, Butler AJ, Kosmoliaptsis V, et al. Liver transplantation outcomes from controlled circulatory death donors: SCS vs in situ NRP vs ex situ NMP. Ann Surg. 2022;275(6):1156–64. https://doi.org/10.1097/SLA.0000000000005428.

46. Mohkam K, Nasralla D, Mergental H, et al. In situ normothermic regional perfusion versus ex situ normothermic machine perfusion in liver transplantation from donation after circulatory death. Liver Transpl. 2022;28(11):1716–25. https://doi.org/10.1002/lt.26522.
47. Watson CJE, Gaurav R, Butler AJ. Current techniques and indications for machine perfusion and regional perfusion in deceased donor liver transplantation. J Clin Exp Hepatol. 2023;14(2):101309. https://doi.org/10.1016/J.JCEH.2023.101309.
48. Hessheimer AJ, de la Rosa G, Gastaca M, et al. Abdominal normothermic regional perfusion in controlled donation after circulatory determination of death liver transplantation: outcomes and risk factors for graft loss. Am J Transplant. 2022;22(4):1169–81. https://doi.org/10.1111/AJT.16899.
49. Watson CJE, Hunt F, Messer S, et al. In situ normothermic perfusion of livers in controlled circulatory death donation may prevent ischemic cholangiopathy and improve graft survival. Am J Transplant. 2019;19(6):1745–58. https://doi.org/10.1111/ajt.15241.
50. Brubaker AL, Sellers MT, Abt PL, et al. US liver transplant outcomes after normothermic regional perfusion vs standard super rapid recovery. JAMA Surg. 2024;159(6):677–85. https://doi.org/10.1001/jamasurg.2024.0520.
51. Savier E, Lim C, Rayar M, et al. Favorable outcomes of liver transplantation from controlled circulatory death donors using normothermic regional perfusion compared to brain death donors. Transplantation. 2020;104(9):1943–51. https://doi.org/10.1097/TP.0000000000003372.
52. Muller X, Mohkam K, Mueller M, et al. Hypothermic oxygenated perfusion versus normothermic regional perfusion in liver transplantation from controlled donation after circulatory death: first international comparative study. Ann Surg. 2020;272(5):751–8. https://doi.org/10.1097/SLA.0000000000004268.
53. Imai D, Hallesy J, Rathi R, et al. Normothermic regional perfusion in controlled donation after circulatory death: growing evidence for liver transplantation. Clin Transpl. 2026;40(2):e70463. https://doi.org/10.1111/CTR.70463.
54. Bekki Y, Croome KP, Myers B, Sasaki K, Tomiyama K. Normothermic regional perfusion can improve both utilization and outcomes in DCD liver, kidney, and pancreas transplantation. Transplant Direct. 2023;9(3):E1450. https://doi.org/10.1097/TXD.0000000000001450.
55. Schlegel A, van Reeven M, Croome K, et al. A multicentre outcome analysis to define global benchmarks for donation after circulatory death liver transplantation. J Hepatol. 2022;76(2):371–82. https://doi.org/10.1016/J.JHEP.2021.10.004.

Recipient Selection and Outcomes in Heart and Lung Transplantation from Donation After Circulatory Death Donors

14

Prakash M. Ludhani and Kumud K. Dhital

Introduction

The continued non-converging disparity between the demand for thoracic organ transplantation and availability of suitable donor organs has placed significant pressure on clinicians to further expand the donor pool largely by adopting flexibility with established donor selection criteria. Over the past two decades, the most impactful of these strategies has been to utilise donor hearts and lungs from donation after circulatory death (DCD). Contemporary advances in donor organ preservation, re-establishing in situ regional perfusion in the donor on a need-to basis through extra-corporeal circulation, and the availability of multiple ex situ platforms for organ preservation and reconditioning have enabled increasing adoption of this donation pathway. Results of DCD solid organ clinical transplants are excellent with outcomes comparable to those achieved using donation after brain death (DBD) donors.

DCD thoracic transplantation introduces unique physiological challenges related to warm ischaemic injury, ischemia-reperfusion injury, inflammatory activation, and graft recovery. Consequently, careful donor and recipient selection is essential to optimise graft utilisation while minimising peri- and post-operative mobidity. Selection of the DCD donor for heart and lung transplantation, and the relevant techniques are described in a separate dedicated chapter in this publication [1]. Recipient risk stratification must account for urgency status, frailty, pulmonary vascular resistance, degree of renal dysfunction, allosensitisation, existing or anticipated use of mechanical circulatory support, and anticipated ischaemic tolerance.

This review summarises contemporary concepts in recipient selection, perioperative transplantation strategies, and clinical outcomes in DCD heart and lung

P. M. Ludhani · K. K. Dhital (✉)
Institutes of Heart-Lung Transplantation and MCS, Apollo Hospital, Chennai, Tamil Nadu, India

S. P. Kolte et al. (eds.), *Organ Donation After Circulatory Death*,
https://doi.org/10.1007/978-981-92-6377-6_14

transplantation. Current evidence comparing DCD and DBD transplantation is critically reviewed. Contemporary evidence supports the expanding role of DCD thoracic transplantation as a safe and effective strategy to reduce wait-list mortality and increase timely access to this therapy. For appropriate candidates with end-stage heart and/or lung disease, transplantation remains the definitive and most validated clinical option for symptomatic control and survivorship and is limited principally by the shortage of suitable and matching donor organs [2]. While DCD lung transplantation has been practiced sustainably for two decades in many centres and continues to expand steadily across multiple international jurisdictions, modern adult DCD heart transplantation was only reintroduced in 2014 [3–6].

Unlike the DBD scenario, DCD organs are exposed to an obligatory period of warm ischaemia between withdrawal of life-sustaining therapy and reperfusion. This interval significantly increases the risk of primary graft dysfunction (PGD), metabolic exhaustion, endothelial injury, and the need for temporary post-transplant MCS support [7–9]. Current practices therefore rely on various technologies and protocols to mitigate these shortcomings. Options include thoraco-abdominal normothermic regional perfusion (TA-NRP), and a selection of ex situ static and perfusion-based organ preservation and organ reconditioning platforms which are discussed elsewhere in this publication [1, 10, 11].

This review examines recipient selection, transplantation techniques, perioperative management, and reported outcomes for DCD heart and lung transplantation, drawing on international registry data available through to early 2026.

Recipient Selection in DCD Heart Transplantation

Selecting a recipient for a DCD graft requires simultaneous consideration of clinical urgency, the graft's predicted tolerance of warm ischaemic injury, technical complexity of the implant, and the likelihood of meaningful post-transplant survival [12]. The aim should be to select a donor that provides the most recipient-protective strategy, in reality, the experience from mature DCD heart transplant programmes, and particularly from those institutions where utilization of DCD donor organs is standard of care, then any wait-listed patients suitable for DBD donor hearts, are equally suitable for DCD organs.

Candidates typically have end-stage heart failure, on the background of advanced cardiomyopathy (ischaemic, dilated, restrictive, hypertrophic, or arrhythmogenic), LV non-compaction or failed palliation of advanced congenital heart disease, and often in refractory cardiogenic shock [13].

Most centres starting a DCD heart transplant programme preferentially accept patients who are in the ambulatory stages of heart failure (INTERMACS 3–5), who have limited extra-cardiac end-organ dysfunction, non-frail, have only mild pulmonary hypertension, low levels of allosensitisation, and no history of complex redo sternotomy [13].

Features that increase risk include pre-transplant ECMO, significant pulmonary hypertension, in situ durable left-ventricular assist device, marked frailty, advanced renal impairment, high allosensitisation, and re-transplantation. It is reassuring that higher volume and mature DCD programmes are able to deliver excellent outcomes, comparable to the use of DBD donor organs, with selected patients from these high-risk groups [11, 14, 15]. This experience also confirms that there are no additional recipient-related contraindications specifically to the use of DCD donor hearts, even if many centres continue to consider them as being marginal organs. Therefore, as per the DBD practice, older age, advanced frailty, morbid obesity, severe peripheral vascular disease, moderate pulmonary hypertension, significant renal or hepatic dysfunction, and high-risk redo sternotomy are considered relative contraindications and require personalised assessment.

Irreversible multi-system organ failure, active malignancy, severe irreversible pulmonary hypertension, uncontrolled infection, neurological injury incompatible with meaningful rehabilitation, and anticipated lack of compliance with post-transplant surveillance protocol remain absolute contraindications [16].

Recipient Selection for DCD Lung Transplantation

Like the selection of recipients for DCD heart transplantation described above, all recipients who are suitable for DBD donor lungs, are also suitable for lungs from the DCD pathway. Standard indications include end-stage interstitial lung disease, chronic obstructive pulmonary disease, suppurative lung diseases (bronchiectasis and cystic fibrosis), pulmonary arterial hypertension, and chronic hypersensitivity pneumonitis [17].

Recipients with controlled pulmonary pressures, preserved right-ventricular function, limited or no pre-operative ECMO requirement, lower body-mass index, and a stable nutritional state tend to have a low risk profile for receiving DCD donor lungs [17].

Patients with severe pulmonary hypertension need careful planning for intraoperative ECMO support because of the heightened risk of primary graft dysfunction and right-ventricular failure. Similarly, those with primary pulmonary hypertension may even require awake ECMO bridging to lower their peri-operative risks [18].

Donor–Recipient Matching and Allocation Considerations

Donor–recipient matching for DCD heart and lung transplantation remains the same as that for standard DBD donor organs, but with the caveat that the DCD organs have a lower tolerance to ischaemia [12]. In pursuing best outcome, the rationale of choosing a recipient-protective strategy warrants some discipline in limiting the added marginality beyond the fact of utilising DCD organs. It is therefore prudent to limit the cold ischaemic time. For hearts, and particularly in the context of borderline transpulmonary gradient, it is wise to oversize the donor. For lungs, avoid the need for downsizing for fear of prolonged air-leak, avoid oversizing on the background of RV dysfunction to avoid tamponade physiology, and remain extra cautious when considering lungs with congestion, contusion, consolidation, and borderline oxygenation. In practice, DCD organs often prove most valuable for urgent or difficult-to-match candidates who might otherwise wait an unacceptably long time [19].

DCD Heart Transplantation Techniques

The preferred implant technique remains standard bi-caval orthotopic transplantation. Key technical points are to minimise ischaemic time during implantation and use intermittent supplementary cardioplegia as required. If the ischaemic time is a concern, then depending on surgical experience, the cross-clamp can be removed at any stage once the left atrial and aortic anastomoses are complete. The remaining anastomoses can safely be carried out on the beating heart. Adequate time must be devoted to myocardial reperfusion with a slow wean from cardiopulmonary bypass with vasoactive support to ensure RV protection.

The actual donor organ retrieval procedures including TA-NRP, and description of available ex situ platforms for organ preservation, transport and reconditioning, are all discussed in a separate chapter [1].

DCD Lung Transplantation Techniques

Bilateral sequential transplantation, via a clamshell incision or bilateral thoracotomies, is carried out with or without ECMO support depending on the degree of pulmonary hypertension, status of RV function, anticipated ease of exposure and surgical dissection, and whether any concomitant cardiac procedure is planned. Controlled reperfusion, lung-protective ventilation, and adjunct use of nitric oxide are key steps in preventing PGD and unloading the RV [20].

Primary Graft Dysfunction in DCD Transplantation

Primary graft dysfunction remains the dominant early complication following thoracic transplantation. In heart transplantation, the TA-NRP protocol has been associated with a reduction in severe PGD (7.6% versus 19.2%) when compared to that following direct procurement and perfusion (DPP) [11]. A more recent cohort analysis suggests that PGD following DCD heart transplantation with the DPP protocol can be as low as 8% [15]. Reassuringly, there is compelling data suggesting a lower mortality among those with PGD following DCD transplants when compared to those with PGD post-DBD transplants [21].

The overall rate of PGD following DCD lung transplantation in several studies varies from 5–44% and 9–47% respectively for the DCD vs DBD cohorts [24]. Although the rate of early PGD at time 0-h and at 24-h appears to be higher in the

DCD group, the rates equilibrate at 72 h post-transplant when it can be as low as 5–8.5% [22, 23].

Outcomes of DCD Heart Transplantation

Contemporary multi-centre and registry series show that survival after DCD heart transplantation is now comparable to that achieved with DBD organs. Findings from a larger international multi-centre study show cumulative survival of 89.5% and 81.5% at 1- and 3-years respectively post DCD heart transplantation, and lower mortality with TA-NRP vs DPP in subgroup analysis [11]. 1- and 5-year survival of 94% and 88% [n.s] for the DCD group and 87% and 81% [n.s] for the DBD group, respectively, has also been reported by the Sydney group in Australia [15].

Outcomes of DCD Lung Transplantation

DCD lung transplantation is also demonstrating short- and medium-term survival to be comparable to DBD cohorts [22]. Analysis of 7 studies on lung transplantation following donation after circulatory death shows 1-, 3-, and 5-year survival range to be 75–100%, 61–82% and 51–80% respectively for the DCD groups, and 82–91%, 69–83%, and 61–78%, respectively for the DBD groups [24]. A multi-centre Australian experience of DCD lung transplantation has reported excellent survival of 97% and 90% at 1- and 5-years respectively for the DCD group versus 90% and 61% survival over the same timeframe for the DBD group [23].

A Spanish study assessing outcomes of DCD lung transplantation following a period of TA-NRP with in situ establishment of circulation except for the brain, versus direct rapid retrieval of the lungs during selective abdominal NRP (A-NRP), showed there was no difference in post-transplant outcome [25]. This has also been validated by a UK study which confirms the A-NRP technique, that permits selective perfusion below the thoracic aorta, is not detrimental to the rapid procurement of lungs and without jeopardy to post-transplant survival [26].

The Indian Perspective

India has in place a Supreme Court-directed legal framework that permits withdrawal of life-sustaining treatment (WLST) as part of end-of-life care where continued medical care is considered futile. A national multidisciplinary DCD consortium has put in place this background of a robust legislative framework with what can be achieved, and how, in India. It additionally addresses ethical, clinical, financial, procedural, and logistical considerations that are specifically pertinent to India [27].

In Maastricht category III-controlled DCD, the decision for WLST is entirely delinked from any consideration of organ donation for transplantation. For families who express a willingness to pursue donation, the procedure is clearly outlined, including the timing and setting for WLST, consent for antemortem interventions, the mandated no-touch interval, and the contingency that donation may be called off, with the patient returning to the intensive care unit (ICU) if donation does not proceed.

For donation after neurologic determination of death (DNDD), should cardiac arrest occur during the brain death certification process, a comprehensive protocol for DCD Category IV is provided. Additionally, the same document addresses DCD Category V, in which organ donation may be feasible following an unsuccessful cardiopulmonary resuscitation effort after an in-ICU cardiac arrest [27]. More recently, the same DCD consortium has also published a consensus on normothermic regional perfusion as a viable option for recovery of organs donated following circulatory death [28].

Although India boasts third place in the total number of transplants carried out annually, the overwhelming majority of transplants occur through living organ donations. The aim of reversing this practice in favour of utilising deceased donated organs is going to be challenging for a number of reasons. While legislation is no longer a hurdle, there is significant lack of awareness both in the community, and within the medical profession about what the law and the DCD concept really mean. There is ongoing confusion regarding understanding and perception of how any deceased donation pathway is delinked from organ donation and transplantation. Culturally, the DCD option with monitors that show asystole and reflect cessation of circulation in the presence of relatives, may be more readily acceptable.

The relentless task of informing the public from schools through to the workplace, and equally within the medical community remains central. An increase in heart and lung transplantation, with its necessary reliance on deceased donor organs is likely to play a key role in shifting abdominal organ transplants from living donation to deceased donation. Adoption of donation after circulatory death practice represents the most obvious way to increase the number of thoracic transplants.

Conclusion

The DCD pathway has become a valuable source of expanded donor availability in numerous countries with direct increase in heart and lung transplant activity. Survivorship post DCD thoracic transplantation reveals comparable outcomes following DBD transplants. For emerging programmes such as in India, structured DCD pathways represent a practical opportunity to reduce wait-list mortality.

Technical advances in TA-NRP, A-NRP, and increasing options of ex situ devises for preservation, transportation, and reconditioning of donor organs are increasing the safety and quality of organs that are used for clinical transplants. Development of indigenous perfusion platforms, regional retrieval hubs, standardized national protocols, and a dedicated and transparent thoracic transplant registry would substantially accelerate progress. DCD transplantation holds the potential to convert every end-of-life discharge against medical advice into an opportunity to save multiple lives.

Competing Interests The author(s) has no competing interests to declare that are relevant to the content of this manuscript.

Ethics Approval The author(s) declares that this manuscript does not include primary research with human participants.

The author(s) declares that this manuscript does not include primary studies involving animals.

References

1. Ludhani P, Dhital K. Chapter 8: Donor selection and thoracic organ retrieval in donation after circulatory death. In: Bhawane AR, Balwani M, Kute V, Kolte SP, editors. Organ donation after circulatory death: strategies for growth in emerging health systems.
2. Singh TP, International Society for Heart and Lung Transplantation, et al. The international thoracic organ transplant registry of the international society for heart and lung transplantation: 2025 annual report of heart and lung transplantation. J Heart Lung Transplant. 2025;44(12):1857–73. https://doi.org/10.1016/j.healun.2025.04.014.
3. Cypel M, Levvey B, Van Raemdonck D, et al. ISHLT donation after circulatory death registry report. J Heart Lung Transplant. 2015;34(12):1278–82.
4. Snell GI, Levvey BJ, Oto T, et al. Early lung transplantation success utilizing controlled donation after cardiac death donors. Am J Transplant. 2008;8(6):1282–9.
5. Van Raemdonck D, Keshavjee S, Levvey B, et al. Donation after circulatory death in lung transplantation – five-year follow-up from ISHLT registry. J Heart Lung Transplant. 2019;38(12):1235–45.
6. Dhital KK, Iyer A, Connellan M, et al. Adult heart transplantation with distant procurement and ex-vivo preservation of donor hearts after circulatory death: a case series. Lancet. 2015;385(9987):2585–91. https://doi.org/10.1016/S0140-6736(15)60038-1.
7. Iyer A, Chew HC, Gao L, et al. Pathophysiological trends during withdrawal of life support. Circulation. 2016;134(21):1562–74.
8. Williams A, Ahmad A, Trahanas J, et al. Ten-minute asystolic warm ischemic time (AWIT) predicts mortality, and severe primary graft dysfunction in donation after circulatory death hearts recovered with thoraco-abdominal normothermic regional perfusion. J Heart Lung Transplant. 2026;45(4):555–65.
9. Hong Y, Nasin U, Dorken-Gallastagi A, et al. Impact of coronary hypoperfusion during agonal phase on outcomes following donation after circulatory death heart transplantation. J Heart Lung Transplant. 2026;45(2):172–81.
10. D'Alessandro DA, Hoffman JR, Knecht KR, et al. Heart transplantation from controlled DCD donors using thoracoabdominal normothermic regional perfusion. Ann Thorac Surg. 2019;108(5):1450–6.
11. Louca JO, Öchsner M, Bhagra S, et al. Outcomes after donation after circulatory determination of death heart transplantation: an international, multicenter retrospective study. JACC Heart Fail. 2025;13(12):102473. https://doi.org/10.1016/j.jchf.2025.04.003.
12. International Society for Heart and Lung Transplantation. ISHLT consensus statement on donation after circulatory death thoracic transplantation. J Heart Lung Transplant. 2021;40(10):1197–214.
13. Macdonald PS, Dhital KK. Heart transplantation from donation after circulatory death donors. Semin Thorac Cardiovasc Surg. 2019;31(1):75–82.
14. Messer S, Cernic S, Page A, et al. A 5-year single-center early experience of heart transplantation from donation after circulatory-determined death donors. J Heart Lung Transplant. 2020;39(12):1463–75.
15. Joshi Y, Scheuer S, Chew H, et al. Heart transplantation from DCD donors in Australia: lessons learned from the first 74 cases. Transplantation. 2023;107(2):361–71.

16. Kittleson M. Who is the candidate? The heart transplant evaluation process. Methodist Debakey Cardiovasc J. 2025;21(3):13–24.
17. Van Raemdonck D, Keshavjee S, Levvey B, et al. Donation after circulatory death in lung transplantation. J Thorac Dis. 2015;7(8):1471–6.
18. Tudorache I, Sommer W, Kuhn C, et al. Lung transplantation for severe pulmonary hypertension – awake extracorporeal membrane oxygenation for postoperative left ventricular remodeling. Transplantation. 2015;99(2):451–8.
19. Ahmed H, Kulshrestha K, Kennedy J, et al. Donation after circulatory death significantly reduces waitlist times while not changing post-heart transplant outcomes: a united network for organ sharing analysis. J Heart Lung Transplant. 2023;43(3):461–70.
20. Osaki S, Anderson JE, Johnson MR, et al. Donation after cardiac death in lung transplantation. Ann Thorac Surg. 2010;89(6):1735–41.
21. Berg A, Krishnan A, Heng E, et al. Persistent primary graft dysfunction with lower mortality among recipients of donation-after-circulatory-death hearts. J Heart Lung Transplant. 2026. https://doi.org/10.1016/j.healun.2026.07.007.
22. Sabashnikov A, Patil N, Popof A-F, et al. Long-term results after kung transplantation using organs from circulatory death donors: a propensity score-matched analysis. Eur J Cardio Thoracic Surg. 2016;49:46–53.
23. Levvey BJ, Harkess M, Hopkins P, et al. Excellent clinical outcomes from a national donation-after-determination-of-cardiac-death lung transplant collaborative. Am J Transplant. 2012;12:2406–13.
24. Parrilla G, Hunt W, Daneshmand M. Lung transplantation following donation after circulatory death. Transplant Rep. 2022. https://doi.org/10.1016/j.tpr.2022.100110.
25. Minasyan A, de la Torre M, Rodriguez J, et al. Outcomes of controlled DCDD lung transplantation after thoraco-abdominal vs abdominal normothermic regional perfusion: the Spanish experience. J Heart Lung Transplant. 2025;44(5):696–705.
26. Williams L, Hogg R, Roque M, et al. The United Kingdom's experience of controlled donation after circulatory death direct procurement of lungs with concomitant abdominal normothermic regional perfusion with an analysis of short-term outcomes. J Heart Lung Transplant. 2025;44(8):1307–18.
27. Seth A, Mohanka R, Navin S, et al. Organ donation after circulatory determination of death in India: a joint position paper. Indian J Crit Care Med. 2022;26(4):421–38.
28. Seth AK, Mohanka RM, Mani RK, Asthana S, Attawar S, Dhital KK, et al. Consensus statement of the National Consortium on normothermic regional perfusion for organ donation after circulatory determination of death in India. Indian J Transplant. 2026;20(1):23–35.

15 Donation After Circulatory Death vs Donation After Brain Death: Global Perspectives and Relevance to Emerging Health Systems

Abhinav Seth

Introduction

Organ transplantation remains the gold standard treatment for patients with end-stage organ failure, offering the greatest potential for prolonged survival, improved quality of life, and reduced long-term healthcare costs compared with alternative therapies. Advances in surgical techniques, immunosuppressive therapy, organ preservation, and perioperative care have significantly improved transplant outcomes over the past several decades, making transplantation the preferred treatment for carefully selected patients with end-stage kidney, liver, heart, lung, and pancreas disease.

Despite these remarkable advances, the global shortage of donor organs continues to represent one of the greatest challenges in modern healthcare. The demand for life-saving organ transplants far exceeds the available supply, resulting in prolonged waiting times, increased wait-list mortality, and substantial healthcare disparities. Current estimates suggest that less than 10% of the worldwide need for organ transplantation is currently met, leaving millions of patients without access to definitive treatment.

Marked geographic disparities continue to characterize access to kidney transplantation worldwide. Access to transplantation also varies dramatically across different regions of the world. While high-income countries have established robust organ donation and transplantation programs, many low- and middle-income countries continue to face significant barriers, including limited healthcare infrastructure, inadequate organ procurement systems, shortages of trained transplant professionals, financial constraints, and insufficient public awareness regarding organ donation. Consequently, transplantation rates differ by more than tenfold between countries. While countries such as the United States and Spain perform

A. Seth (✉)
J. W. Ruby Memorial Hospital, West Virginia University, Morgantown, WV, USA

S. P. Kolte et al. (eds.), *Organ Donation After Circulatory Death*,
https://doi.org/10.1007/978-981-92-6377-6_15

more than 130 kidney transplants per million population (pmp) annually, transplantation rates remain as low as 12 pmp in India, highlighting profound inequities in access to this life-saving therapy [1]. The disparity is even more pronounced in many low- and middle-income countries, particularly across large parts of Africa, where transplant activity is either extremely limited or entirely absent because of inadequate infrastructure, shortages of trained personnel, limited organ donation systems, financial constraints, and lack of supportive healthcare policies [2]. Furthermore, reliable national transplant data are unavailable for many countries, making it difficult to accurately assess the global burden of end-stage kidney disease, benchmark performance, and develop targeted strategies to improve access. These striking variations underscore the urgent need for international collaboration to strengthen organ donation programs, establish sustainable transplant infrastructure, improve data reporting systems, and expand equitable access to kidney transplantation worldwide.

The persistent imbalance between the demand for and availability of donor organs remains one of the greatest challenges in modern transplantation. This shortage contributes to prolonged waiting times, increased wait-list mortality, and significant deterioration in quality of life for patients with end-stage organ failure. In many parts of the world, the scarcity of transplantable organs has also fueled the growth of illegal organ trafficking, where vulnerable individuals are exploited by criminal networks for financial gain [3]. Beyond its medical consequences, this crisis raises profound ethical, legal, and public health concerns.

The burden of end-stage organ failure continues to rise as the global prevalence of chronic diseases increases. Diabetes mellitus, hypertension, obesity, metabolic dysfunction-associated liver disease, chronic viral hepatitis, and an aging population have all contributed to a growing incidence of kidney, liver, and pancreas failure, resulting in an ever-expanding transplant waiting list. Despite this increasing need, it is estimated that only a small fraction of the global demand for organ transplantation is met each year.

A substantial proportion of potential deceased donors remain unrealized. Estimates suggest that approximately 85%–90% of potential organ donors are ultimately not utilized because of a combination of medical, logistical, societal, and regulatory barriers [4]. These include strict donor eligibility criteria, delayed or missed donor identification, limited critical care and organ procurement infrastructure, inadequate coordination among healthcare systems, and cultural, religious, and social factors that influence consent for organ donation Fig. 15.1. Together, these challenges significantly limit the availability of transplantable organs.

To address this critical shortage, numerous strategies have been developed to safely expand the donor pool. These include increasing living donor transplantation, strengthening national deceased donor programs, implementing split-organ transplantation, expanding paired kidney exchange programs, adopting broader regional and national organ-sharing policies, and increasing the utilization of expanded-criteria and marginal donors. Additional innovations, such as donation after circulatory death (DCD), machine perfusion technologies, improved donor management protocols, and more sophisticated organ preservation techniques, have further

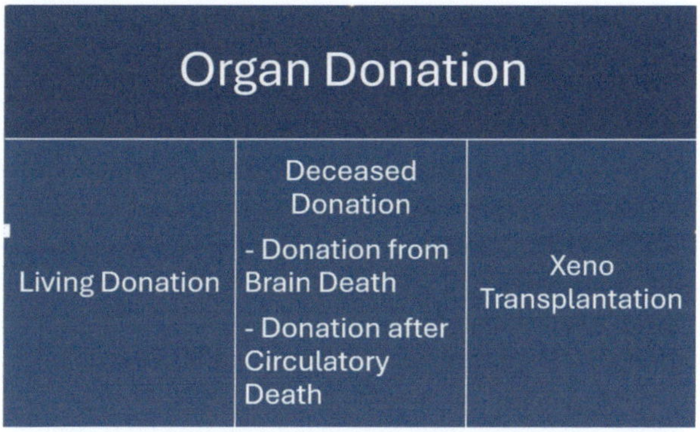

Fig. 15.1 Primary source of organs

enhanced the ability to recover and successfully transplant organs that were previously considered unsuitable [5]. Collectively, these efforts have increased organ utilization and transplantation rates, although the widening gap between organ supply and demand continues to necessitate ongoing innovation and international collaboration.

Organ Donation

Organ donation is the process by which healthy organs or tissues are surgically recovered from a consenting donor and transplanted into a recipient with irreversible end-stage organ failure or severe tissue damage. Organs may be donated by living individuals or recovered from deceased donors following the determination of death according to established medical and legal criteria. Living donation most commonly involves the kidney and a portion of the liver, whereas deceased donation provides the majority of transplantable organs, including the heart, lungs, liver, kidneys, pancreas, and intestine, as well as a wide range of tissues such as corneas, skin, bone, heart valves, tendons, and blood vessels. Every deceased donor can save 8 lives.

Deceased donation occurs after determination of death. Prior to the donation process, the donor is cared for in an ICU or donor care unit (DCU) by the hospital physicians separate from the procurement/transplantation team [5, 6]. It can be Irreversible cessation of the entire brain, including the brainstem (donation after brain death [DBD]) or Irreversible cessation of circulatory and respiratory function (donation after circulatory death [DCD]). Patients who meet the criteria for circulatory death are the one with severe brain injuries in whom brain death criteria are not met and who undergo withdrawal of care (either via advance directive or decision of family members). Informed consent is a must. Life support is withdrawn in the OR/ICU/perioperative area, and the donor is pronounced dead with circulatory cessation. At this point, the procurement team may proceed with organ procurement (usually liver and kidneys) from the deceased donor. The procurement/transplantation team should not be involved in decisions related to the donor's prognosis, withdrawal of care, or the declaration of death.

Expanding *donation after circulatory death (DCD)* programs in emerging healthcare systems represents one of the most promising strategies for increasing the availability of transplantable organs. Successful implementation requires the establishment of robust ethical and legal frameworks that clearly define the determination of death, ensure a strict separation between end-of-life care and organ donation decisions, and safeguard transparency throughout the donation process. A notable example is the United States, where donation after circulatory death (DCD) has become a major contributor to the deceased donor organ supply.

In the United States, the majority of solid organ transplants are performed using organs recovered from *deceased donors (DD)*. Between 2018 and 2025, deceased donors accounted for approximately *75% of kidney transplants, 94% of liver transplants*, and virtually *all heart, lung, and pancreas transplants*. Consequently, improving access to transplantation depends largely on expanding the deceased donor pool. One of the most effective strategies has been the increased utilization of *donation after circulatory death (DCD)*, in which organs are recovered following the irreversible cessation of circulatory and respiratory function after death has been declared. The expansion of DCD has significantly increased organ availability, reduced waiting-list mortality, and become a critical component of modern organ donation systems, demonstrating how innovation in donor utilization can substantially improve access to life-saving transplantation [7].

In United States, DCD accounted for only 2% of all deceased organ donors in 2000, but by 2025 this proportion had risen to 49%. Similarly, donation after DCD have tripled in United Kingdom in last decade. This remarkable expansion reflects advances in ethical and clinical protocols, improved organ preservation strategies, broader acceptance of DCD practices, and the adoption of technologies such as normothermic perfusion and machine perfusion [8, 9]. The growth of DCD has substantially increased the availability of transplantable organs, particularly kidneys, livers, and lungs, thereby helping to reduce waiting-list mortality and improve access to life-saving transplantation [9]. This demonstrates that, with appropriate ethical safeguards, infrastructure investment, and public trust, DCD can evolve from a limited donation pathway into a central component of a national organ donation strategy [10].

Despite its growing adoption, several challenges continue to limit the widespread utilization of *donation after circulatory death (DCD)*. Compared with organs recovered after *donation after brain death (DBD)*, DCD organs are exposed to a period of unavoidable warm ischemia following the withdrawal of life-sustaining therapy, increasing the risk of ischemia–reperfusion injury, delayed graft function, ischemic cholangiopathy, and, in some cases, inferior early graft performance. Consequently, careful donor selection, optimized preservation techniques, and meticulous recipient management are essential to achieve outcomes comparable to those of DBD transplantation.

In addition, DCD organ procurement is inherently more complex and time-sensitive than DBD recovery. Successful organ retrieval depends on a predictable progression from withdrawal of life-sustaining treatment to irreversible circulatory arrest within a predefined time window. If the interval between withdrawal of life support and circulatory death is prolonged, excessive warm ischemic injury may render the organs unsuitable for transplantation, resulting in unsuccessful procurement attempts [11]. These logistical, ethical, and technical challenges necessitate highly coordinated multidisciplinary teams, standardized clinical protocols, and advanced organ preservation strategies, including normothermic regional perfusion and ex situ machine perfusion, to maximize organ utilization and optimize transplant outcomes.

Kidney Transplant Outcomes in DBD vs DCD Donors Kidney transplantation is the best treatment for end-stage renal disease. Five-year patient survival is 86.3% post kidney transplant as compared to 42.9% for patients remaining on dialysis. A persistent disparity exists between the number of patients awaiting renal transplantation and the availability of suitable donor organs, resulting in prolonged waiting times and increased wait-list mortality. The donor pool can be increased by using DCD kidneys. Although donation after circulatory death (DCD) has the potential to increase organ availability, its adoption remains limited in many countries because of perceived concerns regarding graft quality, legislative and regulatory constraints, and ethical issues surrounding the donation process. A systematic review and meta-analysis by Rijksen et al. demonstrated that donation after circulatory death (DCD) kidney transplantation can safely expand the donor pool. The analysis included 51 studies encompassing 73,454 DCD and 518,229 donation after brain death (DBD) kidney transplant recipients. Although DCD transplantation was associated with higher rates of primary non-function (PNF), delayed graft function (DGF), and a 13% increased risk of graft loss during the first post-transplant year, long-term graft and patient outcomes were comparable to those achieved with DBD kidneys [9]. These findings support the broader implementation of DCD kidney transplantation programs as a safe and effective strategy to increase organ availability while maintaining acceptable long-term outcomes. Similar findings have been reported in the pediatric population (<18 years of age). Kizilbash et al. compared outcomes of 285 donation after circulatory death (DCD) and 1132 donation after brain death (DBD) pediatric kidney transplant recipients who underwent transplantation between 1987 and 2017. Although DCD recipients experienced a higher incidence of delayed graft function (DGF), long-term patient and graft survival were comparable between the two groups [10]. Importantly, despite pediatric candidates receiving priority in organ allocation, DCD kidney transplantation was associated with a significant survival advantage compared with remaining on the transplant waiting list. These findings further support the use of DCD kidneys to expand the pediatric donor pool without compromising long-term transplant outcomes.

Liver Transplants Outcomes in DBD vs DCD Donors The global burden of liver failure has increased substantially over the past decade, with more than one million people worldwide dying from cirrhosis each year [12]. Although liver transplantation remains the definitive treatment for end-stage liver disease, access to this life-saving therapy continues to be severely constrained by the persistent shortage of donor organs [13]. To help address this gap, the utilization of donation after circulatory death (DCD) liver grafts has expanded steadily over the past decade, contributing to increased transplant activity and improved access to transplantation for patients with end-stage liver disease [14]. Although published studies have reported higher rates of primary non-function (PNF), ischemic cholangiopathy, and early graft dysfunction following donation after circulatory death (DCD) liver transplantation compared with donation after brain death (DBD) transplantation [15]. These inferior outcomes were largely attributable to prolonged warm ischemia times, suboptimal organ preservation techniques, and the relatively early stage of surgical expertise and perioperative management during the initial adoption of donation after circulatory death (DCD) liver transplantation. Recent advances in donor selection, organ preservation, and recipient management have led to significant improvements in outcomes. Importantly, despite these increased risks, transplantation with DCD liver allografts provides a significant survival benefit for patients from the time of waitlisting compared with remaining on the transplant waiting list as shown by the study done by Tayloe et al. who published data from DCD donors (Maastricht category 3) [16] Fig. 15.2. They also showed that survival advantage was greatest for patients with more advanced liver disease. Alconchel et al. reported that the introduction of controlled donation after circulatory death (DCD) liver transplantation at a single transplant center in Spain was associated with a 19% reduction in wait-list mortality over a five-year period [17]. In a systematic review and meta-analysis of seven studies and 898 patients published by Manzi et al. showed no difference between the 1-year survival rate and the 1-year graft survival rate between high-utilization and low-utilization centers, reinforcing the rationale that the disadvantages of using the previously called marginal or compromised organs are overcome by the center's experience regarding organ selection and surgical procedures [18]. This underscores the value of expanding the use of DCD organs to address the persistent shortage of donor livers.

Lung Transplant Outcomes in DBD vs DCD Donors Currently, the majority of lung allografts are procured from donors after neurologic determination of death

Maastricht Classification	
Category I (Uncontrolled)	Patients who are brought to the hospital already dead
Category II (Uncontrolled)	Patients who suffer an unexpected cardiac arrest with unsuccessful resuscitation efforts
Category III (Controlled)	Patients with severe, irreversible injuries on life support where treatment is planned to be withdrawn in an ICU or Emergency Department setting
Category IV (Uncontrolled)	Patients who experience a sudden cardiac arrest after being declared brain dead
Category V (Controlled/Uncontrolled)	Patients who experience unexpected cardiac arrest as inpatients (sometimes used specifically to classify organ donation after euthanasia in certain jurisdictions)

Fig. 15.2 Maastricht classification for DCD donors

(donation after brain death [DBD]). However, only approximately 20% of DBD donors yield lungs that meet suitability criteria for transplantation, reflecting the unique susceptibility of the lungs to injury and the stringent selection standards required for successful transplantation [19]. To address the persistent shortage of transplantable lungs, increasing attention has been directed toward the use of donors after circulatory determination of death (DCD). The first successful DCD lung transplant was performed by Robert Love in 1995 [20]. In a multicenter analysis of lung transplantation outcomes comparing donation after circulatory death and donation after brain death performed at 11 lung transplant centers in the United States and Europe by Kashem et al. showed excellent 90-day survival for DCD and DBD recipients, although DCD recipients had relatively lower survival. In their study of 1585 patients, 135 received DCD lungs concluded ex vivo lung perfusion (EVLP) did not affect survival [21]. In a study comparing medium-term outcomes after lung transplantation using 1069 donation after circulatory death (DCD) donors and 17,590 donation after brain death (DBD) donors, Li et al. found that recipients of DCD lungs experienced higher overall mortality and a greater incidence of perioperative complications. However, after excluding lungs that underwent ex vivo lung perfusion (EVLP), overall survival was comparable between the DCD and DBD groups, although the increased risk of early postoperative complications in the DCD cohort persisted [22]. These findings suggest that while DCD lung transplantation can achieve survival outcomes similar to DBD transplantation under selected conditions, further studies are needed to better understand the factors contributing to the higher rate of early complications and to optimize donor selection and perioperative management. The active use of DCD donors is expected to significantly reduce mortality on the waiting list for lung transplantation as shown by Hyun et al. [23].

Heart Transplant Outcomes in DBD vs DCD Donors Heart transplantation using donation after circulatory death (DCD) donors has become increasingly adopted, significantly expanding the donor pool and helping to reduce waiting times for patients requiring heart transplantation [24]. Studies from Europe and Australia suggest noninferior outcomes among recipients of DCD compared with DBD hearts [25, 26]. In a randomized controlled trial published by Schroder et al. showed DCD hearts recovered with the use of ex vivo machine perfusion (EVP) had no significant difference in survival to 6 months compared with recipients of DBD hearts recovered with the use of static cold storage [27]. In one of the largest single center comparison of DCD and DBD heart transplant by Siddiqi et al. comprising 385 heart transplants out of which 122 were DCD transplants (83% of which were recovered with use of NRP) found no significant difference in 1-year recipient survival or in rates of severe primary graft dysfunction (PGD), treated rejection, or cardiac allograft vasculopathy at 1 year after transplantation [28]. There is substantial heterogeneity in the reported incidence of severe primary graft dysfunction (PGD), as defined by the International Society for Heart and Lung Transplantation (ISHLT), with rates ranging from 5.7% to 41% across published studies. Although the incidence of PGD appears relatively high, its long-term clinical significance remains uncertain, as it has not been consistently associated with increased mortality.

Pancreas Transplant Outcomes in DBD vs DCD Donors The number of pancreas transplants performed in both Europe and the United States has steadily declined over the past decade [29]. Utilization of pancreas donation after circulatory death (DCD) remains limited, primarily because of concerns regarding the increased risk of ischemia-related complications, including graft pancreatitis and vascular thrombosis [30]. Consequently, many transplant centers remain cautious about the routine use of DCD pancreas allografts [31, 32]. However, emerging evidence supports the feasibility of DCD pancreas transplantation. In a study by Lim et al., recipients of DCD pancreas transplants had a higher risk of acute graft rejection within the first year after transplantation compared with recipients of donation after brain death (DBD) grafts, but patient survival and overall graft survival were comparable between the two groups [33].

Machine Perfusion for DCD Donors

Equally important is investment in modern organ preservation technologies, particularly *normothermic regional perfusion (NRP)* and *ex vivo machine perfusion*, which improve organ viability, expand donor eligibility, and enhance post-transplant outcomes. Normothermic regional perfusion (NRP) is an in-situ preservation technique in which a closed extracorporeal circuit, similar to an extracorporeal membrane oxygenation (ECMO) system, delivers oxygenated blood to the donor organs before procurement. In contrast, ex vivo machine perfusion is performed outside the donor body and can be conducted under either normothermic or hypothermic conditions. Normothermic machine perfusion maintains the organ at physiological temperature (approximately 37 °C), allowing functional assessment, optimization, and potential therapeutic interventions prior to transplantation, whereas hypothermic machine perfusion reduces metabolic activity by lowering organ temperature. These technologies enable prolonged preservation times, facilitate organ viability assessment, and may expand the utilization of marginal and donation after circulatory death (DCD) organs. This effectively minimizes warm ischemic damage and reconditions the organ. Machine perfusion preserves organ viability by continuously circulating oxygenated blood or specialized preservation solutions through the graft, thereby maintaining cellular metabolism and limiting ischemic injury. This technology has been associated with reduced organ discard rates, improved utilization of donation after circulatory death (DCD) organs, and enhanced post-transplant graft survival. In a retrospective analysis of prospectively collected data on 233 DCD liver transplants performed using in situ normothermic regional perfusion (NRP) or ex situ normothermic machine perfusion (NMP) with livers undergoing static cold storage (SCS) by Gaurav et al. showed NRP and NMP were associated with better early liver function compared to SCS, whereas NRP was associated with superior preservation of the biliary system [34]. A retrospective study by Wisel et al. using data from the Organ Procurement and Transplantation Network/Standard Transplant Analysis and Research (OPTN/STAR) database, including liver transplants performed between 2015 and 2023, demonstrated that the use of machine perfusion in liver transplantation was associated with increased liver utilization rates and improved graft survival among recipients of donation after circulatory death (DCD) liver allografts [35].

Conclusion

The World Health Organization has been tasked with developing a comprehensive global strategy to strengthen organ donation and transplantation systems while promoting equitable access, ethical practices, and international collaboration. Despite remarkable advances in transplantation science and surgical techniques, expanding the donor pool remains one of the greatest challenges in modern medicine. Unlike many other healthcare interventions, organ transplantation depends on the extraordinary generosity and altruism of individuals and families who choose to donate organs, often during times of profound personal loss.

Increasing organ donation is particularly challenging because decisions regarding donation are influenced by a complex interplay of cultural traditions, religious beliefs, ethical values, legal frameworks, socioeconomic factors, and personal preferences. In many societies, misconceptions regarding brain death, concerns about bodily integrity, mistrust of healthcare systems, inadequate public awareness, and limited family discussions surrounding organ donation continue to hinder donor registration and authorization. These barriers are further compounded by disparities in healthcare infrastructure, insufficient donor identification and referral systems, and variability in national policies governing organ procurement and transplantation.

Developing the necessary infrastructure, training multidisciplinary healthcare teams, and creating standardized clinical protocols are essential for sustainable program growth. In parallel, public education campaigns that highlight successful transplant stories, emphasize the safety and ethical integrity of DCD, and address cultural and religious concerns can strengthen public confidence and increase donor registration. Together, these measures can enable emerging healthcare systems to establish effective DCD programs, substantially expand the donor pool, and improve access to life-saving organ transplantation.

Lastly, addressing the global shortage of transplantable organs therefore requires far more than medical or surgical innovation. It demands coordinated international efforts to strengthen public education, foster trust in healthcare systems, engage religious and community leaders, establish transparent and ethical governance, optimize deceased donor identification and organ recovery processes, and improve national transplantation infrastructure. A comprehensive global strategy should promote culturally sensitive approaches that respect individual autonomy while encouraging informed decision-making, thereby creating sustainable and equitable systems capable of meeting the growing worldwide demand for life-saving organ transplantation.

Competing Interests The author(s) has no competing interests to declare that are relevant to the content of this manuscript.

Ethics Approval The author(s) declares that this manuscript does not include primary research with human participants.

The author(s) declares that this manuscript does not include primary studies involving animals.

References

1. The Lancet. Organ donation: lessons from the Spanish model. Lancet. 2024;404(10459):1171.
2. Saidi RF, Hejazii Kenari SK. Challenges of organ shortage for transplantation: solutions and opportunities. Int J Organ Transplant Med. 2014;5(3):87–96.
3. Streit S, Johnston-Webber C, Mah J, Prionas A, Wharton G, Casanova D, Mossialos E, Papalois V. Ten lessons from the Spanish model of organ donation and transplantation. Transpl Int. 2023;36:11009.
4. Organ Procurement And Transplantation Network. National data. Health Resources and Services Administration. https://hrsa.unos.org/data/view-data-reports/national-data. Accessed 15 Jan 2026.
5. Smith M, Dominguez-Gil B, Greer DM, Manara AR, Souter MJ. Organ donation after circulatory death: current status and future potential. Intensive Care Med. 2019;45(3):310–21.
6. Husain SA, Motter JD, Stewart D, Levan ML, Bae S, Parent B, Lonze BE, Sommer PM, Gentry SE, Stern JM, Massie AB, Segev DL, Orandi BJ. Changes in organ donation after circulatory death in the United States. JAMA. 2026;335(12):1087–9.
7. Annual Data Report: Epidemiology of kidney disease in the United States, National Institutes of Health, National Institute of Diabetes and Digestive and Kidney Diseases, Bethesda, MD; 2019.
8. Haase B, Bos M, Boffa C, Lewis P, Rudge C, Valero R, et al. Ethical, legal, and societal issues and recommendations for controlled and uncontrolled DCD. Transpl Dermatol Int. 2016;29(7):771–9.
9. Rijkse E, Ceuppens S, Qi H, IJzermans JNM, Hesselink DA, Minnee RC. Implementation of donation after circulatory death kidney transplantation can safely enlarge the donor pool: a systematic review and meta-analysis. Int J Surg. 2021;92:106021.
10. Kizilbash SJ, Evans MD, Chavers BM. Survival benefit of donation after circulatory death kidney transplantation in children compared with remaining on the waiting list for a kidney donated after brain death. Transplantation. 2022;106(3):575–83.
11. Park H, Jung ES, Oh JS, Lee YM, Lee JM. Organ donation after controlled circulatory death (Maastricht classification III) following the withdrawal of life-sustaining treatment in Korea: a suggested guideline. Korean J Transplant. 2021;35(2):71–6.
12. Leon DA, McCambridge J. Liver cirrhosis mortality rates in Britain from 1950 to 2002: an analysis of routine data. Lancet. 2006;367:52–6.
13. Byass P. The global burden of liver disease: a challenge for methods and for public health. BMC Med. 2014;12:159.
14. Laing RW, Scalera I, Isaac J, Mergental H, Mirza DF, Hodson J, et al. Liver transplantation using grafts from donors after circulatory death: a propensity score-matched study from a single center. Am J Transplant. 2016;16:1795–804.
15. Skaro AI, Jay CL, Baker TB, Wang E, Pasricha S, Lyuksemburg V, et al. The impact of ischemic cholangiopathy in liver transplantation using donors after cardiac death: the untold story. Surgery. 2009;146:543–53.
16. Taylor R, Allen E, Richards JA, Goh MA, Neuberger J, Collett D, Pettigrew GJ, Liver Advisory Group to NHS Blood and Transplant. Survival advantage for patients accepting the offer of

a circulatory death liver transplant. J Hepatol. 2019;70(5):855–65. https://doi.org/10.1016/j.jhep.2018.12.033. Epub 2019 Jan 11.
17. Alconchel F, Cascales-Campos PA, Royo-Villanova M, Martínez-Alarcón L, Febrero B, Martínez-Insfran LA, et al. Abstracts s223 impact of controlled donation after circulatory death (cdcd) on waiting list mortality for liver transplantation in the last 10 years: the spanish experience Surgery and Organ Transplantation, Clinical University Hospital Virgen de la A. Transplantation. 2020;104(S3):S223.
18. Manzi JLL, Oliveira ES, Rombach S, Turra V, Zaragoza S, Bababekov Y, Nydam T, Tector AJ, Vianna R, Abreu P. Comparisons of liver transplant from DCD outcomes in high-utilization centers versus low-utilization centers in the US: a systematic review and meta-analysis. Front Immunol. 2025;16:1564551. https://doi.org/10.3389/fimmu.2025.1564551. PMID: 40416988; PMCID: PMC12098045.
19. Moreno P, González-García J, Ruíz-López E, Alvarez A. Lung transplantation in controlled donation after circulatory-determination-of-death using normothermic abdominal perfusion. Transpl Int. 2024;37:12659.
20. Egan TM, Haithcock BE, Lobo J, Mody G, Love RB, Requard JJ 3rd, et al. Donation after circulatory death donors in lung transplantation. J Thorac Dis. 2021;13(11):6536–49. https://doi.org/10.21037/jtd-2021-13.
21. Abul Kashem M, Loor G, Hartwig M, Van Raemdonck D, Villavicencio M, Ius F, Ghadimi K, Salman J, Chandrashekaran S, Machuca T, Sanchez PG, Subramaniam K, Neyrinck A, Calvelli H, Warnick M, Zhao H, Huddleston S, Osho A, D'Silva E, Ramamurthy U, Pena AL, Salan-Gomez M, Shaffer A, Langer N, Emtiazjoo A, Toyoda Y. A multicenter analysis of lung transplantation outcomes comparing donation after circulatory death and donation after brain death. JHLT Open. 2024;6:100132. https://doi.org/10.1016/j.jhlto.2024.100132. Erratum in: JHLT Open 2025 Nov 05;10:100431. https://doi.org/10.1016/j.jhlto.2025.100431. PMID: 40145031; PMCID: PMC11935477.
22. Li S, Funamoto M, Rabi S, Langer N, Singh R, Michel E, Kreso A, Osho A. Donation after circulatory death (DCD) lung transplant outcomes in the United States. J Heart Lung Transplant. 2024;43:S181.
23. Hyun S, Haam S. Donation after circulatory death in lung transplantation. J Chest Surg. 2022;55(4):283–7.
24. Jawitz OK, Raman V, DeVore AD, et al. Increasing the United States heart transplant donor pool with donation after circulatory death. J Thorac Cardiovasc Surg. 2020;159(5):e307–9.
25. Dhital K, Ludhani P, Scheuer S, Connellan M, Macdonald P. DCD donations and outcomes of heart transplantation: the Australian experience. Indian J Thorac Cardiovasc Surg. 2020;36(Suppl 2):224–32.
26. Messer S, Rushton S, Simmonds L, et al. A national pilot of donation after circulatory death (DCD) heart transplantation within the United Kingdom. J Heart Lung Transplant. 2023;42(8):1120–30.
27. Schroder JN, Patel CB, DeVore AD, et al. Transplantation outcomes with donor hearts after circulatory death. N Engl J Med. 2023;388(23):2121–31.
28. Siddiqi HK, Trahanas J, Xu M, Wells Q, Farber-Eger E, Pasrija C, Amancherla K, Debose-Scarlett A, Brinkley DM, Lindenfeld J, Menachem JN, Ooi H, Pedrotty D, Punnoose L, Rali AS, Sacks S, Wigger M, Zalawadiya S, McMaster W, Devries S, Shah A, Schlendorf K. Outcomes of heart transplant donation after circulatory death. J Am Coll Cardiol. 2023;82(15):1512–20. https://doi.org/10.1016/j.jacc.2023.08.006. PMID: 37793748
29. Stratta RJ, Gruessner AC, Odorico JS, Fridell JA, Gruessner RW. pancreas transplantation: an alarming crisis in confidence. Am J Transplant. 2016;16:2556–62.
30. Cornateanu SM, O'Neill S, Dholakia S, et al. Pancreas utilization rates in the UK - an 11-year analysis Transpl. Dermatol Int. 2021;34:1306–18.
31. Mittal S, Gilbert J, Friend PJ. Donors after circulatory death pancreas transplantation. Curr Opin Organ Transplant. 2017;22:372–6.

32. Berney T, Boffa C, Augustine T, et al. Utilization of organs from donors after circulatory death for vascularized pancreas and islet of Langerhans transplantation: recommendations from an expert group Transpl. Dermatol Int. 2016;29:798–806.
33. Lim T, Adjei M, Crichton E, et al. Comparable outcomes of pancreas transplants from donation after circulatory death compared to brain death donors. Am J Transplant. 2025;25:S198.
34. Gaurav R, Butler AJ, Kosmoliaptsis V, Mumford L, Fear C, Swift L, Fedotovs A, Upponi S, Khwaja S, Richards J, Allison M, Watson CJE. Liver transplantation outcomes from controlled circulatory death donors: SCS vs in situ NRP vs ex situ NMP. Ann Surg. 2022;275(6):1156–64.
35. Wisel SA, Steggerda JA, Kim IK. Use of machine perfusion in the United States increases organ utilization and improves DCD graft survival in liver transplantation. Transplant Direct. 2024;10(12):e1726.

Part VI

Special Populations in DCD Transplantation

Donation After Circulatory Death in Paediatric Patients

16

Abbas Ghazanfar and Arpita Ray Chaudhury

Introduction

Worldwide, Donation after Circulatory Death (DCD) has emerged as a key strategy to expand the organ donor pool. As of 2026, DCD transplantation is rapidly expanding into the primary source of deceased organ donation and transplantation. In the United States, DCD donors now account for nearly 49% of the deceased-donor pool, a massive leap from just 2% at the turn of the century. In the United Kingdom, DCD donation has undergone a historic shift. As of the 2024/25 financial year, DCD donors surpassed Donation after Brain Death (DBD) donors for the first time in UK history [10]. This transition marks a fundamental change in the NHS transplant strategy, moving away from reliance solely on brainstem death cases towards a more proactive, technologically assisted DCD model.

Paediatric deceased donors comprise a small fraction of the global donor pool. They typically represent 3–6% of all deceased organ donors across Western Europe, the UK, and Australia and around 6–8% in the United States and China. This distribution is tracked and compiled through registries like the Global Observatory of Donation and Transplantation (GODT) (https://www.transplant-observatory.org/).

Paediatric recipients comprise a minor fraction of global transplant lists, typically accounting for only 1.5–3.5% of all waitlisted patients internationally. The data compiled by the Organ Procurement and Transplantation Network (OPTN) and the Scientific Registry of Transplant Recipients (SRTR) indicate that children represent roughly 1.5–2% of the United States national waiting list. Similarly, the NHS

A. Ghazanfar (✉)
Department of Renal Medicine and Transplant Surgery, St George's University Hospitals NHS Foundation Trust, London, UK
e-mail: a.ghazanfar@nhs.net

A. R. Chaudhury
Department of Nephrology, North Bengal Medical College, Darjeeling, West Bengal, India

S. P. Kolte et al. (eds.), *Organ Donation After Circulatory Death*,
https://doi.org/10.1007/978-981-92-6377-6_16

Blood and Transplant Annual Activity Report highlights that paediatric patients make up about 3.4% of the active UK waiting list (276 out of 8096 patients), with figures from Kidney Research UK confirming that children account for approximately 1.9% of the kidney pool alone. Across Eurotransplant nations and European registries analysed in Deutsches Ärzteblatt International, child candidates consistently fall around the 2% threshold.

Paediatric Donation after Circulatory Death (pDCD) is both a clinical necessity and a deeply sensitive area of practice. Because the death of a child is rare compared to adults, the paediatric donor pool is small, making every successful pDCD process critical for the hundreds of children currently on transplant waiting lists.

Recent data from 2025 and 2026 show that while pDCD was historically underutilised [3], it is now expanding rapidly due to new ethical guidelines and specialised recovery technologies.

Donor Identification, Assessment and Selection in Paediatric Donation After Circulatory Death (pDCD)

The assessment of a potential pDCD donor involves a multidisciplinary evaluation of the likelihood of death within a timeframe that allows for organ viability.

Clinical Triggers: In the paediatric context, most DCD cases are Controlled DCD (Maastricht Category III), where death follows the planned withdrawal of life-sustaining treatment (WLST). Potential donors are typically children in a Paediatric Intensive Care Unit (PICU) or Neonatal Intensive Care Unit (NICU) with

- *Irreversible neurological injury* that does not meet the strict criteria for neurological death.
- *End-stage respiratory or cardiac failure* where the burden of treatment outweighs the benefit.
- *Planned withdrawal of life-sustaining treatment (WLST)*, including mechanical ventilation or vasoactive support.

General Eligibility: While specific criteria vary by jurisdiction, general guidelines include

- *Age*: Neonates to 18 years. For neonates, a corrected gestational age >37 weeks and a weight >2.5 kg are standard benchmarks for solid organ donation.
- *Absence of Contraindications*: Absolute contraindications include active systemic malignancy (with rare exceptions for primary CNS tumours) and untreated systemic sepsis (SaBTO guidelines for cancer and microbiology).

Pre-Withdrawal Organ Assessment: Before proceeding, the transplant team performs a comprehensive review:

Table 16.1 Organ selection criteria for pDCD

Organ	Selection criteria and considerations
Kidneys	Most resilient to ischemia. In donors <10–15 kg, kidneys are usually transplanted 'en-bloc' to prevent vascular thrombosis and ensure adequate graft function
Liver	Highly sensitive. Ideal pDCD livers come from donors with a functional WIT ≤30 min. Use of Normothermic Regional Perfusion (NRP) is an emerging technique to "recondition" these grafts
Lungs	Assessed for secretions and oxygenation. pDCD lungs are often evaluated post-recovery via Ex Vivo Lung Perfusion (EVLP) to confirm gas exchange capability
Heart	Selection is highly restrictive and limited to specialised centres. Criteria include age ≤50 (usually much younger in pDCD) and minimal inotropic support prior to WLST

- *Renal*: Serum creatinine, urine output and urinalysis. In small donors, ultrasound is used to assess kidney size for potential en-bloc transplantation.
- *Hepatic*: Liver function tests (AST, ALT, Bilirubin) and coagulation profiles.
- *Cardiac/Pulmonary*: Echocardiography, chest X-rays and arterial blood gas (ABG) analysis.

Medical Suitability and Organ-Specific Selection: The assessment involves a rigorous review of medical history, current physiological status and the reason for the primary injury. In addition, the selection of paediatric organs depends heavily on the donor-to-recipient size match and the cumulative Warm Ischemic Time (WIT) (Table 16.1).

The 'Warm Ischaemic Time' (WIT) Assessment: The viability of pDCD organs is strictly governed by the time elapsed between the drop in physiological parameters and the start of cold preservation.

- *Agonal Phase*: The period from WLST to circulatory arrest is the agonal phase. If this exceeds a specific limit (e.g., 30 min for liver, 60–120 min for kidneys), the organs may be deemed unsuitable.
- *Functional WIT*: Starts when systolic blood pressure drops below 50 mmHg or oxygen saturation drops below 70%. Due to hypoperfusion, organ outcomes are affected.
- *Stand-down Criteria*: If the patient does not progress to death within the agreed timeframe (usually 2 h), the donation process is often 'stood down' to allow the family to continue end-of-life care in a non-surgical environment.

Ethical and Legal Considerations: Decisions surrounding pDCD are among the most sensitive in modern medicine. They require a delicate balance between honouring the family's wishes, ensuring the potential life-saving gift for recipients, and strictly adhering to legal and ethical frameworks. pDCD in the paediatric population is governed by three core principles:

1. *Best Interest of the Patient*: The decision to withdraw treatment must be independent of the decision to donate. Therefore, ownership of the decision remains with the intensivist, not with the organ retrieval or transplant team.
2. *Parental Autonomy*: Parents must be provided with clear, honest information about the possibility that donation may not occur if the agonal phase is prolonged. They also understand that they can withdraw their consent at any time.
3. *Justice in Allocation*: Ensuring that these rare and precious grafts are allocated to the children most in need, often prioritising paediatric recipients for paediatric grafts.

Donor Allocation and Organ Utilisation in Paediatric Donation After Circulatory Death (pDCD)

Organ allocation in pDCD is a rapidly evolving field, driven by the critical need to reduce waitlist mortality, which remains approximately 17% for children awaiting heart transplants in the United States. In the United Kingdom, the 2024/25 NHS Blood and Transplant (NHSBT) data indicate that while pDCD referrals are high (approx. 201 annually), the family consent rate for pDCD remains significantly lower at 23% compared to 57% for Donation after Brain Death (pDBD). Allocation of pDCD organs follows established national protocols (e.g., UNOS in the US and NHSBT in the UK), which prioritise paediatric recipients for paediatric donor organs to ensure size matching and optimal long-term outcomes.

pDCD kidney transplants have historically been associated with delayed graft function (DGF); recent long-term data indicate that patient and graft survival at 10 years are statistically comparable to Donation after Brain Death (DBD) [11]. To further enhance these outcomes, the field is shifting towards the routine use of Hypothermic Oxygenated Machine Perfusion (HOPE) and Normothermic Regional Perfusion (NRP). These technologies allow clinicians to mitigate the 'warm ischemic hit' inherent in DCD, providing a window to assess renal viability and 'recondition' the kidneys before implantation.

To improve organ quality and utilisation, clinicians are increasingly adopting Normothermic Regional Perfusion (NRP). This technique restores oxygenated blood flow in-situ after the declaration of death, allowing the heart and abdominal organs to be functionally assessed under physiological conditions [12, 18].

Recent research highlights a sharp divergence in the adoption of Thoraco-Abdominal NRP (TA-NRP) between the UK and the US. In the United States, TA-NRP is expanding as a viable method for recovering paediatric hearts that would otherwise be discarded due to Warm Ischaemia Time (WIT), with outcomes increasingly matching those of traditional DBD transplants. Conversely, the UK maintains a more cautious stance: while Abdominal NRP (A-NRP) is utilised, a professional moratorium and ongoing ethical debate regarding TA-NRP remain, centred on the 'dead donor rule' and the legal definition of 'irreversible' cessation of circulation [2]. Despite these hurdles, the integration of NRP is seen as the 'next frontier' because it bypasses the weight restrictions of ex-situ machine perfusion devices, which often require donors to be over 30–40 kg, thereby offering hope to the smallest and most vulnerable neonatal and infant recipients [6].

Furthermore, there is a growing trend towards expanding the donor pool by utilising kidneys from very small paediatric DCD donors (infants and neonates), often via en-bloc transplantation. While technically demanding, these grafts offer excellent long-term nephron mass and adaptive growth potential [5]. By integrating real-time biomarker data during perfusion and refining donor-recipient size-matching protocols, the transplant community aims to make DCD kidneys a primary rather than 'alternative' source for paediatric recipients, ultimately reducing the time children spend on dialysis [11].

- *Utilisation Trends*: DCD heart transplantation has seen a significant rise, accounting for 15.2% of all heart transplants in 2023, up from only 3.6% in 2020 [13].
- *Global Expansion*: DCD now accounts for approximately 28% of all deceased-donor activity worldwide as of 2024, reflecting broader acceptance of these grafts.
- *Size Matching*: For paediatric recipients, donor weight and HLA matching (specifically HLA-B and HLA-DR) are critical factors in organ utilisation decisions [8].

Techniques for Transplant in Paediatric Donation After Circulatory Death (pDCD)

The surgical procedures and preservation techniques in DCD are designed to mitigate Ischemia-Reperfusion Injury (IRI). The surgical recovery of paediatric organs through Donation after Circulatory Death (DCD) is a high-stakes race against the clock, demanding a seamless transition from the declaration of death to the initiation of cold preservation. Unlike brain-dead donors, where hemodynamic stability is maintained, the pDCD donor undergoes a period of warm ischemia that can rapidly degrade graft viability. The 'super-rapid' recovery technique is the standard of care, characterised by a swift midline laparotomy and sternotomy followed by immediate cannulation of the distal aorta. In smaller paediatric donors, surgeons may also cannulate the inferior mesenteric vein to ensure a thorough portal flush, which is critical for protecting the biliary tree—a structure particularly vulnerable to ischaemic cholangiopathy in DCD liver grafts.

Precision is as vital as speed; the small calibre of paediatric vessels necessitates meticulous dissection to avoid intimal injury, which would otherwise predispose the graft to post-transplant thrombosis. While traditional rapid recovery focuses on immediate cooling, the emergence of Abdominal Normothermic Regional Perfusion (A-NRP) in paediatric protocols is shifting the paradigm. By utilising a localised extracorporeal circuit to restore oxygenated blood flow post-mortem, A-NRP allows for a period of 'in-situ' resuscitation and functional assessment of the organs. This technique not only mitigates the initial ischaemic insult but also provides the surgical team with a vital window to evaluate the liver's lactate clearance and bile production before committing to transplantation. Ultimately, the success of the pDCD technique hinges on minimising the functional warm ischemic time (fWIT) and employing tailored back-table reconstructions to accommodate the unique anatomical constraints of the small recipient.

- *Procurement*: Once death is declared (following a 'stand-off' period, usually 5 min), rapid cannulation and cold flush are performed.
- *Normothermic Regional Perfusion (NRP)*: This involves establishing an extracorporeal circuit (ECMO) after death to restore oxygenated blood flow to the organs in situ. This enables a functional assessment of the heart and liver prior to procurement [14].
- *Ex-situ Machine Perfusion*: Organs are placed on a device that maintains physiological conditions during transport. For hearts, the Organ Care System (OCS) is used to monitor lactate trends and haemodynamic stability [14].

Recipient Selection and Management in Paediatric Donation After Circulatory Death (pDCD)

Recipient selection from paediatric Donation after Circulatory Death (DCD) donors requires matching protocols that prioritise low-acuity candidates and stringent physiological compatibility to withstand the heightened risks of ischaemic reperfusion injury and delayed graft function (DGF).

- *Liver Recipient Selection*: According to clinical analyses on Paediatric Liver Transplantation, optimal candidates must have stable metabolic function (ideally an International Normalised Ratio *INR <2* and *albumin >3.5 g/dL*) and are strictly non-ICU bound to minimise primary non-function risks. Selection criteria generally exclude re-transplantation candidates to ensure that the strict functional warm ischaemic time (WIT) cap of 30 min is not compromised by intraoperative surgical delays.
- *Kidney Recipient Selection*: Allocation strategies developed by organisations such as NHS Blood and Transplant (NHSBT) place a high priority on geographic proximity and localised matching. This geographic clustering compresses transport times to keep the total cold ischaemia time (CIT) under 12 h, which dramati-

cally improves initial graft function and reduces post-operative dialysis dependence.

- *Heart Recipient Selection*: Clinical guidelines outlined by the NHSBT Heart Donation Assessment dictate that recipient matching is constrained by donor weight thresholds, with standard protocols requiring a donor weight of >50 kg (or >30 kg for very specialised programmes). This restriction is paired with specialised size-mismatch algorithms to protect vulnerable paediatric recipients from right ventricular strain.
- *Lung Recipient Selection*: Standard framework guidelines published by the British Transplantation Society (BTS) dictate that lung candidate selection should mirror standard Donation after Brain Death (DBD) pathways. Selection favours candidates free of extensive prior thoracic surgeries to ensure rapid implantation, often relying on Ex Vivo Lung Perfusion (EVLP) to serve as an objective viability buffer during transit.

Complications and Graft Outcomes in Paediatric Donation After Circulatory Death (pDCD)

While short-term outcomes are favourable, DCD grafts face specific challenges.

Primary Complications

- *Biliary Complications (Liver)*: DCD liver recipients are at higher risk for *Ischemic Cholangiopathy*. Long-term follow-up (>20 years) shows that early management of biliary strictures via percutaneous bilioplasty or surgical revision is vital [17].
- *Delayed Graft Function (Kidney)*: More common in DCD due to warm ischaemia.
- *Acute Rejection*: In paediatric kidney transplants, 1-year rejection rates are approximately *10–18%* [9]. Longer warm ischaemic time (WIT) is a documented risk factor for rejection.

Graft Survival

- *Kidney*: 10-year graft survival is approximately *60%*, often limited by chronic allograft injury such as transplant glomerulopathy [9].
- *Heart*: 1-year survival in DCD recipients is equivalent to that of DBD recipients, even in high-acuity patients [13].

Patient Survival

Patient survival remains high, but long-term success requires managing the 'chronicity index'—a measure of structural injury (fibrosis and atrophy) that predicts late graft failure more accurately than acute inflammatory markers [9].

Paediatric Donation After Circulatory Death (pDCD) in Emerging Health Systems (EHS)

In Emerging Health Systems (EHS) countries, implementing Donation after Circulatory Death (DCD) programmes for paediatric donors offers a highly scalable solution to combat severe organ shortages and expand local transplantation capabilities. This framework is critical given the immense global disease burden of chronic kidney disease (CKD) in developing nations, where over 7.5 million children and adolescents are newly affected by CKD annually. The vast majority of this debilitating disease burden, alongside associated mortality and Disability-Adjusted Life Years (DALYs), is concentrated in lower Socio-Demographic Index (SDI) regions that suffer from an extreme lack of access to life-saving kidney replacement therapy (KRT). While long-term survival rates for paediatric DCD organ recipients closely match traditional brain-death donations, EHS countries have historically underutilised this option [11]. Concurrently, paediatric intensive therapy units (ITUs) in developing countries experience starkly elevated mortality rates ranging between 20% and 38%—a grim contrast to the sub-6% rates typical of high-income nations [15]. A substantial portion of these tragic ITU deaths follow the ethically managed withdrawal of life-sustaining therapy (WLST) or non-resuscitatable cardiac arrests. By establishing structured paediatric DCD pathways, local health systems can ethically bridge the gap between highly intensive care mortality and the critical shortage of size-matched organs, offering a cost-effective, life-saving alternative to children who would otherwise die on prolonged, resource-intensive dialysis [11].

Paediatric Donation After Circulatory Death (pDCD) in India

Paediatric solid-organ transplantation (pSOT) remains an emerging field in India; surveys reveal that both infrastructural facilities are limited to premier institutes and human resources in terms of specialisation are at an incipient stage [1]. As observed in most of the developing LMICs, India experiences a similar barrier profile of expanding transplant across various socioeconomic profiles, like limited access to tertiary-level health care, limited trained paediatric nephrologists and transplant physicians, lack of facilities for dialysis, lack of an effective deceased-donor programme, non-affordability and non-adherence to immunosuppressant drugs. Only 60% of adult or paediatric nephrologists are involved in paediatric transplantation; few centres do >5 transplants a year, and only a few government centres are active in paediatric organ transplantation. Most of the facilities are concentrated in private institutions, while cost is a barrier for many recipients from low socioeconomic backgrounds [16]. In most centres, it has grown under the umbrella of adult organ transplant programmes; dedicated paediatric surgeons are few. Moreover, compared with the developed world, where deceased donation remains the primary source of organ donation, we see very few paediatric BSD declarations in India. As per

NOTTO data, only approximately 5% of paediatric SOTs are performed, and the number of transplants below 6 years or 6–12 years is lower. With increasing awareness and availability of diagnostic facilities, and expansion of government-subsidised dialysis programmes, more need for kidney, liver and other organ transplantation is being appreciated, but no paediatric national waiting list (organ-based) is available, and though the donor crisis is reported frequently in all national or regional meetings, the exact statistics are missing. The scarcity of data on the demand-supply gap dilutes the problem's magnitude, and administrative actions are not pursued. The need for expanding the donor pool, especially in paediatric SOT, remains understated.

Challenges in Paediatric BSD Declaration Paediatric DBD principles apply to infants and children who meet ALL of the following age criteria

(a) Corrected gestational age ≥37 weeks (term neonates and older).
(b) Post-natal age >7 days.
(c) Age <18 years with a clear proximate cause documenting acceptable aetiologies which include (with exclusion of drug-related reversible causes, which is the most common and difficult confounding factor in younger children, demanding therapeutic drug monitoring whenever possible):
    1. Hypoxic-ischaemic brain injury (post-cardiac arrest, near-drowning, severe asphyxia).
    2. Severe traumatic brain injury.
    3. Intracranial haemorrhage (spontaneous, traumatic, or vascular malformation).
    4. Central nervous system infection (meningitis, encephalitis, cerebral abscess).
    5. Brain tumour causing mass effect or herniation.
    6. Metabolic encephalopathy with confirmed irreversible structural brain injury.

Compared to adults, the incidence of metabolic and traumatic brain injury is lower in the paediatric age group, and the waiting period for brain death declaration is longer, e.g. for the age group of 7 days to <1 year: 24 h. Moreover, *as per THOA 1994 and Rules 2014*, brainstem death must be certified by a board of FOUR medical practitioners registered under the Indian Medical Council Act, 1956. At least, TWO of the four examiners must be neurologists, neurosurgeons or paediatric intensivists with documented training in brainstem death determination, with all examiners having ≥5 years post-qualification experience and none belonging to the organ transplant team or having any pecuniary interest in organ donation.

All these requirements make paediatric BSD declaration even more challenging than in adults and human resource-intensive, which will not be resolved in the near future.

Accepting DCD as a viable modality may resolve many of the ethical and legal dilemmas around BSD declaration and will increase the donor pool for younger paediatric recipients. As growth is an important issue in childhood, receiving organs early improves quality of life far more than receiving them after years on the waitlist.

The infrastructural need for DCD transplant practice will include availability of dedicated OT and manpower, with committed human resources like transplant surgeons. In India, the decision to establish transplant surgery as a speciality, rather than having transplant surgery performed by general urosurgeons or hepatobiliary surgeons, may improve manpower. The meta-analysis published by Kute et al. in 2022 [7], showcased in PKT, the 1-year, 5-year, and 10-year graft survival rates were 93% (range, 90–96%; $I^2 = 63.82$, $H^2 = 2.76$, $P < 0.01$), 83% (range, 76–89%; $I^2 = 86.39\%$, $H^2 = 7.35$, $P < 0.01$) and 66% (range, 57–75%; $I^2 = 81.68\%$, $H^2 = 5.46$, $P < 0.01$), respectively. In PLT, the 1-year and 5-year survival rates were 92% (range, 89–95%; $I^2 = 49.96\%$, $H^2 = 2$, $P < 0.04$) and 88% (range, 85–90%; $I^2 = 0$, $H^2 = 1$, $P = 0.72$), respectively, with low heterogeneity in both, suggesting a uniform immunosuppression protocol in practice and an acceptable rejection rate in PKT. Altogether, this information suggests that despite low volume and a limited workforce, the outcomes are promising and comparable to Western outcome data.

Against this backdrop, the Indian Society of Organ Transplantation has noted the relative growth of DCD in the Western world, with outcomes comparable to those of DBD transplants, and has decided to raise awareness amongst the fraternity and bring the issues to the administrative authority for appropriate action.

Competing Interests The author(s) has no competing interests to declare that are relevant to the content of this manuscript.

Ethics Approval The author(s) declares that this manuscript does not include primary research with human participants.

The author(s) declares that this manuscript does not include primary studies involving animals.

References

1. Banerjee A, Bendre AS, Munghate G, Bodhanwala M. The state of paediatric kidney transplantation in India: a survey-based analysis of practices, challenges, and educational needs. J Indian Assoc Pediatr Surg. 2024;29(6):608–11. https://doi.org/10.4103/jiaps.jiaps_102_24. Epub 2024 Nov 5. PMID: 39691928; PMCID: PMC11649050.
2. Brierley J, Pérez-Blanco A, Stojanovic J, Kessaris N, Scales A, Paessler A, Jansen N, Briki A, Gardiner D, Shaw D. Normothermic regional perfusion in paediatric donation after circulatory determination of death-the Oxford position statement from ELPAT. Front Transplant. 2024;3:1320783. https://doi.org/10.3389/frtra.2024.1320783. PMID: 38993761; PMCID: PMC11235291.
3. Eddy LH, Merrick NK, Staniforth CE, Jukes JL, Hill LJB, Mon-Williams M, Bardid F, Murray R. "The system is a bit broken…" a qualitative exploration of barriers in the pathway for diagnosing Developmental Coordination Disorder. PLoS One. 2026;21(3):e0343972. https://doi.org/10.1371/journal.pone.0343972. PMID: 41774703; PMCID: PMC12956065.
4. Foley ME, Vinson AJ, Skinner TAA, Kiberd BA, Tennankore KK. The impact of combined warm and cold ischemia time on post-transplant outcomes. Can J Kidney Health Dis. 2023;10:20543581231178960. https://doi.org/10.1177/20543581231178960. PMID: 37333478; PMCID: PMC10272701.

5. Ghazanfar A, Forgacs B, Campbell B, Pararajasingam R. Successful en bloc renal transplant from a 19-month-old nonheart-beating donor into an adult recipient: case report. Exp Clin Transplant. 2011;9(1):60–2. PMID: 21605025.
6. Kenny LA, Armstrong L, Berman M, Brierley J, Crossland D, Dark J, Gardiner D, Large SR, Manas D, Nassar M, Shaw D, Simpson E. Heart transplantation and donation after circulatory death in children. A review of the technological, logistical and ethical framework. Transpl Int. 2025;38:13801. https://doi.org/10.3389/ti.2025.13801. PMID: 40026599; PMCID: PMC11867792.
7. Kute VB, Rela M, Gulati S, Bhalla AK, Abraham G, Chauhan S, Mishra V, Meshram HS. Current scenarios of pediatric transplants of kidney, liver, heart, and lung in India: systematic review and meta-analysis. Exp Clin Transplant. 2022;20(12):1058–68. https://doi.org/10.6002/ect.2022.0207. PMID: 36718004.
8. Kim JJ, Fuggle SV, Marks SD. Does HLA matching matter in the modern era of renal transplantation? Pediatr Nephrol. 2021;36(1):31–40. https://doi.org/10.1007/s00467-019-04393-6. Epub 2019 Dec 9. PMID: 31820146; PMCID: PMC7701071.
9. Li J, Xie W, Wang Y, Li Z, Xu B, Fu Q, Wu C, Deng R, Su X, He X, Ling L, Liu L, Zhang H, Li J, Wang C. Prognostic impact of rejection and chronicity index on long-term graft outcomes in pediatric kidney transplant recipients. Front Immunol. 2026;17:1737410. https://doi.org/10.3389/fimmu.2026.1737410. PMID: 41939910; PMCID: PMC13046560.
10. ODT NHS BT Annual Report 2024–2025. https://nhsbtdbe.blob.core.windows.net/umbraco-assets-corp/36795/activity-report-2024-2025-final.pdf.
11. Paessler A, Brierley J, Siebelink M, Loukopoulos I, Kessaris N, Stojanovic J. Long-term outcomes of pediatric kidney transplants from DCD and DBD donors: a comparative OPTN study. Transpl Int. 2025;38:14706. https://doi.org/10.3389/ti.2025.14706. PMID: 41140298; PMCID: PMC12548547.
12. Pasrija C, Tipograf Y, Shah AS, Trahanas JM. Normothermic regional perfusion for donation after circulatory death donors. Curr Opin Organ Transplant. 2023;28(2):71–5. https://doi.org/10.1097/MOT.0000000000001038. Epub 2022 Nov 17. PMID: 36409266.
13. Razavi AA, Chen Q, Tam DY, Sallam A, Perez C, Sharew B, Krishnan A, Megna D, Esmailian F, Gunn T, Bowdish ME, Chikwe J, Emerson D, Catarino P. Expanding use of donation after circulatory death heart transplantation to higher acuity recipients. Ann Thorac Surg. 2026;121(2):430–8. https://doi.org/10.1016/j.athoracsur.2025.10.001. Epub 2025 Oct 28. PMID: 41167576; PMCID: PMC13110794.
14. Rajah T, Blitzer D, Silvestry S, Copeland H. Adult cardiac transplantation utilizing donors after circulatory death. Ann Cardiothorac Surg. 2024;13(6):474–86. https://doi.org/10.21037/acs-2024-dcd-0069. Epub 2024 Aug 23. PMID: 39649635; PMCID: PMC11618117.
15. Siddiqui NU, Ashraf Z, Jurair H, Haque A. Mortality patterns among critically ill children in a Pediatric Intensive Care Unit of a developing country. Indian J Crit Care Med. 2015;19(3):147–50. https://doi.org/10.4103/0972-5229.152756. PMID: 25810609; PMCID: PMC4366912.
16. Sethi SK, Sinha R, Rohatgi S, Kher V, Iyengar A, Bagga A. Pediatric renal transplant practices in India. Pediatr Transplant. 2017;21:e12892. https://doi.org/10.1111/petr.12892.
17. Skaro AI, Jay CL, Baker TB, Wang E, Pasricha S, Lyuksemburg V, Martin JA, Feinglass JM, Preczewski LB, Abecassis MM. The impact of ischemic cholangiopathy in liver transplantation using donors after cardiac death: the untold story. Surgery 2009;146(4):543–552; discussion 552–3. https://doi.org/10.1016/j.surg.2009.06.052. PMID: 19789011; PMCID: PMC2790600.
18. Tingle SJ, Thompson ER, Figueiredo RS, Moir JA, Goodfellow M, Talbot D, Wilson CH. Normothermic and hypothermic machine perfusion preservation versus static cold storage for deceased donor kidney transplantation. Cochrane Database Syst Rev. 2024;7(7):CD011671. https://doi.org/10.1002/14651858.CD011671.pub3. PMID: 38979743; PMCID: PMC11232102.

Extended Criteria DCD Donor-Kidney Transplantation

17

Abbas Ghazanfar and Arpita Ray Chaudhury

Introduction to Extended Criteria Donors (ECD)

The persistent discrepancy between the growing waiting list for renal transplantation and the limited supply of deceased-donor organs has necessitated the expansion of the donor pool. Historically, kidney transplantation relied primarily on optimal donation from live and brain death (DBD) donors. To address organ shortages, transplant programmes increasingly utilise extended criteria donors (ECD) and donation after circulatory death (DCD) donors.

Donation after circulatory death (DCD) donors have risen significantly in the UK over the last two decades, from 128 donors in 2005–2006 to 792 in 2025–2026. DCD now accounts for over half (55%) of all deceased organ donations in the UK, driven by clinical developments and end-of-life care pathways managed by NHS Blood and Transplant [ODT, NHSBT data]. Likewise, in the USA, donation after circulatory death (DCD) surged dramatically, climbing from 2% of all deceased donors in 2000 to 49% by 2025. Total annual DCD donors jumped from 118 to 8129 over this period, driven by innovations in organ preservation and a critical need to expand the transplant waitlist pool [US organ registry data]. India lags behind tremendously in DCD transplantation.

The formalised definition of an ECD was established by the Organ Procurement and Transplantation Network (OPTN) in 2002 to identify marginal allografts with a statistically higher risk of failure [6]. By definition, an ECD kidney has a relative risk of graft loss greater than 1.70 compared to a standard-criteria donor (SCD) [6].

A. Ghazanfar (✉)
Department of Renal Medicine and Transplant Surgery, St George's University Hospitals NHS Foundation Trust, London, UK
e-mail: a.ghazanfar@nhs.net

A. R. Chaudhury
Department of Nephrology, North Bengal Medical College, Darjeeling, West Bengal, India

S. P. Kolte et al. (eds.), *Organ Donation After Circulatory Death*,
https://doi.org/10.1007/978-981-92-6377-6_17

An extended criteria donor (ECD) is conventionally defined as any deceased donor aged ≥60 years or a donor aged 50–59 years presenting with at least two of the following three clinical risk factors:

- Long-standing history of hypertension.
- Terminal serum creatinine >1.5 mg/dL (> 132 μmol/L) prior to procurement.
- Death secondary to a cerebrovascular accident (CVA).

When ECD criteria overlap with DCD status—termed ECD-DCD or 'expanded DCD'—the transplanted graft is exposed to dual cellular insults: baseline chronic pre-existing structural damage (arteriolosclerosis, glomerulosclerosis, tubular atrophy) combined with acute warm-ischaemic injury sustained during circulatory arrest and withdrawal of life-sustaining therapy (WLST). Despite these vulnerabilities, when managed with dynamic organ preservation protocols and matched recipient selection, these high-risk grafts yield substantial survival benefits compared to remaining on chronic dialysis. It is important to note that in contemporary practice, the classic binary ECD/SCD distinction has largely been superseded in the USA by the Kidney Donor Profile Index (KDPI) [10]. The KDPI is a continuous percentile scale from 0% to 100% derived from the Kidney Donor Risk Index (KDRI). Table 17.1 shows the differences between the older ECD and current KDPI systems.

Clinical Meaning for Patients Using KDPI The KDPI system assesses 10 donor factors on a continuous scale from 0% to 100%. A lower score indicates a higher-quality organ expected to last longer. Because the older ECD criteria reflect donors with higher clinical risk, an ECD kidney generally corresponds to a KDPI score of 85% or higher.

If a kidney is labelled as an ECD organ or has a KDPI score of 85% or higher, it carries specific trade-offs for a transplant candidate:

- *Shorter Lifespan*: on average, these kidneys do not function as long as kidneys from younger, healthier donors.
- *Faster Access*: patients who agree to accept high-KDPI/ECD kidneys often skip years of waiting on the transplant list.

Table 17.1 Differences between the older ECD and current KDPI systems

Metric	Older system: ECD	Current system: KDPI
Type of measure	Binary category (either 'Standard' or 'Expanded')	Continuous scale (0% to 100%)
Precision	Low (treats a 60-year-old healthy donor the same as an 80-year-old donor)	High (accounts for exact age, weight and health history)
High-risk threshold	Labelled as ECD	Scored as KDPI ≥85%
Allocation use	Historically used to screen willing recipients	Used today to route organs to patients who benefit most

Table 17.2 Modified Maastricht classification for DCD donation

Category	Type	Description	Clinical context and management
Category I	Uncontrolled	Brought in dead (BID)	Out-of-hospital cardiac arrest; unexpected death without successful CPR
Category II	Uncontrolled	Unsuccessful resuscitation	Unexpected in-hospital cardiac arrest where advanced CPR fails
Category III	Controlled	Awaiting cardiac arrest	Planned withdrawal of life-sustaining therapy (WLST) in an ICU setting
Category IV	Controlled	Cardiac arrest after brain death	Unexpected circulatory arrest occurring during or after formal DBD determination
Category V	Uncontrolled/ controlled	In-hospital cardiac arrest (euthanasia)	Circulatory death following voluntary euthanasia or medically assisted dying

Clinical significance: The vast majority of renal transplants performed globally utilise Category III (controlled DCD) donors. This pathway permits prospective monitoring of hemodynamic deterioration, strict control of functional warm ischemia and coordinated surgical recovery. Uncontrolled DCD (Categories I and II) exhibits higher primary non-function (PNF) and delayed graft function (DGF) rates, requiring rapid post-mortem cannulation and machine perfusion strategies. Category V has its own challenges and regulations across various countries

- *Better than Dialysis*: for many candidates—especially older adults or individuals with health complications—receiving a high-KDPI kidney provides a much longer, healthier life than staying on long-term dialysis while waiting for a lower-KDPI organ.

Types of DCD Donors

DCD donors are classified according to the modified maastricht classification [8], which differentiates between uncontrolled and controlled circulatory death [Table 17.2].

Pathophysiological Synergy of Injury in DCD and ECD Donation

When an allograft is exposed to both the structural senescence of an ECD donor and the ischaemic insult of DCD procurement, a cascade of tissue injury occurs. This ‘double-hit’ phenomenon involves distinct physiological mechanisms:

The First Hit: Structural and Cellular Senescence (ECD) An ECD kidney begins with diminished functional reserve. Histologically, these organs exhibit varying degrees of glomerulosclerosis, interstitial fibrosis, tubular atrophy and arteriolar hyalinosis [2].

At the cellular level, the ageing nephron exhibits advanced telomere shortening, chronic low-grade inflammation and upregulated expression of senescence markers.

The baseline capillary density in the peritubular network is reduced, leaving the renal medulla chronically vulnerable to hypoxic insults.

The Second Hit: Ischemic Cascade and Reperfusion Injury (DCD) The controlled DCD process introduces a highly volatile period of donor warm-ischemia time (DWIT). The DWIT is divided into distinct phases that dictate graft viability:

[Withdrawal of Life-Sustaining Treatment (WLST)]
↓ (Phase 1: Agonal phase / time to death)
[Systolic BP < 60 mmHg or SpO2 < 70%]
↓ (Phase 2: Functional warm-ischemia time)
[Asystole / circulatory arrest]
↓ (Phase 3: Stand-off/no-touch period—typically 5 min)
[Declaration of death and incision]
↓ (Phase 4: Cold in situ flush)

(i) *The Agonal Phase (Time to Death—TTD)*: the period from WLST to circulatory arrest is considered as the Agonal phase. As the donor's blood pressure drops below a systolic threshold of 60 mmHg or arterial oxygen saturation falls below 70%, systemic perfusion fails. This initiates functional warm-ischemia time (fWIT).

(ii) *Cellular Hypoxia*: deprived of oxygen, the renal tubular epithelial cells switch from aerobic oxidative phosphorylation to anaerobic glycolysis. ATP depletion occurs rapidly, causing failure of energy-dependent ion pumps (such as Na/K-ATPase).

(iii) *Intracellular Oedema and Intravascular Microthrombi*: sodium and water accumulate within the cytoplasm, causing cell swelling and blebbing into the tubular lumen. Concurrently, localised stasis and the loss of endothelial nitric oxide synthase (eNOS) promote the formation of microthrombi within the peritubular capillaries.

(iv) *Ischemic-Reperfusion Injury (IRI)*: when the organ is reperfused in the recipient, the reintroduction of oxygen triggers a massive burst of reactive oxygen species (ROS) from damaged mitochondria. This activates the innate immune response via Toll-like receptors (TLRs), driving neutrophil infiltration, complement activation and extensive acute tubular necrosis (ATN).

An ECD kidney has minimal intracellular reserves to withstand this ATP depletion and lacks the regenerative capacity to recover from severe ATN. This directly correlates with high rates of delayed graft function (DGF) [1].

Current Practices in DCD and ECD Organ Allocation and Strategies for Improvement

DCD Organ Allocation Organ allocation schemes for DCD kidneys balance utility (maximising post-transplant graft longevity) with equity (maintaining fair access among waiting-list candidates).

Key Allocation Principles The main aim of allocation for ECD-DCD is to make best use of the organ by choosing the right kidney for the right recipient.

- *Ischemia Time Minimisation*: given that prolonged cold storage compounds early warm-ischemic damage, allocation algorithms prioritise expedited local placement to minimise overall cold-ischemic time (CIT).
- *Kidney Donor Profile Index (KDPI)*: in modern allocation systems (such as the UNOS Kidney Allocation System), continuous scoring via the Kidney Donor Risk Index (KDRI) and KDPI has replaced binary ECD metrics. DCD status acts as an independent multiplicative coefficient in KDRI calculations.
- *Dual/En Bloc Allocation*: high-KDPI DCD grafts or organs from extreme-age ECD-DCD donors are frequently routed through dual-kidney allocation algorithms. Transplanting both kidneys into a single recipient doubles the functional nephron mass, thereby overcoming the loss of individual graft tissue.
- *Accelerated Placement Pathways*: to avoid prolonged cold-ischemic accumulation during systemic waitlist offers, regional networks utilise pre-calculated panel-reactive antibody (cPRA) matching and expedited virtual cross-matching protocols.

Current Practices in ECD-DCD Renal Transplantation Successful DCD renal transplantation requires specialised management across three operational phases: donor withdrawal, organ retrieval and preservation and recipient post-operative care.

- *Preservation Shift*: static cold storage (SCS) alone is associated with DGF rates exceeding 50–70% in DCD kidneys. Hypothermic machine perfusion is now widely adopted as the standard of care to mitigate ischaemia-reperfusion injury.
- *Immunosuppressive Management*: recipients of ECD-DCD kidneys frequently experience early tubular injury. Regimens incorporate potent induction agents (e.g., anti-thymocyte globulin [ATG] or IL-2 receptor antagonists) alongside delayed or cautious titration of calcineurin inhibitors (CNIs) to avoid exacerbating acute tubular necrosis (ATN).

Strategies to Improve ECD-DCD Outcomes and Utilisation Addressing high-discard rates in ECD-DCD transplantation requires multimodal interventions throughout organ recovery and recipient management:

- *Strict Ischemic Time Cutoffs*: minimising functional warm-ischaemia while aggressively reducing cold-ischemic times to <12–18 h.

- *Routine Hypothermic Machine Perfusion (HMP)*: applying continuous hypothermic pulsatile perfusion (4–10 °C) reduces DGF risk and provides real-time hydrodynamic evaluation, including renal vascular resistance (R = MAP / flow).
- *Pre-mortem Anticoagulation*: where legally permitted, administering systemic heparin prior to WLST limits microvascular thrombosis within the intrarenal capillary bed during the agony phase.
- *Recipient Risk Matching*: allocating higher-risk ECD-DCD grafts into older recipients (e.g. European Senior Programme 'Old-for-Old' models) balances life expectancy gains against immunologic risk without subjecting younger candidates to high DGF rates.

Normothermic Regional Perfusion (NRP) Normothermic regional perfusion (NRP) employs extracorporeal membrane oxygenation (ECMO) technology to restore oxygenated blood flow to organs in situ immediately following the declaration of death.

Technical Execution

- *Cannulation*: femoral arterial and venous lines are established post-declaration (or pre-mortem where legal framework permits).
- *Cerebral Protection*: comprehensive ligation or balloon occlusion of the supra-aortic vessels (carotid and vertebral arteries) is performed to prevent unexpected cerebral reperfusion.
- *Circulatory Support*: oxygenated, warm (37 °C) autologous blood recirculates through the abdominal organ bed (abdominal NRP / A-NRP) or thoracoabdominal organ bed (TA-NRP) for 1–4 h.

Clinical Benefits

- Restores cellular energy reserves by replenishing adenosine triphosphate (ATP) levels in situ.
- Clears microvascular microthrombi from intrarenal microcirculation prior to cold flush.
- Provides a functional window for direct organ evaluation (e.g. monitoring lactate clearance, macro-perfusion appearance and urine output).
- Significantly reduces post-transplant DGF rates and biliary complications, yielding graft survival outcomes comparable to DBD transplants.

Machine Perfusion: HMP, HOPE and NMP Dynamic ex vivo organ perfusion technologies have largely superseded passive cold storage by providing continuous metabolic support and functional assessment [5, 9]. Table 17.3 compares various machine perfusion systems.

Pre-implantation Biopsy Pre-implantation (zero-hour baseline or wedge) kidney biopsies provide histological evaluation of marginal ECD-DCD grafts, helping clinicians differentiate reversible acute ischaemic injury from irreversible chronic parenchymal sclerosis.

Table 17.3 Comparison of various machine perfusion systems

Feature	Hypothermic machine perfusion (HMP)	Hypothermic oxygenated perfusion (HOPE)	Normothermic machine perfusion (NMP)
Temperature	4–10 °C	4–10 °C	35–37 °C
Perfusate	Hypothermic crystalloid (e.g. KPS-1)	Oxygenated hypothermic solution	Red blood cell-based or acellular oxygen carriers
Mechanism	Decreases metabolic rate; flushes toxic metabolites	Recharges mitochondrial electron transport chain [11]	Restores full physiological metabolic function ex vivo
Viability metrics	Perfusion pressure, intrarenal resistance, flow rates	Resistance parameters + real-time Flavin Mononucleotide (FMN) levels [3]	Urine production, lactate clearance, acid-base homeostasis, renal blood flow
Logistics	Highly portable, widely implemented	Moderately complex, growing clinical adoption	Technically complex, resource-intensive

Scoring Systems The Remuzzi/Karpinski Histological Score evaluates four key tissue compartments on a scale from 0 to 3:

- Glomerulosclerosis (percentage of global glomerulosclerosis).
- Tubular atrophy.
- Interstitial fibrosis.
- Arterial and arteriolar intimal thickening.

$$\begin{aligned}\text{Total Score} &= \text{Glomerulosclerosis} + \text{Tubular Atrophy}\\ &\quad + \text{Interstitial Fibrosis} + \text{Vascular Changes}\end{aligned}$$

Interpretation and Allocation Decision Matrix

- *Score 0–3 (Mild Damage)*: suitable for standard single kidney transplantation.
- *Score 4–6 (Moderate Damage)*: high-risk single transplantation or allocation into dual-kidney transplantation protocols.
- *Score 7–12 (Severe Damage)*: high likelihood of graft failure; frequently leads to organ discard unless offset by favourable machine perfusion dynamics.

Cautionary Note

Frozen section histology is susceptible to sampling artifacts (particularly wedge biopsy superficial subcapsular scarring), processing freeze-artifacts and inter-observer diagnostic variability. Biopsy scores should be integrated alongside donor clinical history and real-time perfusion metrics rather than used as a sole discard criterion.

Dual-Kidney Transplantation (DKT) When an ECD-DCD kidney possesses a low functional nephron mass, transplanting it as a single graft can lead to early functional exhaustion, chronic allograft nephropathy and premature failure. Dual-kidney transplantation (DKT) circumvents this by implanting both kidneys from a single deceased donor into a single recipient [2, 10].

Surgical Techniques for DKT implanting two kidneys requires careful consideration of the recipient's pelvic anatomy, vascular access and overall surgical risk. Two primary techniques are utilised in clinical practice:

- *Unilateral Placement (the Single-Incision Technique)*: both donor kidneys are placed into a single iliac fossa (typically the right side due to the more horizontal and accessible configuration of the common and external iliac veins).
- *Vascular Anastomoses*: in general, the renal vein and artery of the first kidney are anastomosed to the IVC, CIV or proximal EIV and CIA, respectively. This allows for perfusion of the first kidney and addressing any vascular issues before proceeding to the lower kidney by clamping the vessels distal to the first transplanted vessels. The second kidney is positioned inferiorly, with its vessels anastomosed to distal external iliac vessels.
- *Surgical Advantage*: avoids a second incision, preserves the contralateral iliac fossa for future transplants and minimises total operative time.

Bilateral Placement (The Dual-Incision Technique) Each donor kidney is implanted into its respective iliac fossa via separate right and left extraperitoneal Gibson incisions.

- *Vascular Anastomoses*: standard single-kidney vascular reconstructions are performed bilaterally to the external iliac vessels.
- *Surgical Advantage*: anatomically cleaner positioning of each allograft, reducing the risk of mechanical vascular compression or kinking that can occur when crowding two marginal kidneys into a single iliac fossa.

Allocation, Usage and the Challenge of Organ Discard

The allocation of ECD-DCD allografts requires balancing the imperative to maximise organ utilisation against the need to ensure equitable and safe patient outcomes.

The Problem of Elevated Discard Rates In many developed health systems, particularly in the USA, kidneys with a KDPI >85% face extremely high-discard rates, sometimes exceeding 40–50% [10]. In the UK, 18% of kidneys procured from donation after circulatory death (DCD) donors and roughly 8% from donation after brain death (DBD) donors are discarded. For combined expanded criteria donor (ECD) and DCD categories, international and UK cohort analyses indicate that overall discard rates for higher-risk marginal kidneys can exceed 30–50% depending on donor age and organ quality indices, although precise contemporary subgroup-specific discard numbers for combined ECD/DCD definitions fluctuate annually in the UK Transplant Registry.

This high discard rate is driven by several systemic factors:

- *Regulatory Scrutiny*: centre-specific outcomes are closely monitored by regulatory bodies. Fear of negative evaluations can make programmes risk-averse, leading them to decline marginal organs.
- *Logistical Friction*: extended cold-ischemic time (CIT), compounded by prolonged allocation discussions, can render a usable marginal kidney non-viable.
- *Donor-Recipient Longevity Matching*: the 2014 UNOS allocation revisions sought to match high-survival-longevity recipients with high-longevity organs [10]. Consequently, kidneys with a KDPI >85% are preferentially offered to older candidates or those with lower estimated post-transplant survival (EPTS) scores, where the survival benefit of receiving an ECD organ outweighs the risk of remaining on dialysis [10]. The current UK matching system also tries to better utilise organs from ECD donors.

Accelerated Allocation Protocols To combat organ discard, allocation protocols have introduced streamlined mechanisms to bypass standard, labour-intensive match runs for high-risk kidneys:

- *Expedited Placement Pathways*: when an organ is declined by multiple top-tier candidates on a local list, and CIT approaches a critical threshold (e.g., >18–20 h), allocation systems can trigger open, regional or nationwide pooling. This allows any centre with a pre-consented, appropriate candidate to claim the organ immediately.
- *Up-Front DKT Offering*: OPOs can systematically offer high-risk kidneys as dual units from the outset if the donor meets predefined clinical triggers, thereby circumventing the delays associated with first attempting to place them as single grafts [10].

Clinical Outcomes and Immunosuppressive Management

Graft and Patient Survival Characteristics Inherent to the ECD-DCD definition is an inferior long-term graft survival curve compared with standard-criteria donor organs [6, 7]. The average half-life of an ECD allograft is approximately 5–6 years, compared with over 10 years for an SCD graft [6]. However, focusing strictly on allograft survival curves overlooks the core clinical objective of transplantation. For older patients with ESRD (typically aged over 65 years with multiple comorbidities), accepting an ECD-DCD kidney offers a clear, demonstrable survival advantage over remaining on waitlist dialysis [6]. Dialysis carries a high annual mortality rate in elderly patients with cardiovascular comorbidities. Receiving an ECD-DCD organ, despite lower long-term graft survival and higher initial rates of delayed graft function [1], breaks the ongoing toll of dialysis and extends life expectancy [6]. In certain younger patients approaching end of dialysis access due to various reasons, these organs can provide a reasonable option to extend life.

Immunosuppressive Stratification The highly injured endothelial profile and high rate of acute tubular necrosis in ECD-DCD allografts require an intentional, tailored immunosuppressive approach.

Induction Therapy Because these kidneys are highly susceptible to ischaemia-reperfusion injury and are prone to severe DGF, calcineurin inhibitor (CNI) therapy is often delayed post-operatively to protect the recovering renal vasculature. Consequently, potent *depleting antibody induction* is standard care:

- *Rabbit Anti-thymocyte Globulin (rATG)*: administered intra-operatively and over the first few post-operative days. T-cell depletion provides robust protection against early acute rejection while allowing clinicians to safely hold nephrotoxic CNIs until the graft establishes adequate urine output and creatinine clearance. However, in some elderly patients with other comorbidities, it may not be the right option. In the UK, most centres use a standard Basiliximab induction, irrespective of whether the transplant is for SCD or ECD.
- *Maintenance Regimens*: once the allograft recovers from DGF, a standard triple-therapy maintenance regimen is introduced, but with lower targeted exposure levels to mitigate chronic nephrotoxicity and viral complications:
  - *Calcineurin Inhibitors (Tacrolimus)*: maintained at lower target trough levels (e.g., 5–7 ng/mL after month 3) to minimise vasoconstriction of the already compromised afferent arterioles.
  - *Antimetabolites (Mycophenolate Mofetil—MMF)*: standard dosing to provide baseline immunosuppression without nephrotoxicity.
  - *Corticosteroid Taper*: steroids are either slowly tapered to a low maintenance dose (5 mg/day) or avoided entirely via structured steroid-withdrawal protocols in highly HLA-matched, low-immunological-risk recipients.

New Developments and Future Directions

The landscape of ECD-DCD transplantation is undergoing rapid transformation through molecular, cellular and bioengineering innovations:

- *Targeted Ex Vivo Pharmacotherapy*: utilising NMP circuits as isolated delivery platforms for targeted molecular therapies prior to implantation:
  - *siRNA Therapies*: administering small interfering RNA to silence pro-inflammatory cytokines, complement components (C3, C5a) or apoptotic signalling drivers.

  - *Cell Therapies*: infusing mesenchymal stem cells (MSCs) or stem-cell-derived extracellular vesicles into the perfusate to mitigate ischaemic-reperfusion injury and promote endothelial recovery.
- *Mitochondrial Viability Biomarkers*: quantitative measurement of Flavin Mononucleotide (FMN) release during hypothermic oxygenated perfusion (HOPE) acts as a direct surrogate for mitochondrial complex I structural damage and electron transport breakdown [3, 5].
- *Defatting and Metabolic Conditioning*: adding pharmacological cocktails during NMP to stimulate intracellular lipid breakdown and reduce metabolic cellular strain in steatotic or advanced-age ECD grafts.
- *Real-Time Biomarker Panels*: assessing cell-free DNA (cfDNA), microRNAs and metabolic biomarkers in perfusate to objectively predict post-transplant function without relying on frozen biopsies.

Economic and Health System Impact

From a health economics standpoint, kidney transplantation is consistently more cost-effective than long-term maintenance dialysis. In countries where dialysis is heavily subsidised by public funds or represents a significant out-of-pocket burden for families, transitioning patients to a functional kidney transplant saves substantial healthcare resources ([4].

Even after accounting for the higher initial costs of managing delayed graft function, prolonged hospitalisations and machine perfusion consumables [4], the multi-year savings from removing patients from dialysis can be reallocated to expand primary prevention and access to renal replacement therapy. For an emerging health system, a well-regulated, protocol-driven ECD-DCD programme represents a pragmatic path towards achieving self-sufficiency in organ transplantation.

Across India, 804 registered hospitals are active in transplantation, and India is contributing to the 3rd-highest number of transplants in the world because of a large population living with end-organ disease and an active transplant programme that is continuously growing and expanding. As of 03rd March, 2026, according to the data reported by hospitals and transplant centres on the National Registry Portal of the National Organ and Tissue Transplant Organisation (NOTTO), the waitlist for major organs in the country stands at 89,839. In 2025, the number of organ transplants performed in the country was 20,019 (NOTTO data). This huge supply–demand gap needs active attention from transplant professionals as well as the administrative authorities overseeing transplantation in India (NOTTO, ROTTO and SOTTO). To expand the deceased-donor pool, DCD and DCD-ECD may be an important adjunct to the existing programme, while DBD contributes solely to the deceased-donor programme. For a resource-constrained country like India, where a large number of ESRD patients (every year, 200 thousand people are added to the dialysis pool) are on a publicly funded dialysis programme, it may be more cost-intensive than offering transplants to waiting recipients and strengthening the primary prevention programme. In a recently published paper in Transplant

International from Belgium, Darius et al. nicely presented data showing that centrally subsidised HMP support for DCD-ECD kidneys transplanted improved graft and patient survival, increased organ utilisation and reduced public funding expense on dialysis.

As we know, the primary objective of transplantation is to improve the quality of life rather than to increase life span alone; utilisation of DCD-ECD kidneys may be preferentially allocated to a targeted group of recipients on the wait list with relative life expectancy, like the elderly (> 65–70 years, or > 70 years group on wait list). Choosing an RRT for the elderly can be difficult for the family. As people now live longer with kidney disease, the aged population on dialysis in India is growing, and issues with haemodialysis are cardiovascular instability, sudden fluid and electrolyte shifts, need for vascular access and travel to a nearby dialysis centre, whereas with peritoneal dialysis (PD), the issues are peritonitis and, at times, lack of an attending person to do the exchange. Limited survival data from elderly patients on dialysis in India shows a median overall survival of 26.6 months (SE 1.9). Overall 1-year, 2-year and 3-year survival was 78.9% at 1 year, 54% at 2 years and 26.2% at the end of the 3rd year [12]. Another study from rural Karnataka showed 2-year survival of elderly dialysis patients of 26%, probably showing that rural and remote areas may have poorer outcomes. Comparing survival on dialysis by the Jelokas group 5 years earlier, young and elderly patients also showed similar survival, with elderly dialysis patients at 25 months, showcasing only marginal improvement over 5 years [13]. Compared with international data, Latos et al. from the USA reported a survival of 54% among elderly dialysis patients, which is comparable to Indian data: 71% at 1 year and 54.3% at 2 years [14]. Diabetes remains a dominant underlying comorbidity impacting long-term survival, alongside cardiovascular disease, hypoalbuminaemia (poor nutrition) and infectious complications like sepsis, highlighting the need for primary prevention as well as infrastructural improvement. On the other hand, a retrospective cohort of 1. 150 patients >60 years had 5-year graft survival of 86%, and 5-year death-censored graft survival was 82% (94% and 87% respectively in younger adults). Biopsy-proven acute rejection rates were similar between elderly and younger groups (11.3% vs. 10.2%, $P = 0.12$). They concluded that chronological age should not exclude the elderly from the benefit of transplantation [15]. While these data covers only live donor transplants, B. Shi et al. documented a similar survival advantage with deceased kidneys. While recipients of living and standard-criteria donor kidneys acquired an immediate survival advantage compared with dialysis, the recipients of expanded criteria donor kidneys experienced an elevated risk of death for the first 17 months. Compared with remaining on dialysis, elderly KTRs incur an increased risk of early post-transplant mortality but thereafter may anticipate progressively superior survival rates.

Needs for practical implementation once DCD and ECD-DCD

1. Need for Individualisation of Therapy: relatively healthy elderly recipients with fewer comorbidities (lower Charlson Comorbidity Index), minimal frailty, with no history of cancer may be considered for transplantation, while people with

higher comorbidities and shorter life expectancy or with absolute contraindications may be given the option for conservative and/or dialytic therapies.

2. Recipients with a good match (a strong pre-transplant virtual crossmatch-based allocation) may optimise the outcome, increase graft survival, decrease net immunosuppression post-transplant and decrease infection-related mortality. Virtual crossmatch-based allocation is now practised by a few centres in India, which should be adopted nationally across all transplant centres. The 2014 UNOS allocation revisions sought to match high-survival-longevity recipients with high-longevity organs; kidneys with a KDPI >85% are preferentially offered to older candidates or those with lower estimated post-transplant survival (EPTS) scores, where the survival benefit of receiving an ECD organ outweighs the risk of remaining on dialysis [10]. It is a significant challenge to balance the labour-intensive match run required to allocate the organ to the right recipient with the need for expedited allocation. India may address the situation by establishing an appropriate waiting list for the elderly across all regions under ROTTO and SOTTO to expedite the allocation process.
3. Manpower and Logistics: an increase in the number of surgeons in transplant medicine and wider availability of HLA-LABs and advanced diagnostic labs in cities active in transplantation remain priority areas to increase organ availability and address the huge demand-supply gap prevalent in India. There are reports of utilising NMP circuits in a few centres in India for ECD liver transplantation; popularising their use in high-volume centres accepting DCD-ECD organs is an important adjunct to showcasing relatively good outcomes even with compromised organs.

Competing Interests The author(s) has no competing interests to declare that are relevant to the content of this manuscript.

Ethics Approval The author(s) declares that this manuscript does not include primary research with human participants.

The author(s) declares that this manuscript does not include primary studies involving animals.

References

1. Bischof M. Risk factors of delayed kidney graft function following donation after circulatory death – a retrospective cohort study of Swiss kidney transplants. Swiss Med Wkly. 2026;156:Article 5007.
2. Casati C, Colombo VG, Perrino M, Rossetti OM, Querques M, Giacomoni A, Binaggia A, Colussi G. Renal transplants from older deceased donors: use of preimplantation biopsy and differential allocation to dual or single kidney transplant according to histological score has no advantages over allocation to single kidney transplant by simple clinical indication. J Transplant. 2018;2018:1–12. https://doi.org/10.1155/2018/4141756.
3. Bellini MI, Tortorici F, Amabile MI, D'Andrea V. Assessing kidney graft viability and its cells metabolism during machine perfusion. Int J Mol Sci. 2021;22(3):1121. https://doi.org/10.3390/ijms22031121.

4. Darius T. Nationwide hypothermic machine perfusion for ECD and DCD kidney transplantation in Belgium: one-year outcomes and impact on transplant rates and budget impact analysis. Transpl Int. 2025;38:Article 15282.
5. De Beule J, Jochmans I. Kidney perfusion as an organ quality assessment tool—are we counting our chickens before they have hatched? J Clin Med. 2020;9(3):879. https://doi.org/10.3390/jcm9030879.
6. Filiopoulos V, Boletis JN. Renal transplantation with expanded criteria donors: which is the optimal immunosuppression? World J Transplant. 2016;6(1):103–14. https://doi.org/10.5500/wjt.v6.i1.103.
7. Hellemans R, Kramer A, De Meester J, Collart F, Kuypers D, Jadoul M, Van Laecke S, Le Moine A, Krzesinski JM, Wissing KM, Luyckx K, van Meel M, de Vries E, Tieken I, Vogelaar S, Samuel U, Abramowicz D, Stel VS, Jager KJ. Does kidney transplantation with a standard or expanded criteria donor improve patient survival? Results from a Belgian cohort. Nephrol Dial Transplant. 2021;36(5):918–26. https://doi.org/10.1093/ndt/gfab024.
8. Muston BT, Lo W, Eranki A, Boffini M, Loforte A. Cardiac transplantation in controlled donation after circulatory death: a meta-analysis of long-term survival using reconstructed time-to-event data. Ann Cardiothor Surg. 2025;14:1–10. https://doi.org/10.21037/acs-2024-dcd-20.
9. Norton WG, Pearson R, Devlin J, Nicholson ML, Hosgood SA. Normothermic machine perfusion in renal transplantation. Curr Transplant Rep. 2022;9(4):308–17. https://doi.org/10.1007/s40472-022-00378-x.
10. Tanriover B, Mohan S, Cohen DJ, Radhakrishnan J, Nickolas TL, Stone PW, Tsapepas DS, Crew RJ, Dube GK, Sandoval PR, Samstein B, Dogan E, Gaston RS, Tanriover JN, Ratner LE, Hardy MA. Kidneys at higher risk of discard: expanding the role of dual kidney transplantation. Am J Transplant. 2014;14(2):404–15. https://doi.org/10.1111/ajt.12553.
11. van Rijn R, Schurink IJ, de Vries Y, van den Berg AP, Cortes Cerisuelo M, Darwish Murad S, Erdmann JI, Gilbo N, de Haas RJ, Heaton N, van Hoek B, Huurman VAL, Jochmans I, van Leeuwen OB, de Meijer VE, Monbaliu D, Polak WG, Slangen JJG, Troisi RI, Vanlander A, de Jonge J, Porte RJ. Hypothermic machine perfusion in liver transplantation—a randomized trial. N Engl J Med. 2021;384(15):1391–401.
12. Jeloka T, Sanwaria P, Periera A, Pawar S. Survival of elderly dialysis patients is not dependent on modality or "older" age. Indian J Nephrol. 2016;26(1):23–6. https://doi.org/10.4103/0971-4065.157801.
13. Jeloka TK, Jhamnani A. Survival of elderly/dialysis patients—a single Centre study from India. J Assoc Physicians India. 2011;59:412–4.
14. Latos DL. Chronic dialysis in patients over age 65. J Am Soc Nephrol. 1996 May;7(5):637-46.
15. Bhargava V, Meena P, Agrawaal K, Gaur L, Rana D, Bhalla A, Gupta A, Malik M, Gupta A, Kumar D. Outcomes of kidney transplantation in the elderly recipients. Indian J Nephrol. 2021;31(4):370–6. https://doi.org/10.4103/ijn.IJN_289_20. Epub 2021 Feb 16. PMID: 34584353; PMCID: PMC8443107.

18 Donation After Circulatory Death (DCD) Kidney Transplantation in Elderly Patients

Abbas Ghazanfar and Arpita Ray Chaudhury

Introduction to DCD Donation and Global Trends

Donation After Circulatory Death (DCD)—historically termed non-heart-beating donation—has evolved from a secondary organ retrieval pathway into a critical pillar of modern renal transplantation. Historically, solid organ transplantation relied almost exclusively on Donation after Brain Death (DBD). However, driven by an aging end-stage renal disease (ESRD) population, expanding waitlists, and a persistent shortage of donor organs, major transplant networks worldwide have systematically expanded DCD programs over the past two decades [11, 29].

DCD is broadly classified using the modified Maastricht Classification system, which categorizes donors based on the clinical setting and predictability of cardiac arrest:

- *Category I*: Brought dead to the hospital (Uncontrolled)
- *Category II*: Unsuccessful resuscitation following acute cardiac arrest (Uncontrolled)
- *Category III*: Awaiting cardiac arrest after planned withdrawal of life-sustaining therapy (WLST) (Controlled)
- *Category IV*: Cardiac arrest occurring after the formal diagnosis of brain death (Controlled)
- *Category V*: In-hospital cardiac arrest following voluntary euthanasia (Controlled)

A. Ghazanfar (✉)
Department of Renal Medicine and Transplant Surgery, St George's University Hospitals NHS Foundation Trust, London, UK
e-mail: a.ghazanfar@nhs.net

A. R. Chaudhury
Department of Nephrology, North Bengal Medical College, Darjeeling, West Bengal, India

S. P. Kolte et al. (eds.), *Organ Donation After Circulatory Death*,
https://doi.org/10.1007/978-981-92-6377-6_18

Controlled DCD (cDCD, Category III) accounts for the vast majority of abdominal organ transplants in Western nations, as it allows for prospective donor evaluation, surgical team assembly, and planned withdrawal of therapy in an intensive care setting. Conversely, uncontrolled DCD (uDCD, Categories I and II) relies on rapid emergency response and in situ perfusion protocols, and remains largely restricted to specialized centers in countries such as Spain and France [2, 18].

Global Adoption and International Registries

The uptake, operational frameworks, and legislative underpinnings of DCD transplantation vary significantly across international jurisdictions. Table 18.1 summarizes various networks and DCD utilization.

United States Data from the Scientific Registry of Transplant Recipients (SRTR) and the Organ Procurement and Transplantation Network (OPTN) demonstrate an exponential rise in DCD utilization. DCD donations now account for 30–35% of all deceased organ donors nationwide, exceeding 5000 DCD donors annually [11]. Growth in the US has been further accelerated by regulatory shifts that encourage donor service organizations (OPOs) to optimize organ yield and by the rapid clinical adoption of ex vivo Hypothermic Machine Perfusion (HMP) and Abdominal Normothermic Regional Perfusion (A-NRP) [8].

United Kingdom The UK, governed by NHS Blood and Transplant (NHSBT), maintains one of the highest DCD utilization rates globally. DCD kidney transplants consistently account for 35–40% of all deceased donor kidney transplants per-

Table 18.1 Various networks and DCD utilization

Network	DCD type	Prevalence of DCD in deceased kidney transplants (%)	Primary preservation strategies	Key allocation characteristics
United States (OPTN/SRTR)	Controlled (Category III)	~30–35%	HMP standard; rapid adoption of A-NRP	Longevity matching via KDPI/EPTS continuous scoring
United Kingdom (NHSBT)	Controlled (Category III)	~35–40%	Universal HMP; expanding NMP and A-NRP	Fast-track allocation schemes for high-risk/ marginal DCD
Eurotransplant (NL/BE)	Controlled (Category III)	~40–45%	Dual-HMP; oxygenated HMP (HOPE)	ESP ("Old-for-Old") waives HLA matching to reduce CIT
Spain (ONT)	Uncontrolled (Cat I/II) & controlled	~30–35%	In situ A-NRP standard for uDCD	National rapid-response protocol for out-of-hospital arrest

formed across UK centers ([31]; [19]). National guidelines mandate that cDCD be considered in all intensive care units for patients for whom a clinical decision for WLST has been finalized, thereby creating a standardized national pipeline.

Eurotransplant Region Within Eurotransplant (comprising Germany, the Netherlands, Belgium, Austria, Luxembourg, Croatia, Hungary, and Slovenia), utilization patterns are highly heterogeneous due to disparate national legal frameworks:

- *The Netherlands and Belgium*: Active cDCD programs contribute over 40% of their respective deceased donor pools [10].
- *Germany*: The statutory requirement for brain death determination prior to organ retrieval historically prohibited DCD activity, though recent policy debates seek to address this limitation [12]. Spain differs from these countries due to its presumed consent law and digital tools.

Pathophysiology of DCD Allografts and General Transplant Outcomes

The primary physiological challenge of DCD transplantation is the mandatory warm ischemic injury sustained during the retrieval process. Unlike DBD donation—where systemic organ perfusion is maintained via intact circulation until cold cardioplegia and cross-clamping—DCD involves a period of progressive hypoxemia, hypotension, and tissue ischemia prior to organ preservation [32].

Ischemic Phases in DCD Retrieval

- *Agonal Phase Warm Ischemia*: Commences upon the withdrawal of life-sustaining therapy (WLST) and continues until cardiac arrest. A prolonged agonal phase characterized by severe arterial hypoxemia ($SpO2 < 80\%$) and systemic hypotension (systolic blood pressure < 80 mmHg) induces microvascular endothelial swelling, intravascular thrombosis, and intracellular ATP depletion.
- *True Warm Ischemia Time (WIT)*: Measures the duration from circulatory standstill (cardiac arrest) through the mandatory observation period (typically 5 min to confirm death) until the initiation of cold in situ vascular flush or regional normothermic perfusion.

Ischemia-Reperfusion Injury (IRI) and Delayed Graft Function

Upon restoration of blood flow in the recipient, the accumulated warm ischemic damage triggers a severe inflammatory cascade known as ischemia-reperfusion injury (IRI) [16]. Reoxygenation disrupts mitochondrial electron transport chain function, driving the rapid release of reactive oxygen species (ROS), activation of the complement cascade (specifically C3a and C5a), neutrophil infiltration, and massive pro-inflammatory cytokine release (IL-1, IL-6, TNF-α).

- *Delayed Graft Function (DGF)*: Clinically defined as the requirement for renal replacement therapy within the first 7 days post-transplantation. DGF rates in DCD kidney recipients range from 40% to 70%, compared to 20–30% in standard DBD recipients [5, 34].
- *Primary Non-Function (PNF)*: Irreversible failure of the transplanted organ to establish metabolic function, requiring persistent dialysis or immediate re-transplantation. While DGF is significantly elevated in DCD, PNF rates remain low (2% to 5%) provided total warm ischemia times are maintained within strict clinical thresholds (typically true WIT <30 min) [30].

Despite the higher burden of DGF and early acute tubular necrosis (ATN), large registry datasets confirm that long-term death-adjusted graft survival (DAGS) and recipient survival for DCD kidneys are equivalent to those of standard-criteria DBD kidneys [11, 31].

The Elderly Transplant Recipient: Frailty, Comorbidities, and Pre-transplant Workup

As the global incidence of chronic kidney disease increases, candidates aged 65 years and older represent the fastest-growing segment of the renal transplant waiting list worldwide. Managing elderly candidates requires evaluating physiological age and functional reserve rather than chronological age alone.

Frailty, Sarcopenia, and Multimorbidity Frailty is a vulnerable physiological state characterized by diminished physiological reserve and heightened vulnerability to acute stressors. In patients with ESRD, frailty is exacerbated by uremic toxicity, chronic low-grade inflammation, metabolic acidosis, and protein-energy wasting [15].

- *Fried Frailty Phenotype*: Assesses five clinical domains: unintentional weight loss, self-reported exhaustion, low physical activity, slow walking speed, and weak grip strength.
- *Clinical Impact*: Frail elderly kidney transplant recipients suffer significantly higher rates of early post-operative mortality, prolonged hospital stays, 30-day readmissions, and elevated susceptibility to immunosuppressive drug toxicities [14].

Common comorbid conditions in elderly ESRD candidates include:

- Advanced multi-vessel coronary artery disease (CAD).
- Peripheral vascular disease (PVD) and iliac artery calcification.
- Left ventricular hypertrophy (LVH) and heart failure with preserved ejection fraction (HFpEF).

- Type 2 diabetes mellitus and diabetic micro/macrovascular complications.
- Cerebrovascular disease and subclinical cognitive impairment.

Pre-transplant Assessment Protocol for the Elderly To select candidates who will achieve a meaningful survival benefit while minimizing perioperative mortality, elderly patients undergo targeted screening:

Cardiovascular Risk Stratification: Non-invasive stress imaging (dobutamine stress echocardiography or myocardial perfusion scintigraphy) is recommended for all candidates aged>60 years or with long-standing diabetes. Invasive coronary angiography is indicated for abnormalities on non-invasive tests or clinical angina [3].
Vascular Anatomy Mapping: Non-contrast pelvic computed tomography (CT) to quantify iliac artery calcification. Severe circumferential "porcelain iliacs" can preclude safe surgical vascular anastomosis.
Malignancy Screening: Comprehensive age-appropriate cancer screening including colonoscopy, mammography, cervical cytology, prostate-specific antigen (PSA), and low-dose chest CT for patients with significant smoking histories.
Cognitive and Functional Evaluation: Baseline cognitive assessment using the Mini-Mental State Examination (MMSE) or Montreal Cognitive Assessment (MoCA). Cognitive impairment impairs complex post-transplant medication adherence and increases delirium risk.
Immunological Assessment: Evaluation of panel reactive antibody (PRA) levels and human leukocyte antigen (HLA) sensitization status. In elderly candidates, prioritizing a rapid match over precise HLA matching often yields better survival by minimizing pre-transplant dialysis exposure [23].

Expanded Criteria Donors (ECD) and Marginal DCD Organs in the Elderly

To reduce waitlist mortality among older candidates, transplant programs frequently utilize expanded criteria donors (ECD) and high-risk DCD organs.

Defining Marginal and ECD Criteria Historically, an ECD donor was defined by United Network for Organ Sharing (UNOS) guidelines as any donor aged ≥60 years, or a donor aged 50–59 years with at least two of the following clinical metrics:

- Pre-existing history of systemic hypertension.
- Terminal serum creatinine >1.5 mg/dL (> 132 μmol/L).
- Cause of death secondary to a cerebrovascular accident (CVA).

In modern practice, the Kidney Donor Profile Index (KDPI) in the US replaced the binary ECD system. KDPI measures donor quality on a continuous percentile scale from 0% to 100% relative to the prior year's donor pool. Kidneys with a KDPI

>85% represent high-risk marginal grafts that meet or exceed traditional ECD criteria [11].

The "Dual Hit": Combining DCD with Marginal/ECD Characteristics When an organ donor is both advanced in age (or meets ECD/high-KDPI criteria) and donated via the DCD pathway, the resulting graft suffers a compounding physiological insult:

Pre-Existing Structural Damage: Chronic nephron loss, glomerulosclerosis, vascular hyalinosis, and interstitial fibrosis/tubular atrophy (IFTA) associated with donor aging and hypertension.

Acute Ischemic Injury: Severe warm ischemia during the agonal and retrieval phases superimposed on nephrons with reduced repair capacity.

To safely utilize these marginal DCD kidneys without excessive discard rates, specialized strategies are deployed, including continuous machine perfusion dynamics and histological pre-transplant biopsy scoring (e.g., the Remuzzi score). Grafts with moderate scores may be utilized as Dual Kidney Transplants (allocating both kidneys from one marginal donor into a single elderly recipient) to ensure sufficient functioning nephron mass ([27]; [28]).

Donor-Recipient Age Matching and Allocation Strategies

Allocating donor organs requires balancing utility (maximizing graft and patient life-years gained) with equity (ensuring fair access for older or highly sensitized candidates). Table 18.2 summarizes the allocation systems for elderly recipients worldwide.

Table 18.2 Allocation systems across the world for elderly recipient

Allocation system	Primary objective	Age thresholds	HLA matching requirement	Cold ischemia minimization strategy
Eurotransplant Senior Program (ESP)	Regional placement; reduce wait time	Donor ≥65, recipient ≥65	Completely waived	Strict local/regional allocation to minimize transit time
US OPTN (KDPI/EPTS)	Longevity matching across continuous spectrum	Stratified via continuous EPTS/KDPI	Secondary priority for high KDPI	Local/Regional priority for KDPI >85% grafts
UK NHSBT scheme	Tiered longevity matching and equity	Age-stratified recipient tiers	Weighted based on recipient sensitization	Fast-track allocation protocol for marginal/DCD organs

The Eurotransplant Senior Program (ESP) Established in 1999, the Eurotransplant Senior Program ("Old-for-Old") specifically matches donors aged ≥65 years with recipients aged ≥65 years [4].

- *Key Principles*: ESP prioritizes local and regional organ placement to minimize cold ischemia time (CIT) and waives standard HLA-A, -B, and -DR matching requirements.
- *Clinical Outcomes*: The ESP model significantly reduces waitlist time for elderly candidates and limits cold ischemic damage. Although HLA mismatches are associated with a slightly higher incidence of acute rejection, overall patient survival is preserved by shortening pre-transplant dialysis duration [23].

United States Allocation: The KDPI/EPTS System The US OPTN allocation system utilizes the Estimated Post-Transplant Survival (EPTS) score to quantify recipient longevity based on age, candidate time on dialysis, prior solid organ transplants, and diabetes status:

- Recipients with the lowest 20% of EPTS scores (i.e., those with the highest predicted post-transplant longevity, usually younger candidates) are preferentially allocated kidneys with KDPI ≤20%.
- Elderly candidates (who possess higher EPTS scores) are prioritized for high-KDPI kidneys (KDPI >85%), including elderly DCD grafts. This alignment matches expected graft survival with recipient life expectancy [11].

UK Allocation Scheme The NHSBT kidney allocation scheme balances longevity matching with equitable geographical access. High-risk or elderly DCD kidneys are directed through a dedicated non-standard allocation stream, enabling rapid regional placement into older candidates to prevent prolonged CIT [19].

Outcomes of DCD Kidney Transplantation in Elderly Recipients

Evaluating DCD kidney transplantation in elderly recipients (aged ≥65 years) requires assessing short-term complications such as DGF alongside long-term graft durability and overall patient survival.

Delayed Graft Function (DGF) and Primary Non-function (PNF) In elderly recipients receiving DCD kidneys, DGF rates range from 55% to 75% due to the additive effects of recipient vascular stiffness, altered drug clearance, and donor organ warm ischemic injury ([34]; [7]). DGF in elderly recipients often resolves slowly, extending post-operative recovery. However, when total warm ischemia times are carefully restricted (<30 min true WIT), PNF rates in elderly DCD recipients remain between 3% and 6%, comparable to younger recipient cohorts [30].

Graft Survival, Patient Survival, and Functional Outcomes

- *Death-Adjusted Graft Survival (DAGS)*: Multi-center studies confirm that DAGS at 1, 5, and 10 years post-transplant in elderly recipients of DCD kidneys does not differ significantly from elderly recipients of DBD kidneys (1-year DAGS: ~90–93%; 5-year DAGS: ~75–82%) [23, 31].
- *Patient Survival*: Patient survival in elderly DCD recipients is largely governed by cardiovascular disease and severe post-transplant infection rather than primary immunologic graft failure. Death with a functioning graft (DWFG) remains the leading cause of overall graft loss in elderly populations.
- *Renal Function (eGFR)*: Mean estimated Glomerular Filtration Rate (eGFR) at 1 and 5 years post-transplant in elderly DCD recipients typically ranges from 30 to 42 mL/min/1.73 m^2. While lower than function seen in younger cohorts, this level of native clearance removes the need for renal replacement therapy and resolves uremic toxicity.

Survival Benefit: DCD Kidney Transplantation Versus Dialysis in the Elderly

A central clinical decision in nephrology is whether an elderly patient should accept a high-risk or marginal DCD kidney organ offer or remain on maintenance dialysis.

Survival Advantage Analysis Large observational studies and registry evaluations confirm a clear long-term survival advantage for elderly candidates who receive DCD transplants compared to remaining on the waiting list on hemodialysis or peritoneal dialysis [5, 25]:

- *Initial Perioperative Risk*: During the immediate post-transplant period (0–3 months), transplanted elderly recipients experience a transient increase in mortality risk compared to waitlisted control patients. This early risk spike is driven by surgical trauma, anesthesia exposure, perioperative cardiovascular events, and initial high-dose immunosuppressive induction.
- *Survival Crossover Point*: The cumulative survival curves cross at approximately 3–6 months post-transplantation. Beyond this inflexion point, the relative risk of mortality drops significantly below that of dialyzed waitlist candidates.
- *Long-Term Mortality Reduction*: Over a 5-year follow-up period, elderly recipients of DCD kidneys demonstrate a 40–60% reduction in all-cause mortality compared with matched waitlisted candidates who remain on chronic dialysis ([25]; [23]).

Quality of Life and Health Economics Beyond mortality reduction, kidney transplantation offers significant gains in health-related quality of life (HRQoL) for elderly recipients. Physical vitality metrics, cognitive function, cardiovascular health, and personal autonomy improve following the cessation of maintenance dialysis. From an economic perspective, although the initial cost of DCD kidney transplantation is higher due to DGF management and index hospitalization, the procedure becomes cost-effective relative to chronic dialysis within 2–3 years post-transplant [24].

Immunosuppression Strategies in Elderly DCD Recipients

Designing immunosuppressive protocols for elderly DCD recipients requires balancing the risk of allograft rejection against the risks of immunosenescence, severe infection, and pharmacological nephrotoxicity.

Immunosenescence and Immune Function Immunosenescence refers to the progressive age-related dysregulation of the immune system, characterized by:

- Thymic involution resulting in reduced output of naive T-cells.
- Relative expansion of terminally differentiated memory T-cells (CD28null).
- Impaired antigen presentation by dendritic cells and reduced IL-2 production.
- Decreased primary humoral antibody responses by B-cells.

As a consequence of immunosenescence, acute cellular rejection rates are generally lower in elderly recipients. However, when rejection episodes occur, elderly patients demonstrate reduced renal functional recovery and suffer higher morbidity from high-dose pulse corticosteroid rescue therapy [6].

Individualized Immunosuppressive Regimens These include induction and maintenance therapies.

Induction Therapy: Induction therapy protects against acute rejection and reduces severe IRI during early DGF recovery:

- *Interleukin-2 Receptor Antagonists (IL-2RA—Basiliximab)*: Preferred in non-sensitized elderly recipients. Basiliximab provides targeted immunosuppression without systemic lymphocyte depletion, avoiding increases in post-operative opportunistic infection rates.
- *Rabbit Anti-Thymocyte Globulin (rATG)*: Indicated for highly sensitized elderly recipients or cases with prolonged warm ischemia times. Lymphocyte-depleting induction allows for delayed initiation or dose-reduction of calcineurin inhibitors (CNIs), protecting fragile allografts from early nephrotoxicity during recovery from ATN [35].

Maintenance Therapy

- *Calcineurin Inhibitors (CNI)*: Tacrolimus remains the cornerstone of maintenance regimens. However, targeted trough concentrations are kept lower in elderly recipients (5–8 ng/mL in early months; 3–5 ng/mL after 6 months) to mitigate chronic CNI nephrotoxicity, neurotoxicity, and post-transplant diabetes mellitus (PTDM).

- *Antimetabolites*: Mycophenolate Mofetil (MMF) or Mycophenolic Acid (MPA). Dose reductions are frequently necessary in elderly patients due to bone marrow suppression (leukopenia) and gastrointestinal toxicities.
- *Corticosteroid Minimization*: Protocols involving rapid steroid tapering to low maintenance doses (5 mg/day) or complete withdrawal within 7 days are widely implemented in low-immunological-risk elderly recipients to minimize steroid-related osteoporosis, cardiovascular disease, and metabolic instability.

Opportunistic Infection Prophylaxis Elderly recipients receive extended antimicrobial prophylaxis due to their combined net state of immunosuppression:

- *Cytomegalovirus (CMV)*: Valganciclovir prophylaxis for 3–6 months based on donor/recipient serostatus (D+/R- requiring high vigilance).
- *Pneumocystis Jirovecii Pneumonia (PJP)*: Trimethoprim-sulfamethoxazole (TMP-SMX) daily for a minimum of 6–12 months post-transplant.

Advanced Organ Preservation and Optimization Techniques in DCD

The expansion of DCD transplantation in older populations relies on advances in ex vivo machine perfusion and in situ regional preservation designed to mitigate warm ischemia-reperfusion injury (Table 18.3).

Table 18.3 Advanced organ preservation models

Preservation technology	Temperature range	Primary mechanism of action	Clinical benefits in DCD	Current adoption status
Static Cold Storage (SCS)	2–4 °C	Slows cellular metabolism via hypothermia	Low cost; simple setup	Declining usage for DCD organs due to higher DGF risk
Hypothermic Machine Perfusion (HMP)	4–8 °C	Vascular flushing; continuous dynamic flow	Decreases DGF rates vs SCS; allows viability assessment	Standard of care in UK, US, and Eurotransplant networks
Hypothermic Oxygenated Perfusion (HOPE)	4–8 °C	Active oxygenation; recharges mitochondrial ATP	Reduces ROS generation, DGF severity, and acute rejection	Widely adopted in European centers; expanding in US

(continued)

Table 18.3 (continued)

Preservation technology	Temperature range	Primary mechanism of action	Clinical benefits in DCD	Current adoption status
Normothermic Regional Perfusion (A-NRP)	37 °C (In situ)	ECMO-based oxygenated blood recirculation	Reverses agonal ischemia; lowers DGF to DBD levels	Rapidly expanding standard in UK, Spain, France, and US

Hypothermic Machine Perfusion (HMP) and Oxygenated HMP (HOPE) Static cold storage (SCS) alone is insufficient for fragile DCD kidneys. Continuous Hypothermic Machine Perfusion (HMP) at 4–8 °C continuously recirculates an acellular perfusate through the renal vasculature, flushing toxic metabolic waste products, supplying substrate, and allowing real-time assessment of renal vascular resistance and flow parameters [17].

- *Hypothermic Oxygenated Perfusion (HOPE)*: Supplying active oxygenation to the perfusate during low-temperature machine preservation enables mitochondrial electron transport chain re-energization and re-accumulates ATP stores without generating harmful ROS. Clinical trials demonstrate that HOPE significantly decreases DGF rates, reduces acute rejection, and improves early graft function in high-risk DCD organs ([9]; [26]).

Normothermic Regional Perfusion (NRP) Abdominal Normothermic Regional Perfusion (A-NRP) utilizes an extracorporeal membrane oxygenation (ECMO) circuit to restore oxygenated blood flow at physiological body temperature (37 °C) to abdominal organs in situ following the clinical declaration of death and a mandatory standoff observation period [20].

- *Mechanistic Advantages*: A-NRP reverses acute cellular ischemic damage sustained during the agonal phase, restores tissue ATP levels prior to surgical retrieval, and enables functional evaluation of organ viability (assessing lactate clearance, macroperfusion, and acid-base balance) prior to organ recovery.
- *Clinical Impact*: Kidney allografts recovered using A-NRP display lower DGF rates (reducing rates from ~60% down to 20–30%), lower discard rates, and long-term graft survival outcomes comparable to DBD transplants ([21]; [22]).

DCD/ DCD-ECD in Elderly Recipients: Indian Context

In India, as in many low- and middle-income countries, adults aged 18–50 years constitute the largest cohort of patients with end-stage renal disease receiving dialysis. This burden is driven by primary glomerular diseases, early-onset hypertension, and unknown or toxic causes [33]. This pattern informed NOTTO's policy of prioritizing younger and middle-aged patients for wait-listing and setting the maximum recipient age at 65 years. However, mirroring global trends, India is experiencing a rise in lifestyle-related diseases alongside increasing life expectancy. Advances in drug therapy and guideline-directed medical treatment, greater awareness of cardiovascular mortality, and improved access to healthcare are expected to contribute to a disproportionate increase in the number of older adults receiving dialysis. Analysis of elderly patients receiving transplant from living donors from South India [13], documented better death censored graft survival with less acute rejection but patient survival was challenged by existing comorbidities like CAD, and recurrent hospitalization with infection probably related to immune senescence and reactivation of latent infection, necessitating personalized and softer immunosuppression protocol in this age group, along with careful selection of recipient with less frailty and comorbidity burden. The study from North India [1] reiterated similar hope of comparable death censored graft survival and patient survival at 5 years in elderly group with similar incidence of biopsy-proven acute rejection when compared to a younger cohort. Urinary tract infection was the most common infectious complication. Sepsis was the primary cause of death in both groups. These observations translated in removal of capping of 65 years from prospective wait-listing with expectation of increase in older patients in waitlist. Here lies the relevance of discussing the future policy adoption for India where a separate elderly waitlist registry may be created to facilitate organ allocation like Euro-Senior program where older recipient may receive a prioritized local and regional allocation of graft from older donors arising from neuro-ICU with metabolic challenges, to decrease CIT and match the expected graft survival and patient survival with advantage of better quality of life for the recipients compared to the waitlisted patients on dialysis.

Dr. Ghazanfar presented Western evidence showing a survival advantage of Donation After Circulatory Death (DCD) transplantation over dialysis in older adults. He outlined three allocation models: the Euro transplant Senior Program, the US Organ Procurement and Transplantation Network system based on Kidney Donor Profile Index(KDPI) and Estimated Post-Transplant Survival (EPTS) scores, and the NHS Blood and Transplant system. The first two priorities rapid allocation without weighting HLA matching, whereas the NHSBT model combines rapid regional allocation with HLA matching. As several Indian centers have begun using virtual crossmatch-based allocation, both approaches could be piloted at selected advanced centers before a national policy is adopted. Economic sustainability is also crucial for India as a low- and middle-income country because outcomes with DCD kidneys from expanded criteria donors may be compromised by higher rates of primary non-function and delayed graft function when static cold storage is used. Normothermic regional perfusion may increase costs, but it could reduce delayed graft function to rates comparable with those seen after donation following brain death.

Careful recipient selection (CAD and cardiovascular risk assessment, infection screening including latent tuberculosis, malignancy screening, frailty assessment), individualized immunosuppression (with a relatively lower target level for CNI with minimum steroid exposure) and strategic infrastructure enhancement with trained and motivated workforce may minimize the initial hiccups obvious with implementation of a new policy.

Competing Interests The author(s) has no competing interests to declare that are relevant to the content of this manuscript.

Ethics Approval The author(s) declares that this manuscript does not include primary research with human participants.

The author(s) declares that this manuscript does not include primary studies involving animals.

References

1. Bhargava V, Meena P, Agrawaal K, Gaur L, Rana D, Bhalla A, et al. Outcomes of kidney transplantation in the elderly recipients. Indian J Nephrol. 2021;31:370–6.
2. Dominguez-Gil B, Ascher N, Capron AM, Cantarovich F, Gastaldello K, Matesanz R, et al. Expanding controlled donation after circulatory death: policy considerations and global perspectives. Kidney Int. 2021;99(5):1062–70. https://doi.org/10.1016/j.kint.2020.12.026.
3. Dudley C, Harden P, Roderick P. Assessment and preparation of elderly candidates for renal transplantation. Transplant Rev. 2019;33(3):145–52. https://doi.org/10.1016/j.trre.2019.03.002.
4. Frei U, Noeldeke J, Machold-Fabrizii V, Arbogast H, Margreiter R, Fricke L, et al. Prospective age-matching in elderly kidney transplant recipients—5-year results of the Eurotransplant Senior Programme. Nephrology Dialysis Transplantation. 2008;23(2):722–8. https://doi.org/10.1093/ndt/gfm670.
5. Gill J, Rose C, Lesage J, Joffres Y, Gill J. Use and outcomes of kidneys from donation after circulatory death donors in elderly recipients. Clin J Am Soc Nephrol. 2016;11(12):2239–47. https://doi.org/10.2215/CJN.03880416.
6. Heinbokel T, Elkhal A, Liu G, Edtinger K, Tullius SG. Immunosenescence and European Senior Programme—the challenge of transplanting elderly patients. Transpl Int. 2013;26(3):242–53. https://doi.org/10.1111/tri.12002.
7. Hetzel GR, Klein B, Brausen C, Voiculescu A, Grabensee B. Delayed graft function in elderly renal transplant recipients: risk factors and prognostic impact. Transplant Proc. 2018;50(4):1021–8. https://doi.org/10.1016/j.transproceed.2018.01.042.
8. Husain SA, King KL, Pastan S, Patzer RE, Cohen DJ, Radhakrishnan J, et al. Association between decline in donor kidney utilisation and donor age, KDPI, and DCD status. Am J Transplant. 2019;19(4):1045–56. https://doi.org/10.1111/ajt.15132.
9. Jochmans I, Brat A, Davies L, Hofker HS, van de Leemkolk FE, Leuvenink HG, et al. Oxygenated hypothermic machine perfusion of kidneys donated after circulatory death: a randomised controlled trial. Lancet. 2020;396(10263):1665–74. https://doi.org/10.1016/S0140-6736(20)32411-1.
10. Kers J, Boffa C, Jochmans I, Hunter JP. Donation after circulatory death in Europe: historical trends and current allocation practices. Curr Opin Organ Transplant. 2018;23(3):325–32. https://doi.org/10.1097/MOT.0000000000000529.
11. Lentine KL, Smith JM, Miller JM, Bradbrook K, Larkin L, Weiss S, Handarova DK, Temple K, Israni AK, Snyder JJ. OPTN/SRTR 2021 annual data report: kidney. Am J Transplant. 2023;23(2 Suppl 1):S21–S120. https://doi.org/10.1016/j.ajt.2023.02.004.
12. Mainz K, Schmidt M, Schulte U. Legal obstacles and ethical considerations regarding donation after circulatory death in Central Europe. J Med Ethics. 2022;48(9):612–8. https://doi.org/10.1136/medethics-2021-107432.

13. Mohamed Ali AA, Abraham G, Khanna P, Reddy YN, Mehrotra A, Mathew M, Sundararaj S, Jasmine R. Renal transplantation in the elderly: South Indian experience. Int Urol Nephrol. 2011 Mar;43(1):265–71.
14. McAdams-DeMarco MA, King EA, Luo X, Haugen C, DiBrito S, Shaffer A, et al. Frailty, length of stay, and 30-day readmission after kidney transplantation in elderly recipients. Ann Surg. 2017;265(4):808–14. https://doi.org/10.1097/SLA.0000000000001712.
15. McAdams-DeMarco MA, Law A, Tan J, Salter ML, Walston J, Segev DL. Frailty, post-transplant outcomes, and cognitive function in older kidney transplant recipients. J Am Soc Nephrol. 2015;26(9):2243–9. https://doi.org/10.1681/ASN.2014070718.
16. McKenney C, Torabi J, Todd R, Akhtar MZ, Tedla FM, Shapiro R, Florman SS, Holzner ML, van Leeuwen LL. Wasted potential: decoding the trifecta of donor kidney shortage, underutilization, and rising discard rates. Transplantology. 2024;5(2):51–64. https://doi.org/10.3390/transplantology5020006.
17. Moers C, Smits JM, Maathuis MH, Treckmann J, van Gelder F, Napieralski BP, et al. Machine perfusion or cold storage in deceased-donor kidney transplantation. N Engl J Med. 2009;360(1):7–19. https://doi.org/10.1056/NEJMoa0802289.
18. Molina M, Guerrero A, Ruiz P. Results of uncontrolled donation after circulatory death kidney transplantation: the Spanish experience. Transpl Int. 2019;32(8):801–11. https://doi.org/10.1111/tri.13421.
19. Mumford L, Watson CJ, Johnson RJ. Assessment of the UK national kidney allocation scheme: impact on DCD and marginal donor utilization. Am J Transplant. 2020;20(6):1589–98. https://doi.org/10.1111/ajt.15760.
20. Oniscu GC, Randle LV, Muiesan P, Butler AJ, Currie IS, Perera MT, et al. In situ normothermic regional perfusion in donation after circulatory death donors: the UK experience. Am J Transplant. 2014;14(11):2546–53. https://doi.org/10.1111/ajt.12920.
21. Padilla MD, Coll E, Fernandez-Pello S, Dominguez-Gil B. Abdominal normothermic regional perfusion in controlled donation after circulatory death: outcomes in renal transplantation. Transplantation. 2021;105(6):1282–90. https://doi.org/10.1097/TP.0000000000003513.
22. Pearson R, Hunter J, Watson C. Normothermic machine perfusion and regional perfusion in kidney transplantation: A clinical review. Curr Transplant Rep. 2021;8(2):112–23. https://doi.org/10.10007/s40472-021-00325-1.
23. Peters-Sengers H, Homan van der Heide JJ, Heemskerk MB, ten Berge IJ, Berger SP, van der Pant KA, et al. Similar survival for kidneys from donors after circulatory death and donors after brain death in elderly recipients. J Am Soc Nephrol. 2017;28(1):341–52. https://doi.org/10.1681/ASN.2015091054.
24. Pippias M, Jager KJ, Kramer A, Leivestad T, Sanchez MB, Caskey FJ, et al. Burden of kidney replacement therapy in the elderly: a European perspective. Nephrology Dialysis Transplantation. 2018;33(8):1412–22. https://doi.org/10.1093/ndt/gfx341.
25. Rao PS, Schaubel DE, Guidinger MK, Andreoni KA, Wolfe RA, Merion RM, et al. A comprehensive risk quantification score for deceased donor kidneys: the Kidney Donor Risk Index. Transplantation. 2009;88(2):231–6. https://doi.org/10.1097/TP.0b013e3181ac620b.
26. Ravaioli M, De Pace V, Angeletti A, Comai G, Vasuri F, Baldassarre M, et al. Hypothermic oxygenated machine perfusion (HOPE) for kidney transplantation from donors after circulatory death: A clinical trial. Sci Rep. 2020;10(1):16342. https://doi.org/10.1038/s41598-020-73330-8.
27. Remuzzi G, Cravedi P, Perna A, Dimitrov BD, Turturro M, Locatelli G, et al. Long-term outcome of renal transplantation from older donors: A prospective, multicenter, randomized study using pre-transplant biopsy scoring. Ann Intern Med. 2006;144(11):793–800. https://doi.org/10.7326/0003-4819-144-11-200606060-00005.
28. Rigotti P, Capovilla G, Di Bella C, Silvestre C, Donato P, Luini B, et al. Dual kidney transplantation from expanded criteria donors: long-term results in elderly recipients. Transplantation. 2014;97(12):1241–6. https://doi.org/10.1097/TP.0000000000000010.

29. Saeb-Parsy K, Bradley JA, Pettigrew GJ. Donation after circulatory death kidney transplantation: Progress, challenges, and opportunities. Kidney Int. 2016;89(6):1201–10. https://doi.org/10.1016/j.kint.2016.01.025.
30. Siddiqi N, Boffa C, Watson CJ, Pettigrew GJ. Primary non-function and delayed graft function in DCD kidney transplantation: risk factors and outcomes. Transpl Int. 2021;34(5):890–901. https://doi.org/10.1111/tri.13852.
31. Summers DM, Johnson RJ, Allen J, Fuggle SV, Collett D, Watson CJ, Bradley JA. Analysis of factors that affect outcome after transplantation of kidneys donated after cardiac death in the UK: a cohort study. Lancet. 2015;376(9749):1303–11. https://doi.org/10.1016/S0140-6736(10)60827-6.
32. Thuong AM, Ruiz A, Evrard P. New classification of donation after circulatory death donors: definitions and terminology. Transplant Proc. 2016;48(8):2485–9. https://doi.org/10.1016/j.transproceed.2016.06.040.
33. Kalra V, Agarwal D, Anis Y. Profiling of kidney disease undergoing hemodialysis. Int J Res Med Sci. 2025;13(6):2398–403.
34. Weber M, Farney AC, Rogers J. Delayed graft function in donation after circulatory death kidney transplantation: pathophysiology and clinical interventions. Curr Opin Organ Transplant. 2020;25(1):34–41. https://doi.org/10.1097/MOT.0000000000000721.
35. Wiseman AC. Immunosuppression in the elderly transplant recipient: balancing risk of rejection and infection. Curr Transplant Rep. 2015;2(3):221–8. https://doi.org/10.1007/s40472-015-0063-2.

Part VII

Training, Public Engagement and Future Directions in DCD

Training Framework in Donation After Circulatory Death Transplantation

19

Jumana Yusuf Haji and Shrikanth Srinivasan

Introduction

Organ donation after circulatory determination of death (DCD) is one of the most complex, time-sensitive, and ethically nuanced frontiers in modern transplant medicine. Every step before transplant from donor identification to organ preservation demands precision, coordination, and absolute clarity. In this evolving landscape, hesitation, lack of protocol, or fragmented training can directly impact organ viability and transplant outcomes. Clinicians today often encounter DCD in isolated fragments—guidelines, case discussions, or observational exposure—without ever experiencing a structured, end-to-end understanding of the process. The absence of hands-on exposure to techniques like normothermic regional perfusion (NRP) further limits confidence in real-world implementation.

Training should include a theoretical overview along with a focused, protocol-driven, simulation-backed program that equips clinicians with the technical, clinical, ethical, and logistical expertise as well as the skills required to execute DCD with precision and coordination.

Training guidelines for a donation after circulatory death (DCD) normothermic regional perfusion (NRP) program require a multidisciplinary approach focusing on specialized surgical techniques, perfusion management, and strict adherence to ethical protocols. Effective programs often utilize simulation-based training to prepare teams for rapid, high-stakes procedures.

Brain-stem death allows for sustained organ perfusion via ventilation, whereas donation after circulatory death (DCD) occurs following cardiac arrest, creating

J. Y. Haji (✉)
Fortis Hospital Mulund, Mumbai, Maharashtra, India
e-mail: ecmo@drjumana.in

S. Srinivasan
Manipal Institute of Critical Care Medicine, Manipal Hospitals, New Delhi, Delhi, India

S. P. Kolte et al. (eds.), *Organ Donation After Circulatory Death*,
https://doi.org/10.1007/978-981-92-6377-6_19

urgency for organ retrieval due to potential ischemic damage. Both BSD and DCD require Form 8 certification and Form 10 consent in India. DCD is time-sensitive and needs meticulous teamwork and innovations like hypothermic oxygenated perfusion (HOPE) and normothermic regional perfusion (nRP) to improve organ preservation. A successful DCD program in India requires specialized training for medical teams, including proficiency in perfusion technology, logistics, and consent management.

DCD programs thrive in nations that permit families to withdraw life support from terminally ill patients when further medical intervention becomes futile. They also flourish in regions backed by robust emergency medical services (EMS) for out-of-hospital cardiac arrests. When paramedical teams initiate high-quality cardiopulmonary resuscitation (CPR) within minutes of an arrest, and a well-coordinated ambulance network ensures swift hospital transfer, the vital organs remain oxygenated. While this rapid response maximizes the chances of saving the patient, DCD serves as a viable, life-saving alternative if resuscitation ultimately fails [1].

Key Training Components for DCD NRP Programs

NRP program in India would require pathways which are supported with multidisciplinary training. The training should cover technical, ethical, and legal aspects.

Clinical training parameters aim facilitate improvement in tissue hypoxia and viability of organs. Technical domain which includes knowledge of perfusion technologies from set up to troubleshooting is necessary. Finally, there is a logistic domain which would teach the team members use of checklists, mandatory consents, and time keeping documentation (Table 19.1).

Table 19.1 Key training components of a DCD NRP program

DCD NRP Training Modules Matrix

Module	Target Audience	Core Learning Objectives	Hands-on & Assessment Methods
1. Legal, Ethical, & Regulatory	• Intensivists • Surgeons • Coordinators	• Mastery of the "Dead Donor Rule" • Strict auditing of the 5–10 min "no-touch" window • Legal protocols for WLST	• Video audit case reviews • Family communication role-play • Written compliance examination
2. Perfusion & Circuit Mechanics	• Perfusionists • Intensivists • Anaesthetists	• ECMO circuit design & priming for NRP • Prevention of cerebral reperfusion • Goal-directed biochemical management	• Mechanical pump failure dry-runs • Real-time blood gas analysis drills • Balloon inflation verification tests
3. Surgical Cannulation Pathways	• Transplant Surgeons • Theatre Nurses	• Rapid median sternotomy & vessel ligation (TA-NRP) • Direct aortic/caval cannulation (A-NRP) • Minimising warm ischemic time (fWIT)	• Perfused cadaver/tissue wet labs • High-speed surgical mock drills • Minimum 5 cases as second-surgeon
4. In-Situ Organ Assessment	• Transplant Surgeons • Perfusionists	• Evaluation of "beating heart" contractility • Tracking liver lactate clearance trends • Quantifying real-time bile production	• Echocardiography (TEE) interpretation • Serial blood-gas biomarker tracking • Organ viability scoring checklists
5. Crisis Simulation & Flush	• Full Multidisciplinary Recovery Team	• Troubleshooting massive line clots/air emboli • Coordinated team communication under stress • Seamless transition from NRP to cold flush	• High-fidelity team-based simulation • Unannounced circuit emergency drills • Objective Structured Clinical Exams

Multidisciplinary Team Training (Table 19.2)

Training must involve surgeons, perfusionists, nursing staff, intensive care specialists, and transplant coordinators. Multidisciplinary buy-in and communication and understanding of the new protocol are essential. This requires simulation training which ensures improved communication, teamwork behaviors, and team attitudes in high-risk perioperative environments [2, 3].

Prioritizing simulation education during the implementation phase allows for the vital integration of multidisciplinary teams. These sessions are structured around four key educational pillars: mastering crisis resource management, strengthening team collaboration, aligning staff with local protocols, and facilitating hands-on skills acquisition. By simulating real-world scenarios, team members can safely master complex workflows before engaging in live clinical environments.

Table 19.2 DCD NRP training modules matrix

Module	Target audience	Core learning objectives	Hands-on and assessment methods
1. Legal, ethical, and regulatory	Intensivists Surgeons Coordinators	Mastery of the "Dead donor rule" Strict auditing of the 5–10 min "no-touch" window Legal protocols for WLST	Video audit case reviews Family communication role-play Written compliance examination
2. Perfusion and circuit mechanics	Perfusionists Intensivists Anaesthetists	ECMO circuit design and priming for NRP Prevention of cerebral reperfusion Goal-directed biochemical management	Mechanical pump failure dry-runs Real-time blood-gas analysis drills Balloon inflation verification tests
3. Surgical cannulation pathways	Transplant surgeons Theater nurses	Rapid median sternotomy and vessel ligation (TA-NRP) Direct aortic/caval cannulation (A-NRP) Minimising warm ischemic time (fWIT)	Perfused cadaver/tissue wet labs High-speed surgical mock drills Minimum 5 cases as second-surgeon
4. In situ organ assessment	Transplant surgeons Perfusionists	Evaluation of "beating heart" contractility Tracking liver lactate clearance trends Quantifying real-time bile production	Echocardiography (TEE) interpretation Serial blood-gas biomarker tracking Organ viability scoring checklists
5. Crisis simulation and flush	Full multidisciplinary recovery team	Troubleshooting massive line clots/air emboli Coordinated team communication under stress Seamless transition from NRP to cold flush	High-fidelity team-based simulation Unannounced circuit emergency drills Objective structured clinical exams

Simulation and dry-runs should cover machine setup, surgical techniques, and troubleshooting scenarios (Fig. 19.1). Simulations include rapid cannulation of femoral vein and arteries on mannequins or femoral cutdown and direct cannulation on cadaveric models (Fig. 19.2). Practicing rapid entry, exposure of the aorta, and cannulation on cadavers or models must also be advocated. Troubleshooting dry-runs include practicing scenarios such as equipment failure before actual donor attendance [4].

Standard protocols must be followed for heparin administration to prevent thrombosis, and management of functional warm ischemic time (fWIT), 5-min no-touch observation period after circulatory arrest before commencing NRP and specific protocols exist for DCDD category IV (cardiac arrest during brain death declaration) [5].

DCD NRP training essentials as per steps included in the Indian position paper are shown in (Fig. 19.3) [6].

The training requirements for all personnel are different, and the two main stake holders would be the critical care/emergency medicine and the surgical teams.

Emergency medicine personnel pathway training is important in European countries like Spain where the policy is "opt out." In these countries, the DCD and NRP planning and execution take place in the emergency department for out-of-hospital arrests and uncontrolled Maastricht category donors. In India, currently, the focus is on developing DCD and DCD NRP protocols in-hospital ICU patients as part of end of life care pathway [6, 7].

Intensivists must fulfill comprehensive clinical, legal, and operational training criteria to participate in donation after circulatory death (DCD) with

Fig. 19.1 Circuit set up and circulation simulation

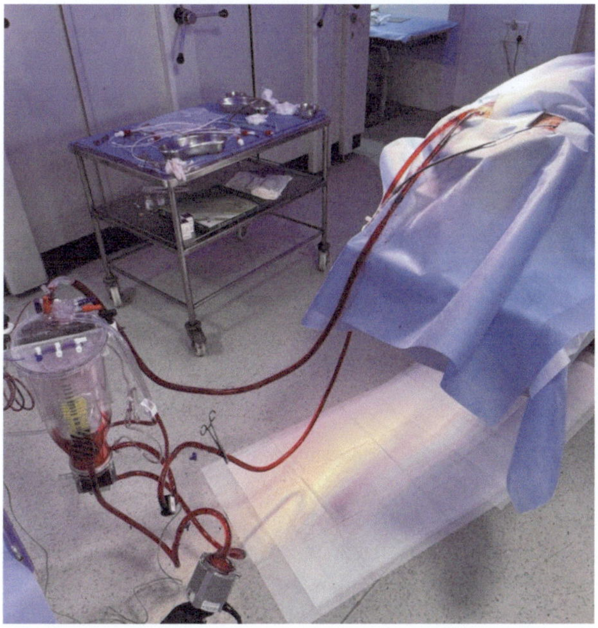

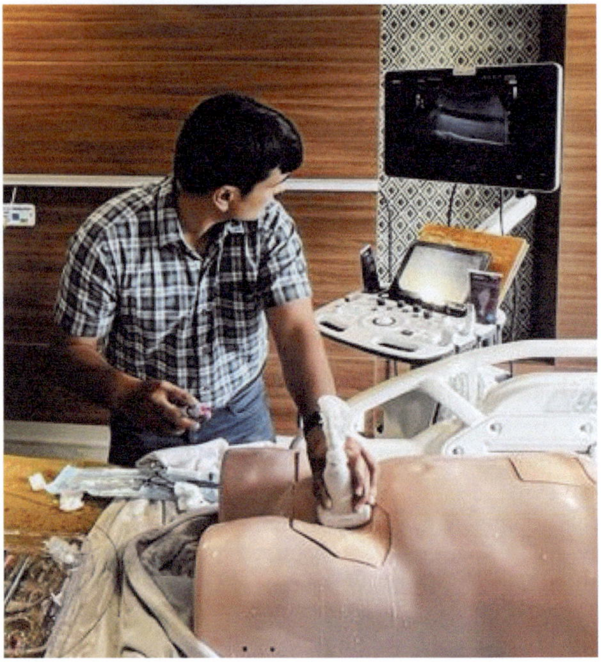

Fig. 19.2 Simulations of rapid cannulation of femoral vein and arteries on mannequins

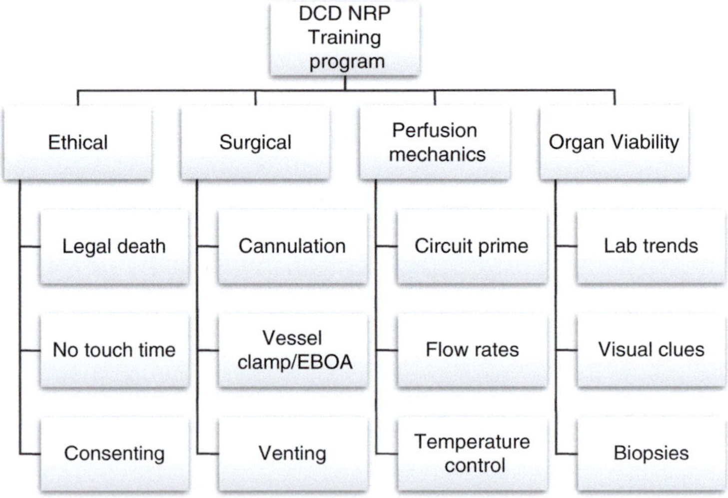

Fig. 19.3 DCD NRP program modules included in the Indian consensus statement

normothermic regional perfusion (NRP). Because their role bridges the transition from end-of-life care to organ preservation, training focuses heavily on ethical boundaries, strict protocol adherence, and advanced extracorporeal management [8].

Because NRP revives the organs in situ at normal body temperature, surgeons must be trained in live, working-bench diagnostics. Depending on the organs to be retrieved, the training differs.

Training for thoracic surgeons covers evaluating a beating heart inside the donor's chest, assessing real-time contractility, checking structural integrity via transesophageal echocardiography (TEE), and transitioning to an ex-vivo device if necessary [9].

For abdominal surgeons, the training centers on monitoring continuous bile production from the liver, tracking clearing lactate levels through blood gases, and evaluating overall macro-perfusion across the liver and kidneys to determine whether an organ is safe to transplant.

Ethical and Legal Training

Strict education on the "dead donor rule," ensuring death is declared based on irreversible cessation of circulatory function before perfusion begins. There must be clear separation between clinical care teams and procurement teams. Education regarding the consent process with donor families is mandatory for every step of the process (7–,9).

Surgical Skill Acquisition

- *Technique Specialization:* Specific training on thoraco-abdominal (TA-NRP) or abdominal (A-NRP) techniques [10].
- *Aortic Occlusion:* Training includes techniques for aortic occlusion to compartmentalize circulation.
- *Collateral Vessel Management:* Management of collateral vessels is required to prevent inadvertent cerebral perfusion.

Perfusion Management

- *Normothermic Conditions:* Training on maintaining near-physiological normothermic conditions (35.5–37.5).
- *Flow and Monitoring:* Training on monitoring flow rates, and managing blood gases and hemodynamics during the perfusion period.
- *Organ Viability Assessment.*

Program Implementation Best Practices (Fig. 19.4)

- *Phased Development:* Programs are often developed in phases: research/ethics review, simulation training, and clinical implementation.
- *"Dry-Runs":* Essential for familiarizing the team with the OR setup, equipment, and troubleshooting potential issues before live cases.
- *Debriefing:* Conducting, consistent post-procedure debriefings to identify areas for improvement.

If there are lessons to be learnt from pilot programs, the important takeaways for setting up a successful NRP program in India would include the following points.

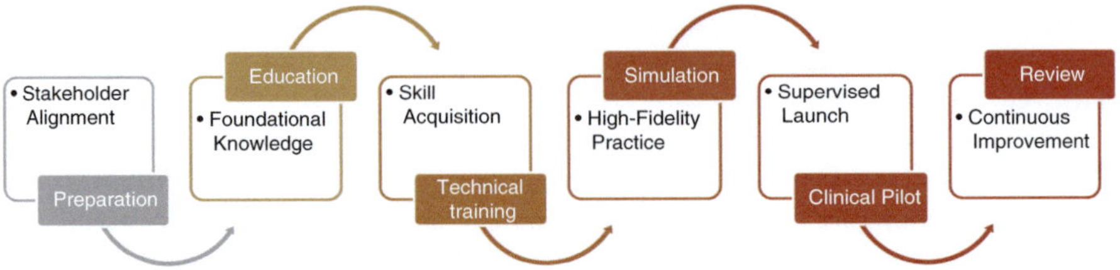

Fig. 19.4 Program implementation for best practicesm

Stringent *selection criteria* and rapid ECMO deployment are pivotal for favorable outcomes.

DCD and NRP remain in its infancy in India, with no published national data or literature currently available on its utilization and outcomes. Its application will be largely limited to adult patients experiencing in-hospital cardiac arrest (IHCA), primarily within private sector hospitals with case reports of successful OHCA occasionally being reported. The absence of a national cardiac arrest registry further hampers the understanding of out-of-hospital cardiac arrest (OHCA) epidemiology and outcomes in the country. As a result, data-driven decision-making, standardized protocols, and broader implementation of DCD NRP or EDCD in OHCA remain significant challenges.

The implementation of EDCD for out-of-hospital cardiac arrest (OHCA) in India is confronted by a host of unique and complex challenges. These begin at the community level, where public awareness of cardiac arrest and the importance of immediate response remain low. Bystander CPR rates are low, and the absence of a robust and integrated emergency medical services (EMS) system is the need of the hour for effective implementation. According to data from NITI Aayog (2020), although 91% of hospitals reported having in-house ambulances, only 34% employed trained paramedics to assist in these services.

Additional hurdles such as timely transport of patients to ECMO-capable centers still persist. Compounding the issue is the extremely limited number of hospitals equipped with ECMO facilities that offer 24/7 readiness and support. EDCD is a time-sensitive intervention, and its success depends on the integrity of every step in the chain of survival—from arrest recognition and early CPR to rapid transport and timely ECMO initiation.

The whole process begins with *patient selection*, which should be guided by either a national consensus statement or institution-specific protocols. These protocols must emphasize the fundamental determinants of favorable outcomes—namely, a witnessed cardiac arrest with high-quality bystander CPR, an estimated low-flow time of less than 60 min, and appropriate consideration of age limits and comorbidities. Additionally, well-defined *termination rules* or "off-ramps" must be established to avoid futile interventions—this includes excluding patients presenting with severe acidosis. Finally, *medicolegal protection* is crucial; hospitals must implement consenting protocols, standardized documentation, and legal safeguards for clinicians performing EDCD. Together, these measures create a foundation for safe, ethical, and outcome-driven EDCD practice.

Interdisciplinary *coordination* and EMS-hospital integration are essential.

Training, *simulations, and protocols SOPs with checklists* foster consistency and safety even in low-volume centers.

Pilot *data* (such as from established transplant centers) will be critical for cost–benefit evaluation and scalable deployment.

Awareness

In order to establish an India, focused roadmap that looks at offering EDCD to the first patient to converting it into a sustainable network, the following aspects need to be considered.

Pre EDCD-Preparation

Piloting the Program

Following adequate preparation, identification of hospitals that already maintain adequate veno arterial (VA) ECMO case volumes and demonstrate proficiency in cannulation during cardiac arrest scenarios becomes the next priority. Initially, these centers should be located in Tier 1 metropolitan cities, allowing for concentrated expertise and resource availability before scaling the model to other regions. Comprehensive training programs are essential, featuring in situ simulation drills that emphasize critical performance metrics such as ECMO initiation time, cannulation efficiency, management of massive transfusion protocols, and rapid troubleshooting of complications like pump failure. Each session should conclude with a debriefing focused on achieving shorter, reproducible time targets, using wall-clock metrics to benchmark progress. The pilot hubs must operate as fully equipped ECMO centers, offering 24/7 access to perfusion services, cardiovascular surgical backup, and an intensive care unit capable of providing advanced care. Finally, the foundation of each program should rest on a dedicated EDCD core team and a fully stocked EDCD kit tailored to the institution's workflow. This combination of infrastructure, training, and readiness should form the cornerstone of an effective, sustainable EDCD initiative in India.

Standardizing ECMO Initiation

To ensure consistency, safety, and optimal outcomes in EDCD programs, it is essential to *standardize clinical care* across all participating centers. A clearly defined *cannulation standard operating procedure (SOP)* should be followed, emphasizing ultrasound-guided femoral-femoral (fem-fem) access, predetermined cannula size selection, appropriate heparin bolus administration strategies. Checklists must be integrated into every procedural step to promote efficiency and reduce errors during high-stress scenarios. Following successful cannulation, a comprehensive *post-cannulation care bundle* should be initiated. This includes serial arterial blood gas (ABG), heparinisation (ACT), and lactate monitoring every 30–60 min and temperature and ECMO setting management continuously.

Training and credentialing as of now, there are 20 ELSO-registered ECMO centers in India. However, based on anonymous data obtained from ECMO equipment dealers and personal communications, approximately 54 centers are actively performing ECMO. A web-based survey revealed that the overall practice of E-CPR in India remains low, with less than 10% of centers reporting its use. Given the stark contrast between the vast population and the limited number of ECMO centers, there is a significant gap in training and awareness among critical care physicians, surgeons, nurses, and perfusionists.

Developing robust *training and credentialing frameworks* is central to the success of any program which depends on the competence and coordination of its personnel. A *tiered training pathway* ensures that all team members acquire the appropriate level of expertise for their specific roles within the DCD + NRP process.

Level 1 training should include all intensive care unit (ICU) and emergency medical services (EMS) personnel, focusing on fundamental competencies such as recognizing EDCD eligible patients and understanding team roles. *Level 2 training* targets ECMO nurses and perfusionists, emphasizing technical mastery of the ECMO console, interpretation and response to alarms, anticoagulation management, and system troubleshooting under real-world conditions. *Level 3 training* is designated for cannulators—typically cardiac surgeons or critical care physicians—and focuses on advanced procedural skills such as vascular ultrasound guidance, percutaneous cannulation techniques, and rapid management of complications, such as circuit failure.

A structured *credentialing matrix* should outline minimum supervised case requirements, mandatory participation in morbidity and mortality (M&M) reviews, annual in situ simulation drills, and maintenance of individual logbooks to document procedural exposure and competencies. Establishing *regional simulation centers* can further enhance training consistency by pooling expert faculty and standardized scenarios, allowing for periodic multi-institutional joint drills involving EMS, perfusion, transplant coordinators, and ICU teams. This collaborative approach ensures uniform skill development, fosters interdepartmental coordination, and promotes a culture of continuous improvement.

Financial Viability

ECMO practice in general is considered to be resource-intensive. In Indian context, the use of ECMO is associated with a substantial financial burden.

Establishing financial sustainability and efficient procurement systems is vital to making EDCD programs viable and scalable in India. A detailed *cost model* should be developed to outline the full spectrum of per-case expenditures, including disposables (circuits, cannulas, oxygenators), blood products, staff overtime or out-of-hours (OOH) call-ins, and ancillary resource utilization such as imaging, ICU stay, and medications.

Quality Metrics and Research

Establishing a robust *data, quality assurance (QA), and research framework* is crucial to demonstrate the clinical and economic value of E-CPR in the Indian healthcare context. A *national DCD NRP registry* should serve as the backbone of this framework, systematically capturing comprehensive data on each case—including patient demographics, case mix, no-flow and low-flow durations, dispatch-to-ECMO initiation timelines, procedural complications, utilisation of organs, and outcomes of DCD and NRP recipients. This centralized database will enable benchmarking across institutions and facilitate nationwide outcome comparisons.

There should be a debrief after every consideration for DCD NRP. Aggregated multicenter findings should be analysed and published periodically to validate outcomes, share best practices. By aligning clinical governance, research, and policy evidence, India can build a transparent, data-driven DCD NRP program that continuously evolves to improve organ quality and organ pool.

Phased Implementation of Program

A *phased implementation strategy* is essential to ensure that DCD NRP implementation in India progresses in a structured, evidence-driven, and sustainable manner.

Phase 0 (3–6 months) should focus on groundwork—developing standardized clinical protocols, establishing formal agreements with EMS agencies, conducting in situ multidisciplinary drills, securing an adequate inventory of ECMO circuits and disposables, and addressing legal and ethical frameworks such as consent and medicolegal protection. Every hospital capable of initiating ECMO should have a multidisciplinary ECMO personnel identified and an ECMO director appointed with responsibility of overseeing training pathways and program evaluation. The program should also include coordinators and financial SPOC.

> *Phase 1 (Year 1)* marks the *pilot implementation stage*, centered around 4–6 high-volume metropolitan hospitals capable of providing round-the-clock ECMO and cardiac services. Each center should target well-selected DCD NRP cases under stringent inclusion criteria, ensuring meticulous data collection and outcome auditing. This phase serves to refine workflows, validate feasibility, and identify operational bottlenecks through rigorous performance evaluation.
>
> *Phase 2 (Years 2–3)* involves *regional expansion* by replicating successful pilot models in state capitals and establishing a *hub-and-spoke network*. In this model, peri-urban "spoke" hospitals focus on early stabilization and rapid transport, while central "hubs" handle cannulation and definitive management. This distributed system enhances access while maintaining procedural quality.

Phase 3 (Years 3–5) represents *mature system integration*, featuring donor hospitals that become centers of optimal donor management with a centralized system of organ allocation increasing the reach of organ donation to non-transplant centers in densely populated metros.

Effective *adaptation of DCD NRP implementation to India's diverse healthcare landscape* requires a nuanced and inclusive approach that recognizes variations in infrastructure, geography, and patient population. The most practical strategy is to *initiate programs in high-readiness private tertiary centers*, which often have existing ECMO capacity, round-the-clock staffing, and strong institutional support. These centers can serve as early *demonstration hubs*, generating outcome data and refining workflows. A key step is to establish *public–private partnerships* by pairing these private hubs with nearby *government medical colleges*, which can function as training and research collaborators. Once the protocols, logistics, and skill sets are validated, the knowledge can be systematically transferred to the public sector for broader accessibility and scalability.

Ethical Barriers

Obtaining informed consent in DCD patients pre-mortem emergency situations poses a significant challenge. Due to the ethical concerns, there should be provision for the formulation of an ethics consultation service to help families and staff deal with the invariable value conflicts and stresses which are very likely to set in.

For in-hospital cardiac arrest (IHCA), patients who are potentially eligible for DCD NRP should be identified in advance and pre-consented, ensuring timely initiation if the need arises.

In the case of out-of-hospital cardiac arrest (OHCA), there is a need for government-led guidelines that empower clinicians to counsel for DCD NRP based on predefined eligibility criteria, allowing for rapid decision-making in time-sensitive scenarios.

The logistics of expedient cannulation, patient selection, and healthcare worker safety have to be weighed against the ethical considerations of providing a therapy of controversial and unknown risks and benefits at a time. Moreover, in India, there exists legal ambiguity regarding advance directives and emergency consent.

Conclusion

The implementation of DCD NRP represents a transformative paradigm shift for organ transplantation in India. By bridging the critical gap between a vast pool of potential donors and a severe shortage of viable organs, NRP holds the potential to significantly alleviate India's organ deficit. However, the successful integration of this advanced technology into the national healthcare fabric depends entirely on the creation of a structured, nationwide training framework.

Moving forward, India's pathway to scaling DCD NRP requires active focus on three interconnected pillars of standardized curriculum development that clearly delineate the training requirements for intensivists, transplant surgeons, perfusionists, and transplant coordinators alike.

It mandates high fidelity, team based dry-runs, and wet labs to master the high-stress, time-critical transition from circulatory death declaration to the initiation of the perfusion circuit. It is essential to align institutional workflows with local regulations to guarantee absolute adherence to the "dead donor rule" and the mandatory "no-touch" observation period, thereby maintaining public trust.

Ultimately, DCD NRP training in India must evolve from isolated institutional initiatives to a centrally regulated, credentialed educational pathway. By equipping clinical teams with both technical mastery and the ethical framework required for regional perfusion, India can establish a highly efficient, sustainable, and trusted organ procurement network that will transform the landscape of deceased organ donation for decades to come.

Competing Interests The author(s) has no competing interests to declare that are relevant to the content of this manuscript.

Ethics Approval The author(s) declares that this manuscript does not include primary research with human participants.

The author(s) declares that this manuscript does not include primary studies involving animals.

References

1. Fischbach C, et al. Application of perfusion technologies to NORMOTHERMIC regional perfusion procedures: State-of-the-art. Curr Transplant Rep. 2025;12(1) https://doi.org/10.1007/s40472-025-00482-8.
2. Hunt F, Johnston C, Coutts L, Sherif A, Farwell L, Stutchfield B, Sewpaul A, Sutherland A, Babu B, Currie I, Oniscu G. From haphazard to a sustainable normothermic regional perfusion service: a blueprint for the introduction of novel perfusion technologies. Transplant Int. 2022;35:10493. https://doi.org/10.3389/ti.2022.10493.
3. Patten E, Miller C, Wong P, Cochrane L, Jarden R. Interprofessional perioperative simulation team training non-technical skill measurement and outcomes: a scoping review. J Interprofession Care. 2025;40:1–21. https://doi.org/10.1080/13561820.2025.2562074.
4. DeVries S, Quintana E, Harris T, et al. Thoracoabdominal normothermic regional perfusion: how I teach it. Ann Thoracic Surg. 2024;118:564–8.
5. Institute of Medicine (US) Committee on Non-Heart-Beating Transplantation II: The Scientific and Ethical Basis for Practice and Protocols. Non-Heart-Beating Organ Transplantation: Practice and Protocols. Washington (DC): National Academies Press (US); 2000. APPENDIX F, Non-Heart-Beating Donation Protocols. Available from: https://www.ncbi.nlm.nih.gov/books/NBK225012.
6. Sheth A, Mohanka R, Haji JY, Dhital K, Banker A, Sharma A, Kumar A, Mirza DF, Mehta D, Dhandapani K, Hote MP, Thomas P, Pandit RA, Mani RK, Attawar S, Kolte SP, Shrinivasan S, Gupta S, Mathur SK, Kota V, Shroff S. Consensus statement of the national consortium on normothermic regional perfusion for organ donation after circulatory determination of death in India. Indian J Transplant. 2026;20(1):23–35. https://doi.org/10.4103/ijot.ijot_81_25.

7. Seth AK, Mohanka R, Navin S, Gokhale AGK, Sharma A, Kumar A, Ramachandran B, Balakrishnan KR, Mirza DF, Mehta D, Zirpe KG, Dhital K, Sahay M, Simha S, Sundaram R, Pandit RA, Mani RK, Gursahani R, Gupta S, Kute V, Shroff S. Organ donation after circulatory determination of death in India: a joint position paper. Indian J Transplantat. 2022;16(1):26–41. https://doi.org/10.4103/ijot.ijot_61_21.
8. Jochmans I, Hessheimer AJ, Neyrinck AP, Paredes D, Bellini MI, Dark JH, Kimenai HJAN, Pengel LHM, Watson CJE, ESOT Workstream 04 of the TLJ (Transplant Learning Journey) project. Consensus statement on normothermic regional perfusion in donation after circulatory death: report from the European Society for Organ Transplantation's Transplant Learning Journey. Transpl Int. 2021;34:2019–30. https://doi.org/10.1111/tri.13951.
9. Croome K, Bababekov Y, Brubaker A, Montenovo M, Mao S, Sellers M, Foley D, Pomfret E, Abt P. American Society of Transplant Surgeons Normothermic Regional Perfusion Standards: Abdominal. Transplantation. 2024;108(8):1660–8. https://doi.org/10.1097/TP.0000000000005114.
10. Funamoto M, Pierson RN, Nguyen JH, D'Alessandro DA. Surgical and logistical concerns for ex vivo-based perfusion strategies for "donation after circulatory death" multiorgan recovery. JTCVS Tech. 2021;11:49–56. https://doi.org/10.1016/j.xjtc.2021.11.005. PMID: 35169736; PMCID: PMC8828966.

Myths and Facts About Donation After Circulatory Death: An Indian Perspective

20

Ashish Sharma and Amit Sharma

Introduction

Organ transplantation stands as one of modern medicine's greatest achievements—a procedure that transforms terminal diseases into renewed life. Yet the promise of transplantation remains unfulfilled for hundreds of thousands of patients worldwide who wait, often in vain, for a suitable organ. In India alone, the gap between organ supply and demand is staggering: approximately 258,000 organs are needed annually, yet fewer than 20,000 transplants occur each year [1].

Donation after circulatory death (DCD)—organ recovery following the irreversible cessation of circulatory and respiratory functions—represents a significant opportunity to expand the donor pool. Unlike donation after brain death (DBD), where organs are retrieved while circulation is maintained using mechanical ventilation and cardiovascular support while the heart continues beating under mechanical ventilation, DCD involves procurement after cardiac arrest has been confirmed and a mandated observation period has elapsed.

Globally, DCD has emerged as a vital pathway for increasing organ availability. Countries like the Netherlands, Belgium, and the United Kingdom now derive a substantial proportion of their deceased donors from DCD programs. The USA has witnessed steady growth in DCD donations over the past two decades [2]. Yet in India, DCD remains virtually non-existent as a systematic practice, constrained by legal ambiguities, infrastructural challenges, and—perhaps most significantly—a dense thicket of myths and misconceptions.

This chapter systematically examines the myths surrounding donation after circulatory death, contrasting them with evidence-based facts drawn from global

A. Sharma (✉)
Department of Renal Transplant Surgery, PGIMER, Chandigarh, India

A. Sharma
Dr. Rajendra Prasad Government Medical College, Tanda, Kangra, Himachal Pradesh, India

S. P. Kolte et al. (eds.), *Organ Donation After Circulatory Death*,
https://doi.org/10.1007/978-981-92-6377-6_20

research and clinical experience. Special attention is given to the Indian context, where cultural, religious, legal, and infrastructural factors create unique challenges and opportunities. The goal is to provide healthcare professionals, policymakers, and the general public with accurate information that can inform decisions about organ donation and help save lives.

Historical Context and Evolution of DCD

The Origin of Organ Transplantation

The deceased donor organ transplantation began with donation after circulatory death till the concept of brain death was formulated. Early transplants relied on kidneys procured from donors whose hearts had stopped beating—what we would now classify as DCD. Throughout the 1960s, as surgical techniques improved and immunosuppression became available, the demand for donor organs grew. However, the lack of sophisticated preservation methods meant that organs deteriorated rapidly after circulatory arrest, limiting transplant success rates.

The Brain-Death Revolution

The introduction of the brain-death concept in 1968, formalized by the Harvard Committee's landmark report, fundamentally transformed organ donation [3]. Brain death allowed for the legal declaration of death while circulation continued under mechanical support, providing optimal conditions for organ preservation. Donation after brain death (DBD) quickly became the dominant paradigm worldwide. For several decades, DCD largely receded from practice. The superior organ quality achievable with DBD, combined with expanding DBD programs, seemed to make DCD unnecessary.

The Renaissance of DCD

By the 1990s, however, the landscape had changed. The gap between organ supply and demand continued to widen. Improved critical care paradoxically reduced the number of brain deaths, as better neurosurgical interventions—such as decompressive craniectomy—saved patients who might previously have progressed to brain death. Simultaneously, medical and ethical acceptance grew for withdrawing life-sustaining treatment in patients with catastrophic injuries who would never recover meaningful neurological function.

These converging factors sparked renewed interest in DCD. The Maastricht classification, developed in 1995 and updated in 2016, provided a standardized framework for categorizing DCD donors [4]:

- *Category I*: Dead on arrival (uncontrolled).
- *Category II*: Unsuccessful resuscitation (uncontrolled).
- *Category III*: Anticipated cardiac arrest following withdrawal of life-sustaining treatment (controlled).
- *Category IV*: Cardiac arrest in a brain-dead donor (uncontrolled or controlled).

This classification helped standardize practices and facilitated research comparing outcomes across different DCD categories.

Global Growth of DCD Programs

Today, DCD accounts for a significant and growing proportion of deceased organ donations in many countries. In the United Kingdom, DCD donors represented over 40% of all deceased donors by 2020 [5]. The Netherlands has achieved DCD rates approaching 10 donors per million population [6]. Belgium, Australia, and Canada have established robust programs. Between 2008 and 2016, DCD activity in Europe progressively increased, with over 12,115 DCD organs transplanted during that period—including 8972 kidneys, 1943 livers, 782 lungs, 404 pancreas, and 14 hearts [7].

The Indian Context: Current Status and Challenges

Legal Framework

India's legal framework for organ transplantation is primarily governed by the Transplantation of Human Organs Act (THOA), 1994, as amended in 2011, and the Transplantation of Human Organs and Tissues Rules, 2014. This legislation recognizes brain death as legal death for the purpose of organ donation and establishes procedures for brain-death certification.

While the Act's provisions for DBD were elaborate, defining protocols to be followed for declaring brain death, same was not true for DCD. This has created legal ambiguity around organ recovery following circulatory death. The lack of explicit legal provisions for withdrawal of life support meant that physicians faced significant uncertainty when considering this pathway. Unlike brain death—where certification procedures, committee composition, and documentation requirements are clearly specified—there is no defined protocol in THOA 2014 for determining death following circulatory arrest or for the subsequent organ retrieval process.

Deceased Donation Statistics

India's deceased organ donation rate remains extremely low by international standards. As of January 2026, the country achieved approximately 0.8 deceased donors per million population in 2024, compared to 49.7 per million in the USA, 28.7 in France, and 20.9 in the United Kingdom. Even other developing economies like Brazil (17.38) and China (4.71) significantly outperform India [8].

In 2023, India recorded 1028 deceased organ donations—a number that, while representing progress, falls far short of addressing the enormous need. Telangana led with 200 donations, followed by Karnataka (178), Tamil Nadu (176), Maharashtra (149), and Gujarat (146) [9].

Nearly all of these donations followed brain death. DCD, as a systematic program, effectively does not exist in India, though isolated programs have been carried out, most notably at the Post Graduate Institute of Medical Education and Research (PGIMER) in Chandigarh, which has pioneered DCD in the Indian context.

The PGIMER Chandigarh Experience

PGIMER Chandigarh documented its first DCD kidney transplant in 2011, whereas some such transplants had happened before the THOA 1994 had come into existence [10]. The donor was a 51-year-old woman with terminal interstitial lung disease whose family decided against further treatment. Following cardiac arrest, her kidneys were retrieved with a warm ischemia time of 90 min—significantly longer than the ideal 60-min window. The outcomes were sobering: One kidney never functioned, and the other achieved only suboptimal function. This experience highlighted the critical importance of minimizing warm ischemia time and implementing organ preservation strategies during the retrieval process.

Subsequently, PGIMER refined its approach, incorporating continuous cardiopulmonary resuscitation (CPR) during the interval between cardiac arrest and organ retrieval to maintain some blood flow to the organs. An automated CPR machine was acquired, along with a double-balloon catheter for rapid cooling. By the time of the most recent reports, 19 DCD donors had been retrieved at PGIMER, with outcomes improving as techniques evolved [11].

Cultural and Religious Considerations

India's religious and cultural diversity creates a complex landscape for organ donation in general and lack of awareness regarding brain death might not make DCD easier to understand. While most major religious traditions do not explicitly prohibit organ donation—and many actively support it as an act of charity—various beliefs and practices still create hesitation.

Concerns about the integrity of the body after death, beliefs about reincarnation, and anxieties about disturbing the journey of the soul can all influence families' decisions. The concept of death itself is understood differently across traditions, and the idea of removing organs immediately after the heart stops may feel especially transgressive to some families.

Additionally, deeply ingrained suspicions about medical institutions—concerns about premature declaration of death, organ trafficking, and preferential treatment for wealthy recipients—create significant barriers to consent.

Infrastructural Limitations

Even if legal and cultural barriers were addressed, India faces substantial infrastructural challenges in implementing DCD programs. The country has a critical shortage of intensive care unit (ICU) beds and ventilators. Many hospitals lack the capacity to maintain potential brain-dead donors long enough to complete the certification process, let alone to implement the rapid-response protocols required for DCD.

Successful DCD demands immediate availability of operating theaters, surgical teams, and organ preservation equipment. The warm ischemia clock begins ticking the moment circulation ceases, leaving no room for delays. Outside major metropolitan centers and a handful of well-resourced institutions, this infrastructure simply does not exist.

Myths and Facts: A Systematic Examination

The following sections address common myths about donation after circulatory death, presenting evidence-based facts that can educate professionals changing their understanding and attitude toward DCD.

Myth 1: Organ Quality from DCD Donors Is Inherently Poor and Unsuitable for Transplantation

The Myth in Detail

A pervasive belief holds that organs retrieved after circulatory death are fundamentally inferior to those from brain-dead donors. The reasoning seems intuitive: Once the heart stops, organs are deprived of oxygenated blood, causing cellular damage that must inevitably compromise function. According to this view, DCD organs represent a last resort—acceptable only when no DBD organs are available—and recipients should expect worse outcomes.

The Facts

Extensive global research demonstrates that DCD organs can achieve excellent long-term outcomes, though the picture is nuanced and varies by organ type.

Kidneys Kidney transplants from DCD donors show comparable long-term survival to those from DBD donors, despite higher rates of delayed graft function (DGF)—a temporary period when the transplanted kidney does not immediately produce urine, requiring dialysis support. DGF rates in DCD kidney transplants range from 40–80%, compared to 15–30% for DBD kidneys [12].

However, DGF in DCD transplants does not appear to carry the same negative prognostic implications as DGF in DBD transplants. Studies consistently show that 5-year and 10-year graft survival rates are similar between DCD and DBD kidney transplants [13]. Registry data from the United Kingdom indicates 10-year graft survival of approximately 74% for first-time DCD kidney recipients [14].

Livers DCD liver transplantation carries higher risks than kidney transplantation, primarily due to the liver's greater sensitivity to ischemic injury. Rates of primary non-function (PNF) and ischemic cholangiopathy—a form of bile duct damage that can lead to graft loss—are elevated in DCD liver recipients.

However, careful donor and recipient selection, minimization of ischemia times, and newer preservation techniques have significantly improved outcomes. A systematic review and meta-analysis found that while DCD liver transplants have higher rates of biliary complications and slightly lower graft survival, patient survival rates are comparable to DBD transplants. The development of the UK DCD Risk Score and similar tools allows transplant teams to identify higher-risk grafts and make informed decisions [15]. New technologies like normothermic regional perfusion have further reduced these risks comparable to DBD donors.

Lungs Paradoxically, DCD lungs may actually tolerate ischemia better than DBD lungs. The lungs can maintain oxygen exchange even after circulatory arrest, as long as ventilation continues, and they can be retrieved in good condition with appropriate techniques. Multiple studies have demonstrated equivalent or even superior outcomes for DCD lung transplants compared to DBD transplants, with comparable rates of primary graft dysfunction and bronchiolitis obliterans syndrome [16, 17].

Hearts DCD heart transplantation was long considered impossible, as the heart was believed to be irreversibly damaged by the warm ischemia following circulatory arrest. However, pioneering work beginning in Australia in 2014 demonstrated that DCD hearts could be resuscitated using ex situ machine perfusion and successfully transplanted [18]. By 2016, 14 DCD heart transplants had been performed in UK [19], and the number has expanded rapidly contributing substantially to heart transplant activity across several countries. The *International Society for Heart and Lung Transplantation (ISHLT)* reported in 2025 that DCD heart transplantation has reached its 10-year milestone and now accounts for *up to 30% of heart transplant volumes* in some programs. Early and medium-term outcomes are promising, though long-term data remain limited [20].

The Key Variables Organ quality in DCD depends critically on minimizing warm ischemia time—the interval between circulatory arrest and cold perfusion of the organs. Controlled DCD (Maastricht Category III), where withdrawal of life-sustaining treatment is planned, and surgical teams are prepared, allows for much shorter warm ischemia times than uncontrolled DCD following unexpected cardiac arrest. Outcomes from controlled DCD approach nearly match those from DBD.

Relevance to India The perception of inferior organ quality has contributed to reluctance among Indian transplant surgeons to pursue DCD. However, with appropriate protocols to minimize warm ischemia—including pre-positioning of surgical teams, use of rapid cooling techniques, and potentially normothermic regional perfusion or ex situ perfusion—excellent outcomes are achievable. The PGIMER experience demonstrates that with experienced teams, learning curves can be surmounted, and good outcomes can be achieved.

Myth 2: DCD Means Patients Will Be Allowed to Die or Killed for Their Organs

The Myth in Detail

Perhaps the most dangerous myth surrounding DCD is the fear that it creates an incentive to hasten death—that physicians will withdraw treatment prematurely, or that patients will be declared dead before they have truly died, in order to harvest organs. This fear is particularly acute in India, where trust in medical institutions is often fragile and suspicions about organ trafficking are widespread.

Some version of this concern affects families in all countries, but it takes particular forms in India. Anecdotal accounts of organ trafficking, often amplified by media coverage and Bollywood films depicting criminal organ trade, have created deep-seated anxieties. Families may fear that consenting to organ donation will lead to inadequate treatment, premature withdrawal of care, or premature declaration of death.

The Facts

Complete Separation of Decisions The ethical foundation of DCD rests on the absolute separation between the decision to withdraw life-sustaining treatment and the decision to donate organs. The decision to withdraw treatment must be made entirely on the basis of the patient's best interests and wishes, without any consideration of organ donation potential. Only after such decision is reached made, and clearly communicated to the family, does the conversation about donation begin.

This separation is enshrined in guidelines worldwide. The physicians involved in the care of the potential donor are entirely separate from the transplant team, and transplant professionals are not involved at all in the process of withdrawal of life support. The family's decision about donation does not influence the timing or manner of treatment withdrawal.

Strict Death Determination Protocols DCD requires rigorous confirmation of death before organ retrieval can proceed. After circulatory arrest, a mandatory observation period (typically 2–5 min, varying by jurisdiction) ensures that circulation has irreversibly ceased [21]. During this period, the patient is monitored to confirm the absence of pulse, blood pressure, and respiratory effort. The determination of death is made by physicians who are entirely independent of the transplant team. The same safeguards that prevent conflicts of interest in brain-death determination apply to circulatory death.

No Acceleration of Death Withdrawal of life-sustaining treatment is a well-established ethical and legal practice that long predates any consideration of organ donation. It is performed when continued treatment is judged to be futile or contrary to the patient's wishes and interests. The decision is made by the treating team in consultation with the family, based on the clinical circumstances.

DCD does not require any intervention that accelerates death. The patient is allowed to die naturally following withdrawal of treatment. Organ retrieval occurs only after death has been confirmed according to well-established criteria.

The "Dead Donor Rule" All organ donation from deceased donors—whether DBD or DCD—is governed by the "dead donor rule," which stipulates that the donor must be dead before organ retrieval begins, and that the act of retrieval must not cause death. DCD protocols are specifically designed to ensure compliance with this rule [22].

Global Experience Countries with established DCD programs have implemented robust ethical safeguards. Decades of experience in the United Kingdom, the Netherlands, Belgium, Australia, and elsewhere demonstrate that DCD can be practiced ethically without compromising patient care or public trust. Indeed, rates of family consent for organ donation remain comparable or higher in countries with active DCD programs, suggesting that the practice has not undermined public confidence.

Relevance to India Addressing this myth requires transparent communication about DCD protocols, public education about the separation of treatment decisions from donation decisions, and robust regulatory oversight to ensure that safeguards are followed. The involvement of independent ethics committees, clear documentation requirements, and visible family presence during the withdrawal process can all help build trust.

Myth 3: DCD Is Illegal in India and Cannot Be Practiced Under Current Laws

The Myth in Detail

A common belief among healthcare professionals and the public is that DCD cannot legally occur in India because the law only recognizes brain death for the purpose of organ donation. According to this view, any attempt to retrieve organs following circulatory death would violate the Transplantation of Human Organs Act and potentially expose physicians to criminal liability.

The Facts

Legal Ambiguity Rather Than Prohibition The legal status of DCD in India is better characterized as ambiguous than as prohibited. The THOA of 1994 introduced brain death as a legal concept specifically for enabling organ transplantation, but it did not thereby exclude organ donation from other forms of death determination.

Circulatory death (cessation of heartbeat and breathing) remains the traditional and universally accepted criterion for death. It is the basis for death certification in the vast majority of deaths in India and worldwide. There is no legal provision that prohibits organ retrieval following death determined by circulatory criteria.

The Challenge of Withdrawal of Treatment The more significant legal uncertainty pertains to the withdrawal of life-sustaining treatment—a prerequisite for controlled DCD (Maastricht Category III). Indian law does not explain clearly when and how on when and how treatment may be withdrawn from patients who are not brain dead but who have no prospect of meaningful recovery.

However, the Supreme Court of India, in the landmark Aruna Shanbaug case (2011) and subsequent rulings [23, 24], has recognized the validity of passive euthanasia—the withdrawal of life-sustaining treatment in certain circumstances—while rejecting active euthanasia. The Court has established that treatment withdrawal may be permissible when continued treatment is futile and contrary to the patient's best interests, subject to appropriate safeguards including judicial approval in contested cases. These rulings provide a legal foundation for the withdrawal of treatment that could, in principle, enable controlled DCD.

Uncontrolled DCD For uncontrolled DCD (Maastricht Categories I and II)—where cardiac arrest occurs unexpectedly in emergency settings—the legal position is clearer in some respects. There is no prohibition on organ retrieval following death determined by circulatory criteria, provided appropriate consent is obtained. The challenge is primarily logistical rather than legal: retrieving organs within the necessary timeframe requires resources and protocols that few Indian institutions possess.

The Path Forward Legal experts and transplant professionals have called for amendments to the THOA or new guidelines that explicitly address DCD. Such reforms could clarify the legal status of controlled DCD, establish procedures for treatment withdrawal in the context of potential organ donation, define standards for death determination following circulatory arrest, and specify consent requirements.

In the absence of legislative reform, individual states or institutions or government bodies like NOTTO could develop protocols consistent with existing law. The PGIMER Chandigarh experience demonstrates that DCD can be practiced in India, albeit on a limited basis [10, 11].

Relevance to India Healthcare professionals should understand that DCD is not explicitly prohibited by Indian law, and that existing legal frameworks may accommodate the practice with appropriate protocols. However, the absence of clear guidelines creates uncertainty that has understandably discouraged broader adoption. Advocacy for legal clarification should be a priority for the transplant community.

Myth 4: Religious Beliefs in India Prohibit DCD and Organ Donation Generally

The Myth in Detail

India's extraordinary religious diversity—with significant Hindu, Muslim, Christian, Sikh, Buddhist, and Jain populations, among others—is sometimes cited as a fundamental barrier to organ donation. The myth suggests that most religious traditions in India prohibit the removal of organs after death, and that DCD in particular would violate religious teachings about the integrity of the body, the process of death, and the journey of the soul.

The Facts

Major Religions Support Organ Donation In reality, none of India's major religious traditions explicitly prohibit organ donation, and most actively support it as an act of compassion and charity.

Hinduism Hindu teachings emphasize the impermanence of the physical body and the immortality of the soul (atman). The body is understood as a vessel that the soul leaves at death. Many Hindu scholars have endorsed organ donation as an act of daan (giving)—one of the highest virtues in Hindu tradition. The Bhagavad Gita's teaching that "the soul is not killed when the body is killed" (Chap. 2, Verse 22) provides theological grounding for the view that organ removal does not harm the deceased [25].

Some families express concern about the impact of organ removal on the soul's journey or on future incarnations. However, authoritative Hindu voices have generally rejected such concerns, emphasizing that the soul's destiny depends on karma (accumulated actions during life), not on the condition of the body after death.

Islam Islamic jurisprudence (fiqh) has extensively debated organ donation, and the consensus of major Islamic scholarly bodies supports transplantation as permissible (halal) when it serves to save another life. The Islamic Fiqh Academy of the Organisation of Islamic Cooperation and numerous national fatwa councils have endorsed organ donation [26].

The principle of necessity (darurah) allows actions that would otherwise be prohibited when they are necessary to preserve life. Saving a life is considered one of the highest values in Islam, consistent with the Quranic teaching that "whoever saves a life, it is as if they have saved all of humanity."

Some Muslims express reservations about brain death as a criterion for death, preferring the traditional criterion of cardiac arrest. For these communities, DCD—where death is determined by circulatory criteria—might actually be more acceptable than DBD.

Christianity All major Christian denominations support organ donation as an act of love and charity consistent with the command to love one's neighbor. The Catholic Church has repeatedly affirmed the morality of organ donation. Protestant and Orthodox churches generally hold similar positions.

Sikhism Sikh teachings emphasize seva (selfless service) and the giving of life to help others. The Sikh community has generally been supportive of organ donation.

Buddhism Buddhist perspectives vary, but many Buddhist teachers have endorsed organ donation as an act of generosity (dana) that expresses compassion for the suffering of others. Some Buddhists prefer that organs not be removed immediately after death, believing that consciousness may not depart the body instantly. This concern might actually favor controlled DCD with appropriate waiting periods over rapid retrieval after brain death.

Jainism Jain teachings on non-violence (ahimsa) and non-attachment to the body have been interpreted by some scholars as supporting organ donation as a supreme act of giving.

The Role of Cultural Practice While religious doctrine generally supports organ donation, cultural practices and folk beliefs may create hesitation. Concerns about the appearance of the body for funeral rites, beliefs about the need for bodily integrity in the afterlife, and general discomfort with medical interventions after death can all influence family decisions.

However, it is important to distinguish between religious teachings and cultural attitudes. The former generally support organ donation; the latter may create barriers that can be addressed through sensitive communication.

The Critical Role of Religious Leaders Engagement with religious and spiritual leaders can be powerful in addressing misconceptions. Statements from respected religious authorities endorsing organ donation can carry significant weight with hesitant families. In India, involving local religious leaders in public education campaigns has shown promise in some regions.

Relevance to India Healthcare professionals should be equipped to address religious concerns with accurate information about the positions of major faiths. Families should be reassured that organ donation is consistent with their religious traditions and that appropriate measures will be taken to treat the donor's body with dignity and respect.

Myth 5: The Heart Can Restart After Death Is Declared, Making DCD Unsafe

The Myth in Detail

A concern frequently raised about DCD is the possibility of autoresuscitation—the spontaneous return of circulation after cardiac arrest, without any external intervention. If the heart could restart after death has been declared, and organ retrieval has begun, this would represent a catastrophic ethical violation: the removal of organs from a living person.

This fear is amplified by popular culture representations of people being declared dead only to "wake up" later, and by occasional media reports of such occurrences. The concern is particularly acute for DCD because the waiting period between circulatory arrest and death determination is relatively brief—typically 5 min or less.

The Facts

Autoresuscitation Is Extremely Rare The phenomenon of autoresuscitation—sometimes called the "Lazarus phenomenon"—has been documented in the medical literature, but it is extremely rare [27]. A systematic review identified only 38 cases in the literature over several decades, most occurring in patients receiving cardiopulmonary resuscitation where brief cessation of CPR was followed by return of circulation.

Importantly, documented cases of autoresuscitation have virtually all occurred within the first 2 min after cessation of circulation and the majority within 10 s. No confirmed case has been reported after a properly observed 5-min no-touch period in controlled DCD. No convincing case of autoresuscitation has been documented more than 5 min after cessation of circulation.

The Waiting Period Provides a Safety Margin DCD protocols require a mandatory observation period (often called the "hands-off" or "no-touch" period) between the cessation of circulation and the declaration of death. During this period, the patient is monitored continuously for any signs of return of circulation, breathing, or consciousness.

The duration of this waiting period varies internationally, ranging from 2 to 10 min depending on jurisdiction. However, 5 min has emerged as a widely accepted standard that balances safety against the need to minimize warm ischemia. The choice of 5 min is based on the absence of documented autoresuscitation beyond this interval and on consensus among medical and ethical experts.

Irreversibility Is the Key Criterion The legal and ethical definition of death requires that the cessation of circulatory and respiratory functions can be irreversible. Some critics have argued that "irreversibility" cannot be determined during the waiting period—that if circulation could potentially be restored through CPR or other interventions, then cessation is not truly irreversible.

However, the accepted interpretation of irreversibility in the DCD context is "will not" rather than "cannot" restart. Once a decision has been made not to attempt resuscitation—because the patient has requested no CPR, or because the treating team has determined that resuscitation would be futile or contrary to the patient's interests—then the cessation of circulation will not be reversed. The intervention that could theoretically restore circulation will not be undertaken.

This interpretation has been endorsed by major medical and ethical bodies internationally. It is consistent with the routine practice of death determination in non-donation contexts, where patients are declared dead without any waiting period after circulation ceases if no resuscitation is to be attempted.

Additional Confirmatory Tests DCD protocols require additional confirmatory tests before death is declared, such as electrocardiographic (ECG) confirmation of asystole, arterial line monitoring showing absent pulsatile flow, or echocardiographic confirmation of absent cardiac activity. These tests provide additional assurance that circulation has irreversibly ceased.

Global Safety Record The extensive international experience with DCD has not produced credible reports of autoresuscitation occurring during organ retrieval. The safety record of DCD programs over decades of practice provides empirical reassurance that protocols are adequate to ensure that donors are truly dead before organ retrieval begins.

Relevance to India DCD protocols in India should incorporate mandatory waiting periods (5 min is recommended) and continuous monitoring for any signs of return of circulation. Clear documentation of the death determination process is essential.

Myth 6: DCD Is Only Relevant for Kidneys and Cannot Provide Other Vital Organs

The Myth in Detail

A common misconception holds that DCD can only yield kidneys—that other organs, particularly the liver, heart, and lungs, are too sensitive to the warm ischemia inherent in DCD and cannot be successfully transplanted.

The Facts

DCD Yields Multiple Organ Types While kidneys were the first and remain the most common organs transplanted from DCD donors, the scope of DCD has expanded dramatically to include livers, lungs, pancreas, and even hearts.

Kidneys Kidneys tolerate warm ischemia relatively well and have been the mainstay of DCD transplantation. Outcomes are excellent, as discussed above.

Livers DCD liver transplantation is now well-established, accounting for a significant proportion of liver transplants in countries with active DCD programs [15]. While outcomes require careful donor and recipient selection, thousands of patients have received life-saving liver transplants from DCD donors.

Lungs DCD lungs have emerged as particularly promising. Because the lungs can maintain oxygenation even after circulatory arrest (as long as ventilation continues), they tolerate the DCD process well. Some studies suggest that DCD lung outcomes match or exceed DBD lung outcomes [17].

Pancreas DCD pancreas for islet cell transplantation or whole-organ transplantation have been successfully used, though volumes are smaller than for kidneys or livers.

Hearts The most recent frontier in DCD has been cardiac transplantation. Using normothermic regional perfusion (NRP) or ex situ machine perfusion, DCD hearts can be resuscitated and assessed for viability before transplantation. Since the first

DCD heart transplant in Australia in 2014, the practice has expanded globally, with promising early results.

Machine Perfusion Is Transforming DCD The development of machine perfusion technologies—both normothermic (warm) and hypothermic (cold)—has been a game-changer for DCD [28]. These technologies allow organs to be preserved, assessed, and even resuscitated outside the body, extending the window for transplantation and enabling the use of organs that would previously have been discarded.

Normothermic regional perfusion (NRP), where the donor's abdominal (and sometimes thoracic) organs are perfused with warm oxygenated blood using extracorporeal membrane oxygenation (ECMO) after death, allows for assessment of organ function and minimization of ischemic injury. Ex situ machine perfusion allows organs to be transported while being continuously perfused and monitored, enabling more distant sharing and longer preservation times [29].

These technologies have dramatically expanded the potential of DCD and are being increasingly adopted worldwide.

The Numbers Are Growing In Europe, between 2008 and 2016, DCD programs transplanted not only 8972 kidneys but also 1943 livers, 782 lungs, 404 pancreas, and 14 hearts. These numbers have continued to grow since [7].

Relevance to India While India's DCD efforts to date have focused exclusively on kidneys, the potential for expanding to other organs exists as infrastructure and expertise develop. The global trend toward machine perfusion offers opportunities to leapfrog some of the logistical challenges that have constrained DCD in resource-limited settings.

Myth 7: Families Are Not Given Time to Say Goodbye in DCD

The Myth in Detail

A concern sometimes raised by families—and by healthcare professionals uncertain about DCD—is that the urgency of organ retrieval will prevent families from having adequate time to say goodbye to their loved ones. The fear is that the dying process will be rushed, that family presence will be excluded, and that the dignity of death will be sacrificed to the demands of organ procurement.

The Facts

Family Presence Is Central to DCD Well-designed DCD protocols explicitly prioritize family presence and support during the withdrawal of life-sustaining treatment. The decision to withdraw treatment is made with the family, and the family is encouraged to be present during the dying process.

In controlled DCD, there is typically no conflict between family presence and organ procurement. Withdrawal of treatment occurs in the ICU or a designated withdrawal room, often with family members at the bedside. The family has time to say goodbye. Only after death has occurred and been confirmed does the patient's body move to the operating theater for organ retrieval.

The Waiting Period Provides Time for Closure The mandatory waiting period between circulatory arrest and death determination—typically 5 min—provides additional time for families to absorb what has happened. This period, while brief, can be a meaningful moment of closure.

Flexible Protocols Accommodate Family Needs Experienced DCD programs recognize that families have different needs and preferences. Some families wish to remain with their loved one until the moment of death; others prefer to say goodbye before withdrawal of treatment and leave before death occurs. Protocols should be flexible enough to accommodate these preferences.

When Withdrawal Occurs In some countries, treatment is withdrawn in the operating theater to minimize warm ischemia time. While this approach optimizes organ quality, it may feel uncomfortable to families who associate operating theaters with active treatment rather than dignified death. Other models withdraw treatment in the ICU or a dedicated withdrawal room, with rapid transfer to the operating theater after death.

The choice of location should balance the competing considerations of organ preservation and family experience. In India, where family presence at the time of death carries particular cultural significance, withdrawal in a setting that allows family presence is likely to be preferred. Involvement of social workers, counselors, and spiritual care providers can help support families through the process.

Communication Is Key The most important factor in ensuring family comfort with DCD is clear, compassionate communication from the healthcare team. Families should understand the process, know what to expect, and feel that their loved one's dignity is being protected throughout.

Myth 8: DCD Will Lead to Neglect of Resuscitation and Treatment Efforts

The Myth in Detail

A related fear is that the existence of DCD programs will create incentives to inadequately resuscitate patients or to prematurely abandon treatment. If organs can be retrieved after cardiac arrest, might emergency responders or physicians be tempted to give up on resuscitation efforts earlier than they otherwise would, in order to preserve organs for transplantation?

The Facts

Strict Separation Is Mandated All DCD protocols mandate strict separation between resuscitation/treatment decisions and organ donation considerations. The team providing treatment and making decisions about resuscitation must be entirely separate from the transplant team. Treatment decisions must be made without any consideration of donation potential.

For uncontrolled DCD following failed resuscitation, standard resuscitation protocols must be followed. The decision to cease resuscitation must be made according to established medical criteria—typically after a defined period of unsuccessful CPR without return of spontaneous circulation—without reference to organ donation.

For controlled DCD following withdrawal of life-sustaining treatment, the decision to withdraw must be made solely on the basis of medical futility and patient/family wishes. The possibility of organ donation must not influence the timing or nature of treatment withdrawal.

Regulatory Oversight In countries with established DCD programs, regulatory bodies provide oversight to ensure that protocols are followed, and that conflicts of interest are avoided. Medical records are reviewed, outcomes are monitored, and any concerns are investigated.

No Evidence of Compromised Care The extensive international experience with DCD has not produced evidence that resuscitation efforts are being compromised, or that treatment is being withdrawn inappropriately. Studies of end-of-life care practices have not found differences in treatment patterns between potential donors and non-donors.

Public Trust Depends on Integrity DCD programs recognize that their viability depends entirely on public trust. Any perception that patient care is being compromised for organ procurement would be catastrophic for donation rates. This understanding creates strong incentives to maintain the highest ethical standards.

Relevance to India Trust in medical institutions is a significant challenge in India, and fears about compromised care are real. Building DCD programs in India will require visible, credible safeguards—clear protocols, independent oversight, transparent documentation, and commitment to family communication.

Myth 9: India Lacks the Infrastructure for DCD and Cannot Implement Such Programs

The Myth in Detail

A fatalistic view holds that DCD, while perhaps appropriate for wealthy Western countries with advanced healthcare systems, is simply not feasible in the Indian context. The challenges are too great: inadequate ICU capacity, shortage of ventilators, lack of trained personnel, poor coordination between hospitals and organ procurement organizations, and insufficient operating theater availability for rapid response.

The Facts

Challenges Are Real But Not Insurmountable The infrastructural challenges facing DCD in India are significant and should not be minimized. However, they are not fundamentally different from the challenges facing deceased organ donation generally, and India has made measurable progress in building its brain-death donation program despite similar constraints.

Controlled DCD May Be More Feasible Than Uncontrolled While uncontrolled DCD following unexpected cardiac arrest requires extremely rapid response—often within 30 min or less—controlled DCD following planned withdrawal of treatment allows for advance preparation. Surgical teams can be assembled, operating theaters prepared, and recipient patients identified before withdrawal occurs.

In settings with limited emergency response capacity, controlled DCD may actually be more feasible than brain-death donation, which requires ICU capacity to maintain the brain-dead donor for extended periods while organ allocation and surgical logistics are arranged.

The PGIMER Model Offers Lessons PGIMER Chandigarh has demonstrated that DCD can be performed in India, albeit on a limited scale, and with some learning curve [10]. Key elements of their approach include:

- ICU teams prepared to continue CPR using automated devices while arrangements are made for organ retrieval.
- Pre-positioned surgical teams ready to move quickly.
- Use of rapid cooling techniques including double-balloon catheters.
- Use of normothermic machine good perfusion for assessment of DCD organs.

These lessons can inform the development of DCD protocols at other Indian institutions. In fact, at least, two other institutes in the country have performed DCD after this experience.

Technology Can Help Advances in organ preservation technology—normothermic regional perfusion, ex situ machine perfusion—may help address some of India's logistical challenges. These technologies extend the window for organ retrieval and allow organs to be preserved and assessed during transport. While expensive, they may become more accessible over time.

Incremental Progress Is Possible India need not implement comprehensive DCD programs immediately. Incremental progress—beginning with controlled DCD at a small number of well-resourced centers, gradually expanding as experience accumulates—is a realistic pathway. The experience of other countries suggests that DCD programs can be built up over time.

Relevance to India Defeatism about DCD in India is unwarranted. While challenges are real, the potential benefits—significant expansion of the deceased donor pool—justify sustained effort. Investment in infrastructure, training, and protocol development can yield meaningful results.

Myth 10: DCD Is a Western Practice Inappropriate for India's Cultural Context

The Myth in Detail

Some argue that DCD is a product of Western medical ethics and healthcare systems that does not translate to India's distinct cultural context. The imposition of Western practices, according to this view, would be inappropriate and potentially harmful.

The Facts

DCD Is Global While DCD programs are most advanced in Western Europe, North America, and Australia, the practice is spreading globally. Countries in Asia, including Japan [30] and South Korea [31], have developed DCD programs. China has transitioned toward DCD as part of broader reforms of its transplantation system. DCD is not inherently "Western."

Cultural Adaptation Is Possible Successful implementation of DCD in diverse cultural contexts demonstrates that the practice can be adapted to local values and circumstances. The core ethical principles—respect for the dead, informed consent, separation of treatment, and donation decisions—are not culturally specific.

Indian Values Support Organ Donation As discussed above, India's major religious and cultural traditions support organ donation as an act of charity and compassion. The challenge is not that Indian values oppose organ donation, but that cultural practices and public awareness have not yet caught up with the possibilities of deceased donation.

India Can Lead in Its Own Context Rather than simply importing Western models, India has the opportunity to develop DCD approaches suited to its own healthcare system, cultural context, and patient population. This might include particular attention to family involvement, respect for religious practices, and creative solutions to infrastructural constraints. DCD in India should not be conceived as importing a foreign practice but as adapting a global innovation to the Indian context. Indian voices—physicians, ethicists, religious leaders, patients, and families—should shape how DCD is implemented in ways that honor Indian values.

International Best Practices and Lessons for India

Countries with successful DCD programs offer valuable lessons for India.

The United Kingdom

The UK has one of the world's most successful DCD programs, with DCD donors representing over 40% of all deceased donors. Key success factors include:

- Clear national guidelines from the Academy of Medical Royal Colleges and NHS Blood and Transplant.
- Systematic integration of DCD protocols into intensive care unit practice.
- Strong coordination between Specialist Nurses for Organ Donation (SNODs) and hospital staff.
- Public education campaigns that have built awareness and acceptance.

The Netherlands

The Netherlands has achieved among the highest DCD donation rates in the world. Contributing factors include:

- Early adoption and sustained commitment to DCD.
- Investment in rapid-response infrastructure.
- Research and innovation in organ preservation.
- Cultural acceptance of end-of-life decision-making.

Spain

Spain leads the world in overall deceased organ donation rates and has developed both controlled and uncontrolled DCD programs. Key elements include:

- The "Spanish Model" of in-hospital transplant coordinators—often intensivists with additional training—who identify potential donors and manage the donation process.
- Strong legal framework supporting both brain death and circulatory death donation.
- Systematic approach to uncontrolled DCD using normothermic regional perfusion.

Australia

Australia pioneered DCD heart transplantation and has been innovative in machine perfusion technologies. Lessons include:

- Willingness to push the boundaries of what is possible with DCD.
- Investment in research and technology development.
- Integration of DCD into comprehensive deceased organ donation programs.

Recommendations for India

Based on the evidence and international experience reviewed in this chapter, the following recommendations are offered for advancing DCD in India:

Legal and Regulatory Reforms

1. *Clarify the Legal Status of DCD*: Amendments to the Transplantation of Human Organs and Tissues Act 2014 or national guidelines developed by NOTTO should explicitly address organ donation following circulatory death, establishing clear procedures for death determination and consent.
2. *Develop Guidelines for Withdrawal of Life-Sustaining Treatment*: Building on Supreme Court rulings recognizing passive euthanasia, clear clinical and legal guidelines for treatment withdrawal should be developed.
3. *Establish National DCD Protocols*: The National Organ and Tissue Transplant Organisation (NOTTO) should develop and promulgate standardized protocols for DCD, covering all aspects of the process from identification of potential donors through organ retrieval till the amendments in law are carried out.

Institutional Development

4. *Begin with Controlled DCD at Selected Centers*: A small number of well-resourced tertiary care centers should be designated as pilot sites for controlled DCD, with intensive support for protocol development, training, and monitoring.

5. *Invest in Infrastructure*: Critical investments include ICU capacity, ventilator availability, operating theater readiness for rapid response, and organ preservation equipment.
6. *Train Transplant Coordinators*: Transplant coordinators play a critical role in DCD. Training programs should prepare them for the unique challenges of DCD, including time-sensitive decision-making and family communication.
7. *Build Intensivist Capacity*: Intensivists are key to DCD. Training should be provided through professional societies and medical councils.

Public Education and Trust-Building

8. *Launch Public Awareness Campaigns*: Sustained public education about deceased organ donation, including DCD, should address myths and misconceptions while respecting cultural and religious sensitivities.
9. *Engage Religious and Community Leaders*: Partnerships with religious leaders can help communicate that organ donation is consistent with India's faith traditions.
10. *Ensure Transparency*: Public trust depends on transparency about DCD practices and outcomes. Data should be collected and reported systematically.

Research and Innovation

11. *Establish Outcome Registries*: Systematic collection of outcome data from DCD transplants will enable continuous quality improvement and build the evidence base.
12. *Pursue Technology Adoption*: Normothermic regional perfusion and ex situ machine perfusion technologies should be evaluated for adoption in India.

Conclusion

Donation after circulatory death represents a significant opportunity to expand organ availability in India, where the gap between supply and demand costs tens of thousands of lives annually. More than 100,000 people are currently on the US organ wait list alone, and the global need is staggering. In India, the disparity is even more acute.

The myths surrounding DCD—concerns about organ quality, fears about premature death determination, religious objections, and assumptions about impracticability—can be addressed with evidence and appropriate protocols. Global experience demonstrates that DCD can be practiced safely and ethically, yielding organs with excellent long-term outcomes for recipients.

India faces particular challenges: legal ambiguity, infrastructural constraints, cultural complexity, and a healthcare system struggling to meet basic needs. Yet these challenges are not insurmountable. With legal clarification, institutional investment, public education, and commitment from the transplant community, India can develop DCD programs that save lives while honoring the dignity of donors and their families.

The path forward requires action on multiple fronts: legislative reform to clarify the legal framework, protocol development to guide clinical practice, infrastructure investment to enable rapid response, training to build clinical capacity, and public engagement to build trust and awareness.

Each organ transplanted from a DCD donor represents a life saved—a patient removed from the waiting list, freed from dialysis, rescued from heart failure, spared from the progressive deterioration of end-stage organ disease. In a country where the need so vastly exceeds the supply, the moral imperative to explore every avenue for expanding organ availability is clear.

DCD is not a replacement for brain-death donation but a complement to it—another pathway through which the gift of life can be given. India's transplant community, policymakers, and public have the opportunity to embrace this pathway, learning from global experience while adapting to Indian realities.

The facts support DCD. The myths, carefully examined, dissolve under the light of evidence. What remains is a choice: to act on the evidence and save lives, or to allow misconceptions to perpetuate a preventable tragedy.

Competing Interests The author(s) has no competing interests to declare that are relevant to the content of this manuscript.

Ethics Approval The author(s) declares that this manuscript does not include primary research with human participants.

The author(s) declares that this manuscript does not include primary studies involving animals.

References

1. Cadaveric organ donation: Indian perspective - Indian J Forensic Community Med [Internet]. [cited 2026 Jun 5]. Available from: https://ijfcm.org/archive/volume/11/issue/2/article/14700.
2. Husain SA, Motter JD, Stewart D, Levan ML, Bae S, Parent B, et al. Changes in organ donation after circulatory death in the United States. JAMA. 2026;335(12):1087–9. https://doi.org/10.1001/jama.2026.0976. PubMed PMID: 41746614; PubMed Central PMCID: PMC12947068.
3. De Georgia MA. History of brain death as death: 1968 to the present. J Crit Care. 2014;29(4):673–8. https://doi.org/10.1016/j.jcrc.2014.04.015. PubMed PMID: 24930367.
4. Thuong M, Ruiz A, Evrard P, Kuiper M, Boffa C, Akhtar MZ, et al. New classification of donation after circulatory death donors definitions and terminology. Transpl Int. 2016;29(7):749–59. https://doi.org/10.1111/tri.12776.
5. Messer S, Rushton S, Simmonds L, Macklam D, Husain M, Jothidasan A, et al. A national pilot of donation after circulatory death (DCD) heart transplantation within the United Kingdom. J Heart Lung Transplant. 2023;42(8):1120–30. https://doi.org/10.1016/j.healun.2023.03.006.
6. IRODaT – International Registry on Organ Donation and Transplantation [Internet]. [cited 2026 Jun 5]. Available from: https://www.irodat.org/?p=database&c=NL.
7. Lomero M, Gardiner D, Coll E, Haase-Kromwijk B, Procaccio F, Immer F, et al. Donation after circulatory death today: an updated overview of the European landscape. Transpl Int. 2020;33(1):76–88. https://doi.org/10.1111/tri.13506. PubMed PMID: 31482628.
8. International Registry on Organ Donation and Transplantation (IRODaT). Database of Organ Donation and Transplantation Activities. Available from: https://www.irodat.org/?p=database.
9. Sarma B, Dash SK, Ghormade PS, Kumar DAV. Cadaveric organ donation: Indian perspective. 2025. https://doi.org/10.18231/j.ijfcm.2024.012

10. Singh S, Kumar S, Dasgupta S, Kenwar DB, Rathi M, Sharma A, et al. A single-center experience of kidney transplantation from donation after circulatory death: challenges and scope in India. Indian J Nephrol. 2017;27(3):205–9. https://doi.org/10.4103/0971-4065.202843. PubMed PMID: 28553041; PubMed Central PMCID: PMC5434687.
11. Sharma A, Singh S, Panjathia A, Sharma A, Kenwar DB, Patil SKS. Uncontrolled donation after circulatory determination of death: 11-years single center experience in India. Korean J Transplant. 2022;36(1):213. https://doi.org/10.4285/ATW2022.F-3515.
12. Akoh JA. Kidney donation after cardiac death. World J Nephrol. 2012;1(3):79–91. https://doi.org/10.5527/wjn.v1.i3.79. PubMed PMID: 24175245; PubMed Central PMCID: PMC3782200.
13. Kizilbash SJ, Chavers BM, Evans MD. Survival benefit of donation after circulatory death kidney transplantation in children compared with remaining on the waiting list for a kidney donated after brain death. Transplantation. 2022;106(3):575–83. https://doi.org/10.1097/TP.0000000000003733. PubMed PMID: 33654002; PubMed Central PMCID: PMC8408288.
14. Schaapherder AF, Kaisar M, Mumford L, Robb M, Johnson R, de Kok MJC, et al. Donor characteristics and their impact on kidney transplantation outcomes: results from two nationwide instrumental variable analyses based on outcomes of donor kidney pairs accepted for transplantation. eClinicalMedicine. 2022;50:101516. https://doi.org/10.1016/j.eclinm.2022.101516.
15. Schlegel A, Kalisvaart M, Scalera I, Laing RW, Mergental H, Mirza DF, et al. The UK DCD risk score: a new proposal to define futility in donation-after-circulatory-death liver transplantation. J Hepatol. 2018;68(3):456–64. https://doi.org/10.1016/j.jhep.2017.10.034. PubMed PMID: 29155020.
16. Spadaccio C, Salsano A, Altarabsheh S, Castro-Varela A, Gallego Navarro C, Juarez Casso F, et al. Short and long-term outcomes of lung transplantation from brain death vs. circulatory death donors: a meta-analysis of comparative studies. J Heart Lung Transplant. 2025;44(5):708–18. https://doi.org/10.1016/j.healun.2024.12.010. PubMed PMID: 39798936.
17. Hyun S, Haam S. Donation after circulatory death in lung transplantation. J Chest Surg. 2022;55(4):283–7. https://doi.org/10.5090/jcs.22.060. PubMed PMID: 35924534; PubMed Central PMCID: PMC9358165.
18. Sydney SVH. St Vincent's Hospital Sydney [text] [Internet]. St Vincent's Hospital Sydney; [cited 2026 Jun 5]. Available from: https://www.svhs.org.au/newsroom/news/st-vincent-s-hospital-sydney-transplants-first-circulatory-death-human-heart.
19. del Mar Lomero M, Johnson R, Coll E, Jansen N, Antoine C, Procaccio F, et al. Donation after circulatory death: an updated description of the European landscape. Transplantation. 2018;102:S386. https://doi.org/10.1097/01.tp.0000543149.04890.0a.
20. Default [Internet]. [cited 2026 Jun 13]. DCD Heart Transplantation Reaches 10-Year Mark, Now up to 30% of Transplant Volumes. Available from: https://www.ishlt.org/about/news-detail/2025/04/27/dcd-heart-transplantation-reaches-10-year-mark-now-up-to-30-of-transplant-volumes.
21. Seth AK, Mohanka R, Navin S, Gokhale AG, Sharma A, Kumar A, et al. Organ donation after circulatory determination of death in India: a joint position paper. Indian J Crit Care Med Peer-Rev. 2022;26(4):421–38. https://doi.org/10.5005/jp-journals-10071-24198. PubMed PMID: 35656056; PubMed Central PMCID: PMC9067489.
22. den Hartogh G. When are you dead enough to be a donor? Can any feasible protocol for the determination of death on circulatory criteria respect the dead donor rule? Theor Med Bioeth. 2019;40(4):299–319. https://doi.org/10.1007/s11017-019-09500-0. PubMed PMID: 31562590; PubMed Central PMCID: PMC6790209.
23. Aruna Ramchandra Shanbaug vs Union Of India & Ors on 7 March, 2011 [Internet]. [cited 2026 Jun 5]. Available from: https://indiankanoon.org/doc/235821/.
24. Common Cause (A Regd. Society) v. Union of India (2018)—[cited 2026 Jun 5]. Available from https://indiankanoon.org/doc/184449972/. [C allows passive euthanasia, Centre needs to take its cue. The Indian Express [Internet]. 2026 Mar 12 [cited 2026 Jun 5]. Available from: https://indianexpress.com/article/opinion/editorials/sc-allows-passive-euthanasia-centre-needs-to-take-its-cue-10577252/25].

25. Hinduism and Organ Donation. LifeCenter Northwest [Internet]. [cited 2026 Jun 5]. Available from: https://lcnw.org/hinduism-and-organ-donation/.
26. International Islamic Fiqh Academy. Resolutions and Recommendations of the International Islamic Fiqh Academy. Official Edition. Resolution No. 26 (1/4). Available from: Official IIFA Resolutions PDF. Accessed June 2026.
27. Rzeźniczek P, Gaczkowska AD, Kluzik A, Cybulski M, Bartkowska-Śniatkowska A, Grześkowiak M. Lazarus phenomenon or the return from the afterlife—what we know about auto resuscitation. J Clin Med. 2023;12(14):4704. https://doi.org/10.3390/jcm12144704. PubMed PMID: 37510819; PubMed Central PMCID: PMC10380628.
28. Tingle SJ, Thompson ER, Figueiredo RS, Moir JA, Goodfellow M, Talbot D, et al. Normothermic and hypothermic machine perfusion preservation versus static cold storage for deceased donor kidney transplantation. Cochrane Database Syst Rev. 2024;2024(7):CD011671. https://doi.org/10.1002/14651858.CD011671.pub3. PubMed PMID: 38979743; PubMed Central PMCID: PMC11232102.
29. Karimian N, Matton APM, Westerkamp AC, Burlage LC, op den Dries S, Leuvenink HGD, et al. Ex Situ normothermic machine perfusion of donor livers. J Vis Exp JoVE. 2015;99:52688. https://doi.org/10.3791/52688. PubMed PMID: 26067131; PubMed Central PMCID: PMC4542958.
30. Kotani Y. Barriers and solutions for introducing donation after circulatory death (DCD) in Japan. J Artif Organs. 2025;28(3):343–7. https://doi.org/10.1007/s10047-024-01491-7. PubMed PMID: 39812997; PubMed Central PMCID: PMC12373537.
31. Jeong E, Baik S, Park H, Oh J, Lee Y, Lee J m. First organ donation after circulatory death following withdrawal of life-sustaining treatment in Korea: a case report. J Korean Med Sci. 2021;36(23):e171. https://doi.org/10.3346/jkms.2021.36.e171. PubMed PMID: 34128599; PubMed Central PMCID: PMC8203855.